D1706870

Current Techniques in
Interventional Radiology

Edited by

Constantin Cope, MD

Professor of Radiology
Section of Angiography
and Interventional Radiology
Hospital of the University of Pennsylvania
Philadelphia, Pennsylvania

PHILADELPHIA
1995

Current Medicine

Managing Editor: *Lori Bainbridge*
Editor: *Michelle Fitzgerald*
Art Director: *Paul Fennessy*
Designer: *Robert LeBrun*
Illustration Director: *Larry Ward*
Illustrators: *Weisia Langenfeld, Ann Saydlowski, and Larry Ward*
Typesetting Director: *Colleen Ward*
Production: *David Myers and Wendy Feinstein*

ISBN: 1-878132-59-8
ISSN: 1068-3879

Printed in Singapore by Star Standard Industries Pte. Ltd.

5 4 3 2 1

©**Copyright 1995 by Current Medicine**, 20 North Third Street, Philadelphia, PA 19106. All rights reserved. No part of this publication may be reproduced, stored in a retrieval system, or transmitted in any form by any means electronic, mechanical, photocopying, recording, or otherwise without prior written permission of the publisher.

Preface

The concept behind this annual is to demonstrate current interventional techniques in attractive step-by-step illustrations and to present important developments that can be of interest to the practicing interventionist as well as other specialists. The following topics have been chosen either to re-emphasize the best techniques that can be used for performing already well-accepted procedures or to present next year's potential new star.

Parathyroid localization and embolization is usually considered a rare procedure that can only be done in specialized centers because it is time-consuming and may require great catheter skills. Today, however, subselective catheterization of parathyroid glands is a technique that can be potentially performed by most fellowship-trained interventional radiologists, because of significant advances in subselective catheter guidewire technology that has greatly facilitated such procedures. Likewise, the recent introduction of hydrophyllic coating for guidewires and catheters allows the interventionist to advance standard preshaped catheters deeper into vessel arborizations with less chance of causing vascular spasm—a major problem that has often prevented completion of the procedure. The techniques described for embolization of bronchial arteries, uterine arteries, and vascular malformations all depend for their safety and success on prompt and accurate positioning of delivery catheters, which can often be performed only through the use of this new technology.

In the management of both vascular malformations and Oriental cholangiohepatitis, which are given detailed coverage in this book, the interventionist must understand that there is no quick cure for these conditions; these unfortunate patients must be kept as asymptomatic as possible over the long term by simple periodic re-evaluations and basic treatments that will not compromise future access to the lesions.

Interventional management of ostial lesions of the renal artery with percutaneous transluminal angioplasty (PTA) is often unrewarding. Trost and Sos discuss the potential benefits of using metal stents to obtain longer-term patency for this difficult problem.

The past few years have signaled the introduction of transjugular intrahepatic portosystemic shunts (TIPS) on the clinical front. As more centers have become involved with this life-saving procedure, we have also seen an increasing number and variety of mishaps, perhaps often due to the fact that the exact anatomic relationship of the intrahepatic branches of the portal and hepatic veins were not fully understood. The exquisite injection studies provided by Uflacker and colleagues should be of great help to those of us who have difficulty in visually internalizing intrahepatic vascular anatomy.

Mitty and Sterling are pioneering a new field in preventive and emergency interventional management of major obstetric bleeding—a procedure, which in the past, had been found unacceptable to obstetricians because of their concern for excessive radiation exposure to the patient. Efforts to educate our obstetric colleagues about the indications and feasibility of this form of treatment can save a patient from hysterectomy and sometimes even fatal hemorrhage.

Intravascular ultrasound (IVUS) is a new tool that can help us map out with great accuracy the presence and extent of atherosclerotic disease and the therapeutic results obtained following vascular interventions. Because this method is expensive to acquire and run on a fairly routine basis, I have asked Grubbs and Katzen to discuss the many uses of this modality so that readers can decide for themselves its cost-effectiveness in their own clinical practice.

For those of you who are increasingly involved in managing malfunctioning dialysis access grafts, the strategies reported by Sullivan and Besarab, which include frequent screening for stenoses and angioplasty before graft thrombosis occurs, are to be highly recommended because they are both simple and cost-effective.

Kensey has devised and introduced a vascular plug that can apparently arrest postcatheterization bleeding, even in heparinized patients, without the need for external compression. When commercially available, this device should become extremely valuable in the performance of vascular interventional procedures requiring high doses of anticoagulant and thrombolytic drugs or the concomitant insertion of large-diameter therapeutic devices.

Although the standard treatment for vascular thrombosis and embolization continues to be pharmacologic, thrombolytic therapy is expensive because of high drug costs and the necessity of observing the patient in an intensive care unit for 1 day or more. Therefore, there is a great need for developing efficient mechanical means for extracting or pulverizing thrombi to shorten the treatment period. The current use of suction catheters and baskets has limited applicability; more sophisticated rotary, ultrasound, and hydraulic devices are being investigated clinically.

On the nonvascular front, Bell, Yeung, and Ho give a persuasive argument for performing percutaneous gastrostomy and gastrojejunostomy by standard fluoroscopic techniques because of the simplicity, safety, and cost-effectiveness. It is interesting that gastroenterologists and surgeons feel that percutaneous endoscopic gastrostomy (PEG) is the only acceptable technique for performing this procedure, despite its higher cost. These physicians claim that endoscopic inspection of the stomach may yield unsuspected lesions that may change the management of the patient, and that endoscopic inspection is safer than the blind fluoroscopic method. However, paradoxically we are still asked to perform direct percutaneous gastrostomy in the presence of esophageal strictures, ascites, abdominal carcinomatosis, and postoperative gastric remnants—all conditions that put the patient in a higher-risk category!

One of the most useful and accepted interventional procedures certainly continues to be percutaneous drainage of abscesses. Nakamoto and Haaga provide us with a balanced view of accepted puncture and drainage techniques as well as a decision analysis for choosing percutaneous, surgical, or a combination of approaches.

Increasing attention is paid to the management of esophageal and tracheobronchial strictures with various types of metal stents, some of which are coated to prevent tumor ingrowth. Stent placement techniques are well described by Cwikiel and by Rousseau and colleagues, respectively. Because of favorable clinical results, it is anticipated that these procedures will soon be found acceptable for general use in the treatment of malignant strictures.

For those patients with complex patterns of biliary obstruction who require temporary stenting or who have occluded their metal stents, Shlansky-Goldberg describes a simple method with articulated tubes that can be used to decompress several bile ducts through only one entry site.

We continue to witness an avalanche of new techniques and concepts in interventional radiology, many of which are still in the feasibility stages. However, we must realize that testing and evaluating new devices and procedures may be somewhat curtailed in the near future due to anticipated cuts in government and private insurance reimbursements. This may lead to severe hospital budget shortages, which may in some cases temporarily prevent the purchase of even standard catheter-guidewire equipment. Our only defense against this kind of problem is to ensure that all of our new techniques be tested prospectively from the start in as rigorous and disciplined manner as possible, ideally on a multi-institutional basis. Data from such projects could be quickly collected on a national scale through a central computer bank, carefully analyzed for firm evidence of efficacy, cost benefits, and clinical need, and then rapidly submitted to the Food and Drug Administration (FDA) for approval.

Constantin Cope, MD
Professor of Radiology
Section of Angiography and Interventional Radiology
Hospital of the University of Pennsylvania

Contributors

Stuart D. Bell, MB, BS, MRCP, FRCR
Clinical Fellow
Department of Radiology
University of Toronto
    and The Toronto Hospital
Toronto, Ontario, Canada

Anatole Besarab, MD
Medical Director
Thomas Jefferson University
Intermediate Dialysis Unit;
Professor of Medicine
Department of Medicine
Thomas Jefferson University Hospital
    and Jefferson Medical College
Philadelphia, Pennsylvania, USA

Ignatio Bilbao, MD
Clinica Universitaria
Pamplona, Spain

Patricia E. Burrows, MD
Associate Professor
Harvard Medical School
Cambridge, Massachusetts;
Department of Radiology
Children's Hospital
Boston, Massachusetts, USA

Phillippe Cárre, MD
Department of Pneumology
Centre Hospitalier Universitaire
Hopital de Rangueil
Toulouse, France

Byung Ihn Choi, MD
Department of Diagnostic Radiology
Seoul National University Hospital
Seoul, Korea

Wojciech Cwikiel, MD, PhD
Department of Radiology
University Hospital
Lund, Swedan

Luiz C. D'Albuquerque, MD
CETEFI
Specialized Center for Therapy
    of Liver Diseases
Hospital Beneficência Portuguesa
Sao Paulo, Brazil

Alain Didier, MD
Department of Pneumology
Centre Hospitalier Universitaire
Hopital de Rangueil
Toulouse, France

Kenneth E. Fellows, MD
Professor of Radiology
University of Pennsylvania School of
    Medicine;
Radiologist-in-Chief
Department of Radiology
Children's Hospital of Philadelphia
Philadelphia, Pennsylvania, USA

Gerald E. Grubbs, MD
Miami Vascular Institute
Miami, Florida, USA

John R. Haaga, MD
Professor of Radiology,
    Chairman and Director
Department of Radiology
University Hospitals of Cleveland
Cleveland, Ohio, USA

Joon Koo Han, MD
Department of Diagnostic Radiology
Seoul National University Hospital
Seoul, Korea

Chia-Sing Ho, MB, BS, FRCPC
Professor
Department of Radiology
University of Toronto
    and The Toronto Hospital
Toronto, Ontario, Canada

Francis Joffre, MD
Department of Radiology
Centre Hospitalier Universitaire
Hopital de Rangueil, France

Barry T. Katzen, MD, FACR, FACC
Medical Director
Miami Vascular Institute;
Clinical Professor of Radiology
University of Miami School of Medicine
Miami, Florida, USA

Kenneth R. Kensey, MD
Kensey Nash Corporation
Exton, Pennsylvania, USA

Simon Martel, MD
Department of Pneumology
Centre Hospitalier Universitaire
Hopital de Rangueil
Toulouse, France

Harold A. Mitty, MD
Professor of Radiology
Department of Radiology
Mount Sinai School of Medicine
New York, New York, USA

Dean A. Nakamoto, MD
Assistant Professor
Department of Radiology
University Hospitals of Cleveland
Cleveland, Ohio, USA

Johanna Pallotta, MD
Department of Endocrinology
Beth Israel Hospital
Boston, Massachusetts, USA

Jae Hyung Park, MD
Department of Diagnostic Radiology
Seoul National University Hospital
Seoul, Korea

Jim A. Reekers, MD
Department of Radiology
Academic Medical Centre
The Netherlands

Paulo Reichert, MD
CETEFI
Specialized Center for Therapy
of Liver Diseases
Hospital Beneficência Portuguesa
Sau Paulo, Brazil

Herve P. Rousseau, MD
Department of Radiology
Centre Hospitalier Universitaire
Hopital de Rangueil
Toulouse, France

Barry A. Sacks, MD
Department of Radiology
Leonard Morse Hospital
Natick, Massachusetts;
Beth Israel Hospital
Boston, Massachusetts, USA

Richard D. Shlansky-Goldberg, MD
Assistant Professor of Radiology
Hospital of the University of Pennsylvania
Philadelphia, Pennsylvania, USA

Adavio de Oliveira e Silva, MD
CETEFI
Specialized Center for Therapy
of Liver Diseases
Hospital Beneficência Portuguesa
Sao Paulo, Brazil

Thomas A. Sos, MD
Professor of Radiology
Department of Radiology
The New York Hospital
and Cornell Medical Center
New York, New York, USA

Keith M. Sterling, MD
Department of Radiology
Mount Sinai School of Medicine
New York, New York, USA

Kevin L. Sullivan, MD
Associate Professor of Radiology
Department of Radiology
Thomas Jefferson University Hospital
and Jefferson Medical College
Philadelphia, Pennsylvania, USA

David Trost, MD
Assistant Professor of Radiology
Department of Radiology
The New York Hospital
and Cornell Medical Center
New York, New York, USA

Renan Uflacker, MD
Professor of Radiology
Section of Vascular and Interventional
Radiology
Department of Radiology
Medical University of South Carolina
Charleston, South Carolina, USA

Ivan Vujic, MD
Professor of Radiology
Chief
Section of Vascular and Interventional
Radiology
Department of Radiology
Medical University of South Carolina
Charleston, South Carolina, USA

Eugene Y. Yeung, BS, BSC, MRCP, FRCR, FRCPC
Assistant Professor
Department of Radiology
University of Toronto
and The Toronto Hospital
Toronto, Ontario, Canada

Contents

Chapter 1   1

Anatomic Studies of the Liver Applied to the Transjugular Intrahepatic Portosystemic Shunt
Renan Uflacker, Paulo Reichert, Luiz C. D'Albuquerque, Adavio de Oliveira e Silva, and Ivan Vujic

Chapter 2   11

Techniques for Management of Pediatric Vascular Anomalies
Patricia E. Burrows and Kenneth E. Fellows

Chapter 3   29

Radiologic Management of Hemoptysis
Ivan Vujic and Renan Uflacker

Chapter 4   39

Obstetric Embolotherapy
Harold A. Mitty and Keith M. Sterling

Chapter 5   51

Diagnosis and Ablation of Parathyroid Adenomas
Barry A. Sacks and Johanna Pallotta

Chapter 6   67

Uses of Intravascular Ultrasound in Vascular Intervention
Gerald E. Grubbs and Barry T. Katzen

Chapter 7   81

Puncture Site Hemostasis
Kenneth R. Kensey

Chapter 8   87

Interventional Management of Ostial Lesions in the Renal Artery
David Trost and Thomas A. Sos

Chapter 9   103

Review of Devices for Percutaneous Thrombectomy
Jim A. Reekers

Chapter 10   111

Percutaneous Drainage of Postoperative Intra-abdominal Abscesses and Collections
Dean A. Nakamoto and John R. Haaga

Chapter 11   125

Strategies for Maintaining Dialysis Access Patency
Kevin L. Sullivan and Anatole Besarab

Chapter 12   133

Esophageal Stenting
Wojciech Cwikiel

Chapter 13   143

Self-expanding Stents in the Management of Tracheobronchial Stenosis
Herve P. Rousseau, Phillipe Cárre, Francis Joffre, Simon Martel, Alain Didier, and Ignatio Bilbao

Chapter 14   155

Percutaneous Fluoroscopic Gastrostomy and Gastrojejunostomy: Current Status of the Technique
Stuart D. Bell, Eugene Y. Yeung, and Chia-Sing Ho

Chapter 15   173

The Use of Articulated Catheters for Biliary and Pancreatic Obstructions and Difficult T-tube Placements
Richard D. Shlansky-Goldberg

Chapter 16   185

Interventional Management of Recurrent Pyogenic Cholangitis
Joon Koo Han, Jae Hyung Park, and Byung Ihn Choi

Index   197

Anatomic Studies of the Liver Applied to the Transjugular Intrahepatic Portosystemic Shunt

Renan Uflacker

Paulo Reichert

Luiz C. D'Albuquerque

Adavio de Oliveira e Silva

Ivan Vujic

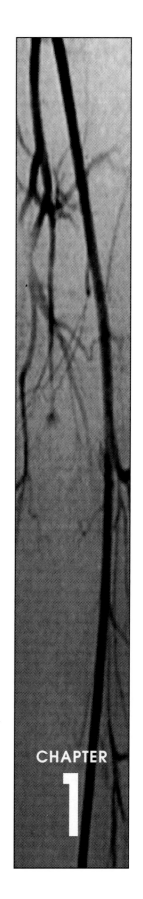

CHAPTER

1

Chronic liver disease may result in cirrhosis, portal hypertension, and the development of esophageal varices and refractory ascites. Variceal hemorrhage is a life-threatening complication of portal hypertension responsible for several thousand hospital admissions worldwide. Despite medical and surgical advances, the management of such problems is still challenging and no single treatment is adequate for all patients [1••]. The most recent development in the treatment of portal hypertension is the transjugular intrahepatic

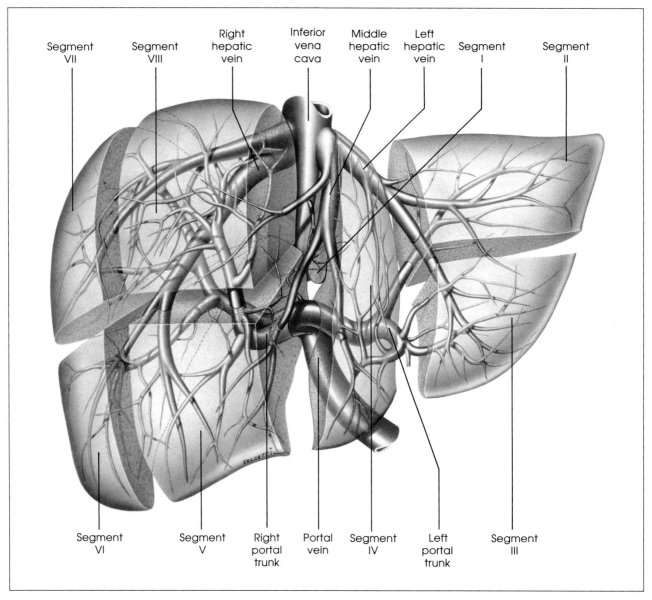

FIGURE 1-1.

The venous anatomy, the portal anatomy, and liver segments. The distance between the vascular structures is increased because of the liver segment separation (Counaud Liver Segments). Note that the main RHV runs along the RHF and is superior and posterior to the portal vein bifurcation and right main portal trunk. As the RHV courses along the RHF, it receives venous branches from segments V and VIII anteriorly and segments VI and VII posteriorly. Segments VII and VIII are mainly drained by an accessory RHV, which is a frequent finding. The MHV mostly drains segment IV, but also part of segments V and VIII. The LHV drains segments II and III. Note that the MHV and LHV are anterior and superior to the left main portal trunk. The caudate lobe, or segment I, has its own draining vein directly to the IVC. (*From* Uflacker R: Atlas of Vascular Anatomy: An Angiographic Approach. Edited by Uflacker R. New York: Thieme Medical Publishers; 1994, in press, with permission).

portosystemic shunt (TIPS) procedure. In this procedure, the portal vein is partially decompressed through a neocommunication between the hepatic and the portal veins using an interposed metallic stent. Preliminary reports suggest that the TIPS procedure is technically feasible, easily repeated, and relatively safe for partial portal vein decompression [1••,2•,3,4••,5•,6••,7, 8•,9••,10–12,13•]. However, some complications have been reported with this procedure. These include shunt occlusion, extraparenchymal puncture and the creation of an intraperitoneal shunt, bleeding caused by transhepatic portal vein catheterization, which is no longer used or necessary, liver-capsule perforation by the transjugular needle and intraperitoneal bleeding, misplacement and migration of the stent, and cardiac perforation. Other complications relate to traversing a hepatic arterial or venous branch or biliary radicle during the parenchymal puncture and stent placement, theoretically causing hemobilia, arteriovenous fistula, liver infarction, bleeding, segmental biliary obstruction, or stent occlusion [10,14–19,20••].

The success and safety of the TIPS procedure depends on a thorough knowledge of hepatic venous and portal anatomy, in addition to a careful and standardized technique. The anatomic basis for performing TIPS is the assumption that the right hepatic vein

(RHV) is located superior and posterior to the portal vein bifurcation. As the RHV courses along the right hepatic fissure, it receives branches from both anterior and posterior segments. In the periphery of the liver, the RHV is located in the middle of the anterior and posterior branches of the right portal trunk, whereas more proximally the origin and the final few centimeters of the RHV are cranial and dorsal to the bifurcation of the portal vein and the right portal trunk (Fig. 1-1). The transparenchymal puncture made to create the intrahepatic shunt is therefore performed from the proximal RHV in a caudal and anterior or slightly medial direction, hitting the portal vein at the bifurcation or at the proximal right portal trunk or less frequently at the proximal left portal trunk (Fig. 1-2) [1••,6••]. Alternatively, the portal vein may be approached from the middle hepatic vein (MHV) or left hepatic vein (LHV) [6••]. Portal vein targeting may be facilitated in certain instances by ultrasound guidance during the procedure or prior placement of a metallic marker by a percutaneous transhepatic approach [21–23]. A femoral venous approach may be alternatively used when anatomic anomalies of the hepatic veins are present [24].

Information concerning the anatomy of the hepatic and portal veins and their relationship with adjacent

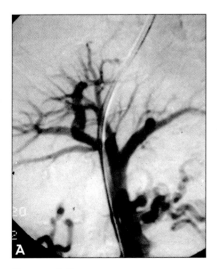
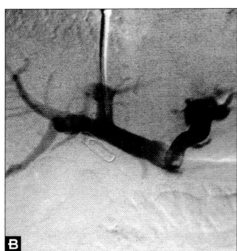
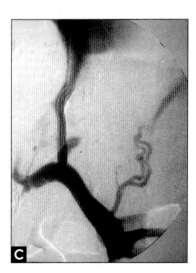

FIGURE 1-2.

A, Portography before stent placement and creation of an intrahepatic portal systemic shunt, demonstrating the portal puncture site on top of the bifurcation of the main right portal trunk. **B**, Portography after puncture on top of the portal bifurcation before stent placement creates a portal systemic shunt. **C**, Portography after puncture of the main left portal trunk and stent placement, approached from the right hepatic vein in a conventional fashion at about 1.5 cm from the IVC. Note a short stent incorrectly postioned in the periphery of the right portal vein in a previous TIPS attempt at another institution.

arterial and biliary structures in this area of the liver is scarce. We studied the vascular and biliary liver anatomy as applied to the TIPS procedure to establish the anatomic basis for its improved success and safety [25••]. We describe the anatomic findings of 25 liver casts, including plastic injections in the hepatic and portal veins, and hepatic artery and bile ducts, with particular emphasis on the anatomic relationships of these structures.

Materials and Methods

Twenty-five macroscopically normal human livers obtained as necropsy specimens in subjects who died from causes unrelated to the liver were used in this study. The group consisted of 18 men's and 7 women's cadavers, with a mean of 58 years of age, ranging from 20 to 70 years of age.

The standard specimen consisted of the liver including the inferior vena cava (IVC) from the right atrium down to the right renal vein, the hepatic pedicle, and part of the right and left diaphragmatic dome. After extensive cleansing with water, measurements were taken. The specimens were dissected with the IVC, common bile duct, portal vein, and proper hepatic artery identification. The cystic duct was also dissected and ligated with sutures. The cranial and caudal aspects

of the IVC were ligated with thick sutures and the vein was catheterized with a large-bore catheter. The vascular elements and bile duct at the hepatic pedicle were each catheterized with a 12-French catheter. Water injections were made to clean the vessels and to verify the existence of perforations and leaking in the liver surface. The right adrenal vein was ligated at this point in the procedure. After correcting the lacerations and leaking with delicate sutures, the injection material was prepared. Acrylic material, called Jet Acrylic Resin (Lang Dental, Chicago, IL), for odontologic application was used for the injection, consisting of 50% powder and 50% fluid (ratio 1:1). In a few cases where the hepatic artery and the bile duct were too small, a more fluid solution was used for injection (ratio 1:2). After injection of the four structures with four different colors, the specimens were left for 1 hour to have the plastic material cured. The corrosion of the organs was made in a tank with 20 L of water and 1 kg of sodium hydroxide or caustic soda (JT Baker Chemical, Phillipsburg, NJ) for 24 hours. After corrosion, the casts were washed thoroughly in running water, carefully cleaned with pincers to take out the organic material still present, and measurements were taken.

In 25 cases, the IVC and the portal veins were successfully injected, although in six cases the artery or the bile duct did not acceptably fill up to the periphery.

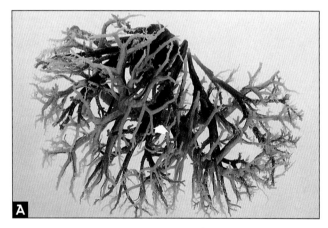

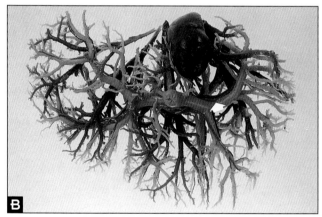

Figure 1-3.

A, Anterior view of a liver cast showing the hepatic veins and IVC in blue, the portal vein in yellow, the hepatic artery in red, and the bile duct in green. Note the relationship of the RHV with the right main portal trunk and the closer relationship of the MHV with the portal bifurcation (*arrow*). The bile duct and hepatic artery are hardly visible in this view. **B,** Posterior view of the liver clearly showing that the puncture from the RHV traverses the main right portal trunk, which has the artery and bile duct of segment VII (*arrow*) located in the path of the intraparenchymal puncture if it is on top of the portal trunk. In this case, the puncture of the right portal trunk should be as posterior as possible. (*From* Uflacker *et al.* (25••), with permission).

The findings related to the anatomy were reviewed. The right and middle hepatic veins, sizes of the casts, distances between the anterior-inferior aspect of the RHV, 1 cm from the ostium at the IVC and the superior-posterior aspect of the portal bifurcation were obtained. The distances between the inferior aspect of the MHV and the superoposterior aspect of the portal bifurcation, anatomy of the portal bifurcation, the relationship of the three elements of the portal triad at the level of the portal bifurcation, and the first 2 cm of the right and left portal trunks were recorded.

Results

MEASUREMENT OF THE ORGANS

The livers were measured laterolaterally and anteroposteriorly before and after the injection and corrosion of the organ. There was a reduction in size of the specimens of about 5% after separation. The sizes of the casts ranged from 21 to 29 cm at the laterolateral axis and from 14 to 21 cm in the anteroposterior axis, with a mean size of 24.5 × 18.0 cm.

THE ANATOMY OF THE RIGHT HEPATIC VEIN

In 16 cases, there was a single RHV of large diameter receiving several tributaries (Fig. 1-3). Two casts showed tributaries with large diameter from segment VIII, reaching the RHV near the IVC.

One case showed two RHVs with similar sizes parallel to each other. In two cases, the RHV had a single short trunk (1 cm), near the IVC but was bifid and had two distal parallel veins with similar sizes.

Six livers showed an accessory RHV caudal and distal, varying from 3 to 6 cm with a mean of 4 cm from the RHV, but parallel to the main vein and posterior to the portal vein bifurcation.

In two cases the RHV was extremely underdeveloped. One of these casts was included in the six casts in which an accessory RHV was found. The other showed several inferior branches parallel to the main RHV.

In a different group of 62 liver casts not included in this series, one case (1.6%) presented three RHVs and the most anterior one was located anterior to the portal vein bifurcation and to the anterior branch of the right trunk (Fig. 1-4).

THE ANATOMY OF THE MIDDLE HEPATIC VEIN

There was a single MHV in all 25 cases. The MHV joined the IVC directly in 20% of the cases and formed a common trunk with the LHV in 80% of the cases.

DISTANCE FROM THE RIGHT HEPATIC VEIN TO THE PORTAL BIFURCATION

The distance from the anterior aspect of the RHV at 1 cm from the IVC and the posterior aspect of the portal bifurcation was measured in a straight line. This

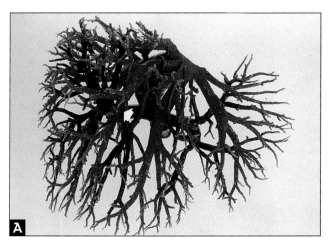

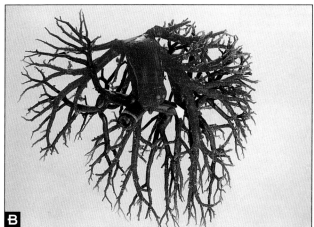

FIGURE 1-4.

A, Anterior view of a liver cast showing three right hepatic veins. The hepatic veins and IVC are red and the portal vein is green. Note that the most anterior hepatic vein is anterior to the right main portal trunk and the portal bifurcation (*arrow*). The middle hepatic vein reaches the IVC independently from the left hepatic vein. **B**, Posterior view of the liver cast showing the main right hepatic vein posterior to the right main branch of the portal vein and portal bifurcation (*arrow*). This anatomic variation is very rare. Note that the portal bifurcation is rather medial. (*From* Uflacker *et al.* (25●●), with permission).

distance ranged from 2.7 to 5.4 cm with a mean of 4.41 cm (Fig. 1-5).

In the cases where there were two RHVs not included in the average distance calculation, the distance was 1.8 cm from the medial branch and 4.2 cm from the lateral branch. The accessory RHVs and the portal bifurcation were very close. The distance between the anterior aspect of the accessory RHVs measured at 1 cm from the IVC and the portal bifurcation was 2.2 to 4.3 cm with a mean distance of 3.1 cm.

DISTANCE FROM THE MIDDLE HEPATIC VEIN TO THE PORTAL BIFURCATION

The distance between the inferior aspect of the MHV at 1 cm from the IVC and the superior-posterior aspect of the portal bifurcation and left portal trunk was measured in a straight line. This distance ranged from 2.4 to 4.5 cm, with a mean of 3.9 cm.

ANATOMY OF THE PORTAL BIFURCATION

In 24 livers, the portal vein presented a very short right trunk and a long left trunk. In almost every specimen, branches to the caudate lobe were seen, arising from the bifurcation of the portal vein or from the first 1 cm of the left trunk.

One liver presented an anomalous variation at the portal bifurcation. The portal vein bifurcated in a larger left trunk and a small right trunk. The left trunk further divided into a real left trunk and branched to segments V and VIII of the right lobe.

RELATIONSHIP OF THE ELEMENTS OF THE PORTAL TRIAD AT THE LEVEL OF THE PORTAL BIFURCATION AND THE FIRST TWO CENTIMETERS OF THE RIGHT AND LEFT PORTAL TRUNKS

In one liver, the portal bifurcation was anomalous. The bile duct and the artery crossed posteriorly to the origin of the portal trunk to segments V and VIII, following a joint path close to the posterosuperior aspect of the portal branch to segments VI and VII.

In another liver, the hepatic artery bifurcated proximally and to the left of the portal bifurcation, giving off one large anterior branch and a smaller branch that crossed posterior to the portal bifurcation and followed a path on the posterosuperior aspect of the right trunk of the portal vein. In one case there was a posterior arterial branch in the first 2 cm of the left portal trunk.

In nine specimens, there were arterial or biliary structures obstructing the first centimeter of the RHV and the portal bifurcation (Figs. 1-5 and 1-6). These biliary and arterial branches were oriented toward segment VII or segments VI and VII. In these cases, there was an intimate relationship between these two bilioarterial structures, but overall the biliary branches were posterior. In general, the biliary and arterial

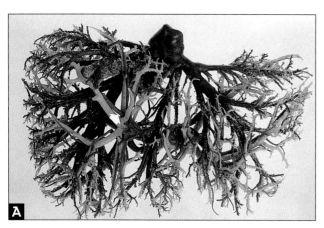 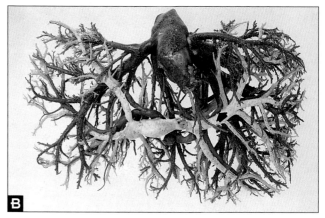

FIGURE 1-5.

A, Anterior view of a liver cast showing the most common relationship of the RHV with the portal bifurcation and main right portal trunk. The hepatic veins and IVC are blue, the portal vein is yellow, the bile duct is green, and the hepatic artery was not injected. Note the presence of a large bile duct coming from segments VII and VIII in the anterosuperior aspect of the right portal trunk (*arrow*). **B**, Posterior view of the liver cast shows the bile duct at the bifurcation of the right main portal trunk, in a possible path for the TIPS puncture. Note that in this case the right bile duct is anterior to the right main portal trunk, on the way of puncture from the MHV. (*From* Uflacker *et al.* (25••), with permission).

structures are close to the superior aspect of the portal trunks and are more frequently anterosuperior.

A portal branch from the right side was found to reach the caudate lobe, arising from segment VIII and parallel to the RHV. In another specimen, portal branches from segments V and VIII with a posterior location also reached the caudate lobe.

Discussion

Richter and collegues [6••] has stated that the best tract for TIPS is not always the shortest possible but rather the most accessible transparenchymal communication. This opinion reflects the fact that either the right or middle hepatic veins were used alternatively for the transparenchymal puncture and shunt creation according to accessibility during the procedure. However, further experience with TIPS has shown that the portal vein may be consistently approached from the RHV in the majority of patients, and this is the approach of choice. The MHV and LHV are reserved for an additional shunt or as an alternative for shunting when an anatomic anomaly is observed [4••].

The RHV approach has been regarded as both safe and simple for performing TIPS with a relatively low number of complications reported [10,14–19,20••]. The liver parenchyma immediately adjacent to the stent shows only minimal focal hemorrhagic changes. Bile ducts and small veins close to the stent are compressed but no evidence of stasis or necrosis is generally observed [26]. The most feared procedure-related complication of TIPS is the creation of a partial intraperitoneal shunt where blood may leak into the peritoneum through the wall of the stent. This has been reported in only one instance to date [14]. Misplacement and migration of the Wallstent has also been mentioned in three recent reports [1••,18,19]. A report of cardiac perforation has been attributed to the permanency of the stiff 10-French introducer sheath placed inside the right atrium after the procedure [17]. Complications related to interposing structures in the puncture pathway have been mentioned as possibilities, and two cases have been recently reported regarding hepatic arterial injury [20••]. Only one description of biliary injury followed by hemobilia has been reported; however, intrahepatic biliary ductal puncture or inadvertent gallbladder puncture has occurred in several patients without sequelae [4••].

The use of an RHV approach allows for the creation of a portosystemic shunt connecting the RHV to the right portal trunk, portal bifurcation, or left portal trunk, including more distal branches of the portal trunks (Fig. 1-2). The variety of sites for portal puncture originated from the RHV approach is a matter of concern, as several vascular and biliary structures are frequently interposed.

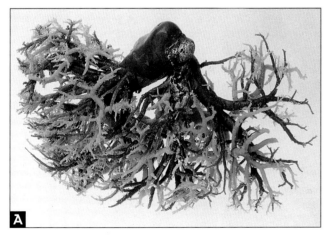

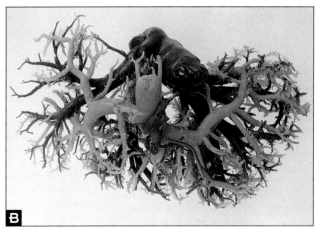

FIGURE 1-6.

A, Anterior view of a liver cast. The hepatic veins and IVC are blue, the portal vein is yellow, the hepatic vein is red, and the bile duct is green. The RHV is short and has a large diameter. The hepatic artery and the common bile duct are hard to see from this view. **B,** Posterior view of the liver cast. The hepatic artery and common bile duct are seen anterior to the portal vein and running around the bifurcation of the portal vein. The right portal trunk shows the artery anteriorly. The right bile duct is not seen because it is either posterior or on the top of the portal trunk. (*From* Uflacker *et al.* (25••), with permission).

The three-dimensional vascular and biliary anatomy and the relationship between these structures as applied to TIPS has never been previously studied using liver casts. It is important to note the constancy of a single, large right hepatic vein in 64% of the patients. Duplicated RHV, accessory RHVs, and an underdeveloped RHV were seen in the remaining 36% of the patients, making the RHV available and adequate caliber for the procedure in the majority of patients. The proximity of the RHV to the portal vein bifurcation makes it suitable for the procedure when compared with the other hepatic veins with a mean distance of 4.41 cm. This finding illustrates the need to use a stent at least 6.5 cm in length to bypass the parenchymal tract. When making this observation, it should be noted that the plastic material used for the cast shrinks approximately 5% to 10%. Furthermore, cirrhotic livers are likely to be smaller than the normal livers used in this study and the actual distance between the two venous systems may be smaller. In only one patient we observed an RHV anterior to the portal vein bifurcation, caused by an uncommon variation in number of the RHVs. This fact, although rare, should be taken into consideration when deciding in which direction the transjugular needle should be used.

The existence of a portal branch to the caudate lobe in the path of the puncture should not raise undue concern for ischemic lesions or bleeding in case of perforation, because of the small size and rare occurrence. The portal bifurcation shows little anatomic variation. In this series, only one patient (4%) would have created any additional difficulty for the TIPS procedure. A more important finding was the relatively high incidence of portal, biliary, or arterial structures in the path between the RHV and the portal vein bifurcation (48%) (Figs. 1-3, 1-5, and 1-6), although there was only one patient (4%) with arterial and biliary structures behind the left trunk. These structures are more commonly anterior to the left portal trunk. The biliary and arterial structures usually run over the anterosuperior aspect of the portal vein bifurcation.

Although only a few complications related to violation of the biliary ducts have been reported [4••] and only two reports of arterial injury around the portal vein bifurcation are available [20••], it would most likely be safer to perform the transparenchymal puncture in the posterior aspect of the portal vein bifurca-

tion and right portal trunk, and never in the superior aspect of the bifurcation or right portal trunk. In most cases, the left portal trunk may be approached safely from either the RHV or MHV because the artery and bile ducts are usually anterior, based on our observations. Patients with cirrhosis may be more prone to develop arterial injuries because of the vicarious enlargement and increased flow in the hepatic artery. In addition, the puncture for the TIPS procedure is performed close to the bifurcation of the hepatic artery and the confluence of the bile ducts, near the liver hilum where these structures are larger.

The mean size of the cast specimens was 24.5 × 18.0 cm. One of the 25 livers (4%) presented two RHVs of similar size, and six livers (24%) had an accessory RHV. Two livers (8%) presented an extremely underdeveloped RHV. In one liver, there was an accessory RHV and in the other there were several inferior vein branches parallel to the RHV. In two (8%), the RHV was bifid with a single trunk, 1 cm in length from the ostium to the confluence of the two parallel branches, both of which were similar in size. The distance from the anterior wall of the RHV measured 1 cm from the IVC and the posterior aspect of the portal bifurcation ranged from 2.7 to 5.4 cm, with a mean distance of 4.41 cm. The distance between the anterior aspect of the accessory RHV measured 1 cm from the IVC and the bifurcation of the portal vein and was significantly smaller than average. The relationship of the structures of the portal triad was extremely variable. The portal bifurcation presented few variations, generating a short right portal trunk and a longer left portal trunk. One liver (4%) presented an anomalous portal bifurcation with the branch to the segments V and VIII originating from the left portal trunk in a way that the arterial and biliary structures might be damaged by the puncture during the TIPS procedure. In 13 patients (52%), the path between the first 1 cm of the RHV and the portal bifurcation was considered to be safe and free of major vascular and biliary structures. In 12 patients (48%), portal, biliary, or arterial structures were identified in the path between the first 1 cm of the RHV and the portal bifurcation.

In two livers (8%), there was one portal branch arising from the right portal trunk parallel to the RHV and in the direction of the caudate lobe (segment I). In one liver (4%), there was an anomalous arterial branch in the path of the puncture.

In nine livers (36%), there were biliary or arterial structures to segment VII or to segments VI and VII in the path of the puncture.

In only one patient (4%), there was an arterial and biliary structure posterior to the left portal trunk in the path of a posterior puncture in the left portal trunk from the RHV. The portal branches to the caudate lobe arise predominantly from the bifurcation of the portal vein or from the first 1 cm of the left portal trunk. These vascular structures would be at risk of puncture when approaching the left trunk of the portal vein from the RHV. The biliary and arterial structures predominantly follow the superior aspect of the portal vein bifurcation. We suggest the TIPS puncture be performed in the back and lower aspect of the right portal trunk; preferably in the posterior aspect and not in the superior wall of the portal vein bifurcation.

Damage to either the hepatic artery or to a major bile duct would carry an increased morbidity and mortality rate in patients with cirrhosis. Aside from the need for knowledge of the anatomic background described here, it is probably warranted to pursue the development of a more flexible, small-gauge coaxial needle-catheter system than presently available, to reduce injuries to the structures that exist in the pathway between the hepatic veins and the portal system [27].

References and Recommended Reading

Recently published papers of particular interest have been highlighted as:

- Of interest
- Of outstanding interest

1.●● Zemel G, Katzen BT, Becker GJ, *et al.*: Percutaneous Transjugular Portosystemic Shunt. *JAMA* 1991, 266:146–149.
One of the first papers describing TIPS and a review of the procedure.

2.● Ring E, Lake JR, Sterneck M, *et al.*: Intrahepatic Portocaval Shunt for Variceal Hemorrhage Prior to Liver Transplantation. *Transplantation* 1991, 52:160–162.
Indication for TIPS in patients undergoing liver transplant.

3. Richter GM, Noeldge G, Roessle M, *et al.*: Evolution and Clinical Introduction of TIPSS, the Transjugular Intrahepatic Portosystemic Stent-Shunt. *Sem Interv Radiol* 1991, 8:331–340.

4.●● LaBerge JM, Ring EJ, Gordon RI, *et al.*: Creation of Transjugular Intrahepatic Portosystemic Shunts with the Wallstent Endoprosthesis: Results in 100 Patients. *Radiology* 1993, 187:413–420.
Most comprehensive follow-up of a large cohort of patients that refers to indicators, technique, and complications in TIPS patients.

5.● Zemel G, Becker GJ, Bancroft JW, *et al.*: Technical Advances in Transjugular Intrahepatic Portosystemic Shunts. *Radiographics* 1992, 12:615–622.
Review of the techniques used in TIPS.

6.●● Richter GM, Noeldge G, Palmaz JC, *et al.*: The Transjugular Intrahepatic Portosystemic Stent-Shunt (TIPSS): Results of a Pilot Study. *Cardiovasc Intervent Radiol* 1990, 13:200–207.
The first important paper written about TIPS in the english language. It deals with technique, variations of the procedure, and short-term follow-up of earlier patients.

7. Noeldge G, Richter GM, Roessle M, *et al.*: Morphologic and Clinical Results of the Transjugular Intrahepatic Portosystemic Stent-Shunt (TIPSS). *Cardiovasc Intervent Radiol* 1992, 15:342–348.

8.● Peltzer MY, Ring EJ, LaBerge JM, *et al.*: Treatment of Budd-Chiari Syndrome with a Transjugular Intrahepatic Portosystemic Shunt. *JVIR* 1993, 4:263–267.
Important new indication for TIPS.

9.●● Conn HO: Transjugular Intrahepatic Portal-systemic Shunts. The State of the Art. *Hepatology* 1993, 17:148–158.
Most comprehensive review of the TIPS procedure, results, complications, and indications under a clinical point of view. First comparison between the two larger series available at the time.

10. Rosch J, Barton RE, Keller FS, Uchida B: Transjugular Intrahepatic Portosystemic Shunt. *Prob Gen Surg* 1992, 9:502–512.

11. Ring EJ, Lake JR, Roberts JP, *et al.*: Using Transjugular Intrahepatic Portosystemic Shunts to Control Variceal Bleeding Before Liver Transplantation. *Ann Intern Med* 1992, 116:304–309.

12. Chalmers N, Redhead DN, Simpson KJ, *et al.*: Transjugular Intrahepatic Portosystemic Stent Shunt (TIPPS): Early Clinical Experience. *Clin Radiol* 1992, 46:166–169.

13.● Radosevich PM, Ring EJ, LaBerge JM, *et al.*: Transjugular Intrahepatic Portotosystemic Shunts in Patients with Portal Vein Occlusion. *Radiology* 1993, 186:523–527.
Shows how the TIPS procedure can be performed in portal vein occlusion.

14. Perarnau JM, Roessle M, Noeldge G, *et al.*: Presented at the III International Meeting of the Society for Minimally Invasive Therapy, Boston, November 1991.

15. Sanchez RB, Roberts AC, Valji K, *et al.*: Wallstent Misplaced During Transjugular Placement of an Intrahepatic Portosystemic Shunt: Retrieval with a Loop Snare. *AJR* 1992, 159:129–130.

16. Darcy MC, Vesely TM, Picus D, *et al.*: Percutaneous Revision of an Acutely Thrombosed Transjugular Intrahepatic Portosystemic Shunt. *JVIR* 1992, 3:77–82.

17. Fit G, Thomson K, Hennessy O: Delayed Fatal Cardiac Perforation by an Indwelling Long Introducer Sheath Following Transjugular Intrahepatic Portocaval Stents (TIPS). *Cardiovasc Intervent Radiol* 1993, 16:109–110.

18. Cekirge S, Foster RG, Weiss JP, *et al.*: Percutaneous Removal of an Embolized Wallstent During a Transjugular Intrahepatic Portosystemic Shunt Procedure. *JVIR* 1993, 4:559–560.

19. Cohen GS, Ball DS: Delayed Wallstent Migration After a Transjugular Intrahepatic Portosystemic Shunt Procedure: Relocation with a Loop Snare. *JVIR* 1993, 4:561–563.

20.•• Haskal ZJ, Pentecost MJ, Rubin RA: Hepatic Arterial Injury After Transjugular Intrahepatic Portosystemic Shunt Placement: Report of Two Cases. *Radiology* 1993, 188:85–88.
First paper to report arterial complications following TIPS.

21. Wenz F, Nemcek AA, Tischler HA, *et al.*: US-guided Paraumbilical Vein Puncture: An Adjunct to Transjugular Intrahepatic Portosystemic Shunt (TIPS) Placement. *JVIR* 1992, 3:549–551.

22. Harman JT, Reed JD, Kopecky KK, *et al.*: Localization of the Portal Vein for Transjugular Catheterization: Percutaneous Placement of a Metallic Marker with Real-time US Guidance. *JVIR* 1992, 3:545–547.

23. Teitelbaum GP, Van Allan RJ, Reed RA, *et al.*: Portal Venous Branch Targeting with a Platinum-tipped Wire to Facilitate Transjugular Intrahepatic Portosystemic Shunt (TIPS) Procedures. *Cardiovasc Intervent Radiol* 1993, 16:198–200.

24. LaBerge JM, Ring EJ, Gordon RL: Percutaneous Intrahepatic Portosystemic Shunt Created Via a Femoral Vein Approach. *Radiology* 1991, 181:679–681.

25.• Uflacker R, Reichert P, D'Albuquerque LC, *et al.*: Liver Anatomy Applied to the Transjugular Intrahepatic Portosystemic Shunt (TIPS). Radiology 1994; 191:1–9.
Demonstrates the anatomy of the liver applied to the TIPS procedure, and the relationships between the vascular biliary structures within liver in the path of the needle.

26. LeBerge JM, Ferrel LD, Ring EJ, *et al.*: Histopathologic Study of Transjugular Intrahepatic Portosystemic Shunts. *JVIR* 1991, 2:549–556.

27. Maynar M, Cabrera J, Pulido-Duque JM, *et al.*: Transjugular Intrahepatic Portosystemic Shunt: Early Experience with a Flexible Trocar/Catheter System. *AJR* 1993, 161:301–306.

Select Bibliography

Haskal ZJ, Pentecost MJ, Rubin RA: Hepatic Arterial Injury After Transjugular Intrahepatic Portosystemic Shunt Placement: Report of Two Cases. *Radiology* 1993, 188:85–88.

LaBerge JM, Ring EJ, Gordon RL, *et al.*: Creation of Transjugular Intrahepatic Portosystemic Shunts with the Wallstent Endoprosthesis: Results in 100 Patients. *Radiology* 1993, 187:413–420.

Uflacker R, Reichert P, D'Albuquerque LC, *et al.*: Liver Anatomy Applied to the Transjugular Intrahepatic Portosystemic Shunt. *Radiology* 1994, 191:1–9.

Techniques for Management of Pediatric Vascular Anomalies

Patricia E. Burrows
Kenneth E. Fellows

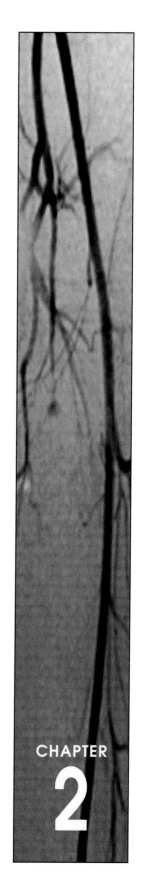

CHAPTER
2

An understanding of the anatomy and pathophysiology of congenital vascular malformations has advanced remarkably in the past 15 years, stimulated by technologic developments allowing new treatment possibilities and by individuals who have refined the scientific medical basis for diagnosing and classifying these complex lesions. A giant step in progress was made by Mulliken and Young [1], whose revolutionary biologic classification of vascular birthmarks led to a logical and now generally accepted system of terminology [2•, 3]. They advocate the principle that two distinct types of vascular abnormalities exist—hemangiomas and malformations—each with distinctive clinical, cellular, hematologic, radiologic, and skeletal differences [1, 2•]. We are no longer limited by a morass of confusing and redundant terms based on poetic description (*eg*, strawberry, port wine, cavernous), Latin nomenclature (*eg*, macula materna, naevus flamieus), and anatomic observation (*eg*, lymphangioma cytoids) [1, 2•]. We must also not be misled by the tendency of some to lump most congenital vascular lesions under the broad term *hemangioma*. As stated by Mulliken and Young [1], "...any strictly histopathological classification without clinical correlation has not proved to be useful in the diagnosis and management of patients with vascular birthmarks."

Hemangiomas are benign vascular tumors, generally having a predictable proliferative phase in the patient between 2 weeks and 18 months of age, and an equally predictable involutionary stage ranging from 2 to 6 years. Because they are self-limited, they usually require no intervention. However, a few hemangiomas do require medical, surgical, or catheter therapy by virtue of their anatomic location (*eg*, orbital) or their pathologic activity (*eg*, platelet trapping, bleeding) [1, 4].

Vascular malformations are congenitally abnormal vessels and vascular connections that are present at birth and grow with the child, often expanding rapidly as vascular spaces fill in response to the hormones of adolescence and pregnancy, trauma, or other stimuli. Vascular malformations have few proliferating cells and do not involute and cannot be encouraged to regress with steroids, irradiation, or other measures effective for hemangiomas [1]. For these reasons, vascular malformations are often problematic, and affected patients are frequently candidates for surgical treatment, interventional therapy, or both.

Vascular Anomalies Clinics

As medical understanding of congenital vascular malformations and hemangiomas has increased, the medical and surgical management of these lesions has similarly expanded. Medical treatment for hemangiomas now offers steroids and interferon alfa therapy [4]. Surgical alternatives to all vascular birthmarks include total or partial excision, debulking, cosmetic reconstruction, and laser therapy. Interventionalists can treat vascular malformations by catheter embolization and sclerosis via arterial or venous routes, or by direct needle puncture. In many cases, a combination of medical, surgical, and radiologic interventions is appropriate.

Because accurate diagnosis of vascular anomalies is critical and because complete consideration of all therapeutic options best serves the patient, a vascular anomalies clinic in which multiple specialists participate is recommended as the best way to evaluate affected children and adolescents [3, 5]. Multiple disciplinary vascular clinics have the advantage of concentrating experience with these relatively rare abnormalities in the hands of those intensely interested in the problem. Clinics also have the potential to improve long-term outcomes by maintaining clinical trials, detailed records, and long-term follow-up.

Core participants in any vascular anomalies clinic should include a plastic surgeon, general surgeon, dermatologist, hematologist, and radiologist. Additional consultants should be available from orthopedic and otorhinolaryngologic surgery and ophthalmology. With all these perspectives represented in one clinic, any patient presenting with a hemangioma or vascular malformation can receive an efficient diagnosis as well as sophisticated recommendations for coordinated therapy and follow-up in one or two convenient visits.

In this scheme, which is operative in many contemporary medical centers, the interventional radiologist has two important functions: 1) to recommend for each patient the most appropriate imaging techniques, such as arteriography, magnetic resonance imaging (MRI), or MR angiography (MRA), required for accurate diagnosis and therapeutic planning; and 2) to suggest the best interventional alternatives for therapy, if any [3,5]. The radiologist is also there to interpret previously performed diagnostic-imaging studies and to participate in patient follow-up and any changes required in treatment plans. Many times, the long-range therapy of a vascular lesion involves a combination of laser therapy, embolization, or other intervention as well as surgery; the radiologist must be present to insure proper selection and sequencing of these procedures. Inasmuch as the radiologist becomes central to preoperative preparation and long-term follow-up, participation in these clinics requires a substantial clinical commitment.

PROCEDURAL SUPPORT

Interventional procedures for treating patients with pediatric vascular anomalies are best performed in a children's hospital, where personnel are comfortable with infants and children and are equipped to handle their needs. Special requirements include heating devices to avoid unnecessary heat loss during anesthesia induction; extra padding under pressure points to avoid skin damage from long procedures under anesthesia; and bladder catheterization. Small femoral arterial-access systems and systemic heparinization are effective in avoiding femoral artery thrombosis, even through lengthy procedures. In general, the smallest catheter size to accommodate the diagnostic and interventional procedure should be used and custom shaping of the catheters is often necessary. The contrast medium should be kept to a minimum and recorded carefully. General anesthesia is useful not only in obtaining patient immobility, but also in altering blood flow. In particular, the use of hypercarbia promotes vasodilation and prevents arterial spasm, which is a frequent problem in children. Following arterial procedures, pedal pulses must be monitored carefully. Femoral artery thrombosis occurs infrequently if the above listed precautions are followed, but when it occurs it should be aggressively treated if possible. Finally, the patients should recover in a unit with consistent nursing personnel who are aware of the nature and possible complications of the procedures.

Specific Lesions

HEMANGIOMAS

These very common, benign vascular tumors in infants and children (Fig. 2-1) rarely require radiologic therapeutic intervention because of their natural history to involute [1]. Large facial hemangiomas near the orbit can cause amblyopia and strabismus by obstructing vision; these are treated by ophthalmologists with oral

or intralesional administration of steroids [4]. Oral hemangiomas can cause bleeding and feeding difficulties in infancy. These are also effectively treated by systemic steroids [6].

The term *alarming hemangiomas* was introduced to describe those lesions that impair normal function or become life-threatening risks by virtue of their extreme size or anatomic location [7]. Examples are giant cutaneous hemangiomas causing a thrombocytopenic coagulopathy (Kasabach-Merritt syndrome); pulmonary hemangiomatosis causing respiratory compromise; diffuse gastrointestinal hemangiomas complicated by severe blood loss; and hepatic hemangioendotheliosis causing infantile congestive heart failure [1, 8••]. If clinical conditions permit, pharmacologic therapy is available for these tumors using corticosteroids, cyclophosphamide, and interferon alfa-2a [8••]. However, these medical therapies when effective usually require weeks to months for results. Occasionally, embolization therapy is needed on an urgent basis, particularly with platelet-trapping hemangiomas and infantile hepatic hemangioendotheliomas.

Kasabach-Merritt Syndrome

Hemangiomas may trap platelets and affect other coagulation factors, but arteriovenous malformations do not.

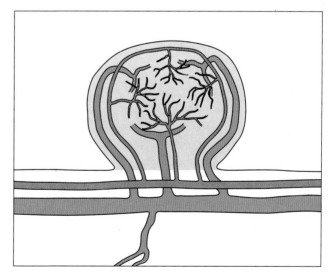

FIGURE 2-1.

The hemangioma is a benign, usually cutaneous tumor of vascular tissue characterized by a central, dense association of capillaries surrounded by peripheral supplying arteries and draining veins distributed in a circumferential pattern. Adjacent vessels are normal, not anomalous, and usually there is no arteriovenous shunting.

Thrombocytopenic bleeding induced by hemangiomas occurs during tumor growth (early infancy) and disappears with tumor involution. Kasabach-Merritt syndrome is a self-limited condition [1]. If medical therapy using prednisone, cyclophosphamide, interferon alfa-2a, and surgical excision are not possible, effective, or timely enough, arterial embolization should be considered [9, 10]. Polyvinyl alcohol or collagen particles (Avitene; MedChem, Woburn, MA) can be used to block a large percentage of the tumoral vessels, thereby preventing further platelet trapping and destruction and hastening involution of the lesion. Recurrence of the coagulopathy after an excellent initial response is frequent, resulting from revascularization of the lesion; repetition of the embolization two or three times may result in a permanent improvement. Alternately, consideration should be given to surgical excision after embolization, if possible.

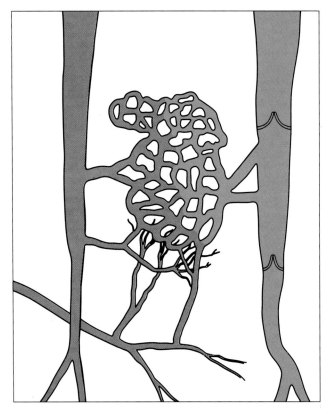

FIGURE 2-2.

An arteriovenous malformation is a congenital network (the nidus) of anomalous vascular channels and connections of variable diameter allowing high-volume arteriovenous shunting that produces enlargement of the afferent arteries and efferent veins. With time, during trauma, or after treatment, adjacent undistended channels often fill and connections to other vessels (collaterals) open.

Infantile Hepatic Hemangioendotheliomas

These usually multiple and benign vascular tumors of the liver affecting infants are immature variants of hemangiomas. As such, they have characteristic proliferative and involutional stages in childhood. Hemangioendotheliomas are frequently complicated by severe congestive heart failure and when medical management of the failure (with digitalis and diuretics) or the tumors (with prednisone, cyclophosphamide and interferon alfa-2a) is ineffective, embolization of hepatic arteries and other collateral vessels supplying these highly vascular tumors is recommended [11•, 12•]. A variety of embolic materials have been successfully used in the treatment of liver hemangioendotheliomas. However, the size of arteriovenous connections in the lesions varies and embolization of small particles to the pulmonary circulation (or systemic circulation by crossing the foramen ovale) may occur. Hepatic artery embolization with 1- to 5-mm coils is an effective alternative [11•]. The aim of the embolization is to reduce hepatic arterial blood flow which will sufficiently relieve high-output cardiac failure; complete obliteration of the abnormal vasculature is unnecessary. The hemangioendotheliomas usually involute sufficiently in the patient by 18 to 24 months of age to preclude further symptomatology. In some patients, embolization of adjacent intercostal and visceral arteries that supply collateral flow to the liver tumors will be necessary to achieve an effective reduction in blood flow [11•, 12•]. Arterial portography should always be performed prior to embolization; if there is tumor supply from the portal circulation, extensive arterial embolization may result in fatal hepatic necrosis [12•]. Vascular malformations can also occur in the liver and cause congestive heart failure in infants. In these cases, medical therapy using steroids, cyclophosphamide, and interferon to reduce the size of the vascular lesion will inevitably fail, leaving either embolization (for diffuse lesions) or surgical excision (for those with a segmental or lobar localization) as the only efficacious therapy [11•].

Arteriovenous Malformations

GENERAL CONCEPTS

Congenitally abnormal connections between arteries and veins, devoid of the usual arteriolar resistance vessels and capillary beds, constitute a common form of combined vascular anomaly termed an *arteriovenous malformation* (AVM). There is a prevalent concept that these malformations have a central confluence or nidus of tortuous vessels where the shunting of arterial blood to veins occurs (Fig. 2-2). Although true and identifiable in small localized AVMs (Fig. 2-2), the nidus is often large or spread out, or there may be multiple nidi in one lesion. It is true that obliteration of the nidus will usually cure the malformation; unfortunately, this is not always possible when the nidi are large or multiple. What can be

said of all AVMs is that none can be cured or permanently controlled by merely blocking the supplying arteries by embolization, surgery, or other means. Collaterals are always available and will always be recruited to reconstitute arterial flow. In fact, mere embolization or surgical ligation of supplying arteries actually makes matters worse. The collaterals that develop are more difficult or impossible to treat because they are small, multiple, and often unreachable (Fig. 2-3).

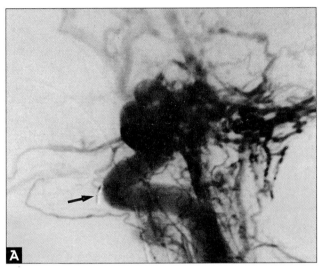

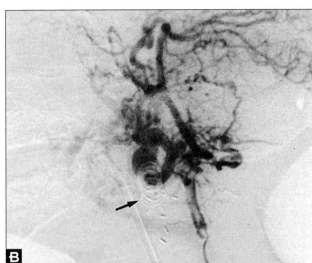

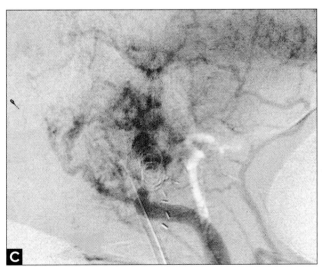

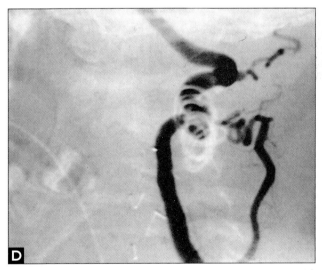

FIGURE 2-3.

A venous embolization. An 18-month-old boy, when in congestive heart failure resulting from a large AVM of the left face and neck, had an ill-advised ligation of the left external carotid artery as a neonate. **A,** Left vertebral arteriogram, lateral view, showing dense filling of the internal jugular vein (*arrow*) periauricular AVM. **B** and **C,** Left vertebral arteriogram before and after coil embolization of the left internal jugular vein, respectively. **B,** Because

there was no direct access to the afferent arteries of the AVM, the left internal jugular vein was embolized with three 12-mm diameter coils (*arrow*). **C,** Venous drainage immediately after embolization is to adjacent small veins of the neck, which reconstitute the distal internal jugular vein. **D,** Repeat left vertebral arteriogram 6 months after jugular embolization. Arteriographically and clinically the AVM has resolved, apparently from venous thrombosis.

In addition, proximal arterial occlusion may result in worsening of ischemia in the adjacent tissues.

As with other vascular malformations, AVMs are present at birth and persist as the child grows, often suddenly enlarging in response to trauma, hormones, or other stimuli. They are often symptomatic, causing pain, overgrowth, ischemia (steal phenomenon through the AVM and venous hypertension), hemorrhage, or heart failure. Clinically, they are frequently recognizable by the presence of a pulsatile mass, increased warmth and sometimes redness, and increased pulse strength in major feeding arteries.

Most AVMs can be managed but not cured by catheter embolization and sclerosis [13, 14, 15•]. At present, cures are mostly the result of combined interventional and surgical treatment. Any therapy, whether to prevent or alleviate hemorrhage or ischemia, or to eradicate the AVM because of pain or heart failure, should be thoroughly planned by all specialists involved.

Embolization of feeding arteries by particles is adequate prior to surgical excision. In patients for whom surgery is not an option, particle embolization produces some initial improvement in symptoms such as pain or bleeding, but the lesion invariably recurs. Therefore the nidus should be embolized whenever possible with a permanent occluding agent, such as tissue adhesive or 100% ethanol [13, 14]. Where the nidus cannot be reached by subselective catheterization, sclerosants may be injected by retrograde or direct cannulation of the nidus after occlusion of the feeding arteries [13, 14, 15•]. Another therapeutic alternative is embolic occlusion of venous outflow from AVMs (Fig. 2-3). This less-common technique may have some efficacy, although experience with this technique is insufficient at this time.

ARTERIOVENOUS MALFORMATIONS OF THE FACE AND NECK

Cervicofacial arteriovenous anomalies are considerably less common than low-flow venolymphatic malformations in the head and neck region and distinctly uncommon when compared with intracerebral AVMs [1]. Although always present at birth, they often go unnoticed for years, hidden by facial muscles or camouflaged by mild cutaneous staining. Because of intrinsic, often high-flow arteriovenous shunting, they invariably become either visible (as a swollen, pulsatile, warm, discolored mass), symptomatic (painful, buzzing, throbbing, or disfiguring) or both [1]. Spontaneous oral hemorrhage or excessive bleeding at the time of tooth extraction are common presentations and are often catastrophic [9, 16, 17].

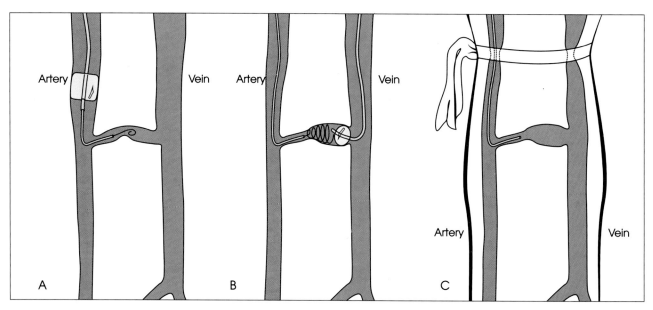

FIGURE 2-4.

Flow-control techniques for occluding AV fistulae and AVM. **A**, An upstream (proximal) balloon catheter placed within the artery proximal to the AVF. The catheters are for use with microcoils, liquid sclerosants, and tissue adhesive. **B**, A downstream (distal) balloon catheter placed in the draining vein, for use with coils, sclerosants, and tissue adhesive. **C**, A tourniquet or manual compression for injection of sclerosants through a catheter or directly through a needle.

The therapeutic options are embolization alone, as palliation of specific symptoms, or in combination with surgical excision or dental extraction. For large AVMs, the operative approach is risky and frequently disappointing because of poor cosmetic result and recurrence. However, it may be the best treatment for a patient with debilitating pain or severe bleeding. The operative procedure to be assiduously avoided is ligation of the external carotid artery. Not only does this maneuver have no long-term benefit, as ipsicontralateral tributaries reconstitute the AVM quickly (Fig. 2-3), but the ligation and subsequent collateralization also preclude future arterial embolization unless the occluded carotid is surgically reconstructed [18•].

Embolization of cervicofacial AVMs requires subselective catheterization of external carotid artery branches, the thyrocervical trunk, and other medium and small arteries. This is usually best accomplished with a coaxial catheter system consisting of a 4- or 5-French guiding catheter and an inner 2- to 3-French delivery catheter, such as Tracker catheter (Target Therapeutics, Los Angeles, CA). The most commonly used embolic materials are polyvinyl alcohol particles (150 to 600 µm) and microcoils. These particles are effective, but large enough to spare vessels to skin and cranial nerves. Gelfoam (Upjohn, Kalamazoo, MI) particles can be used for preoperative embolization if the surgery follows within 24 to 72 hours. Coils and alcohol or other liquid agents can be injected directly

through needles inserted into the AVM after flow has been controlled by arterial embolization or other techniques (Figs. 2-4 and 2-5). Direct injection of embolic material or sclerosing agents into the nidus of the AVM may also be curative [16, 19].

Patients having dental AVMs associated with acute bleeding and loose teeth should undergo embolization immediately prior to tooth extractions, which may be carried out in the angiography room before removing the catheters in case additional embolization is necessary [9]. Intranidal injection of ethanol or tissue adhesive is helpful in completing the hemostasis. If the teeth are not loose, this maneuver including arterial embolization and intranidal injection may result in thrombosis of the malformation and bony healing and may actually obviate the need for dental extractions and radical surgical resections [17, 19]. The surgical alternatives include maxillectomy or mandibulectomy (usually requiring revisions to accommodate growth) and curettage of the AVM to preserve the bony cortex.

Embolization of AVMs in the head and neck can be complicated by stroke, cranial nerve palsies, skin necrosis, infection, blindness, and pulmonary embolism [18•]. These adverse effects can be minimized by careful planning and performance of the procedure. The operator must have an excellent knowledge of craniofacial and spinal vascular anatomy, including the normal supply to the cranial nerves, communications between the external and internal carotid

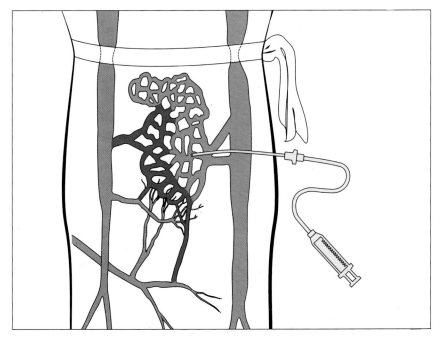

FIGURE 2-5.

Direct sclerosant injection of AVM after arterial embolization and with additional tourniquet flow control.

systems, and anatomic vascular variants. The internal carotid artery should always be studied prior to external carotid artery embolization, not only to determine if it supplies the lesion, but also to define the vascular supply to the globe.

EXTREMITY ARTERIOVENOUS MALFORMATIONS

Arteriovenous malformations involving the extremities may be localized but are usually diffuse, often involving the entire extremity and adjacent trunk (*eg*, Parkes-Weber syndrome). Symptoms include extremity-length discrepancy, congestive cardiac failure, and ischemic pain or ulceration. AVMs involving most or all of an extremity are usually incurable by any means short of amputation [1, 13, 15•]. Rarely, an AVM may be so localized that embolization or complete surgical excision is possible [20]. When one muscle or a muscle group is involved, surgical removal after preoperative embolization may also be curative. Usually, the arteriovenous shunting is extensive and no localized nidus exists; these patients often have high-flow lesions that result in congestive heart failure. The therapeutic alternatives are multiple embolizations and limited resections to minimize flow or amputation of the extremity. Even the latter can be rendered ineffective or impossible if the AVM extends into the chest wall or pelvis.

Arteriovenous malformations involving localized parts of the hands or feet are often amenable to embolization and direct injection of alcohol, after arterial embolization or occlusion of venous outflow to slow flow [13, 14, 15•, 21]. Although there are attendant ischemic complications to such catheter therapy, they are less common and less serious than the 50% complication rate that accompanies surgical attempts to control these lesions [1].

TRUNCAL ARTERIOVENOUS MALFORMATIONS
Thorax and Lungs
Pulmonary arteriovenous malformations often occurring in patients who have Rendu-Osler-Weber syndrome cause cyanosis, clubbing, and polycythemia as well as cerebral infarcts and abscesses, because of the right-to-left shunting and the loss of the normal filter function of the pulmonary vascular bed. Embolization of the pulmonary arterial side of isolated or multiple lesions using either coils or detachable balloons has become the preferred therapy [22]. Another form of pulmonary AVM consisting of tiny microshunts diffusely scattered throughout one or both lungs is not amenable to embolization or other catheter therapy. Lobectomy or pneumonectomy is curative in the rare cases of patients with uninvolved lung parenchyma. These diffuse pulmonary AVMs may be isolated congenital anomalies, but sometimes occur after cavalpulmonary arterial anastomoses in patients with congenital heart disease, and also in association with polysplenia, portal vein thrombosis, and liver cirrhosis [23]. Those lesions associated with hepatic disease may regress after liver transplantation.

Arteriovenous malformations involving the thorax may be limited to the chest wall, but often are part of a large malformation extending into the neck, upper extremities, and the abdominal wall [1]. By virtue of their size alone, they are difficult to treat with either surgery or embolotherapy. If symptoms make therapy imperative, the best hope is flow-reducing preoperative embolization followed by surgical excision. Embolotherapy alone is never sufficient; the extensive collateral connections between intercostal arteries, internal mammary arteries, brachiocephalic vessels, and mediastinal arteries render any embolic gains disappointingly transient.

Abdomen and Pelvis
Vascular malformations located within the gastrointestinal tract are often primarily venous, occurring multiply throughout the gastrointestinal tract and causing chronic gastrointestinal bleeding [24]. These are frequently associated with either Rendu-Osler-Weber syndrome or the Blue-Rubber Bleb Nevus syndrome [1]. Congenital arteriovenous malformations are less common, occurring most frequently in the small bowel where mass lesions may cause acute or chronic hemorrhage, obstruction, or intussusception [1]. The diagnosis in children is usually confirmed by mesenteric arteriography [25, 26]. Even when the diagnosis has been established, the lesions are notoriously difficult to locate intraoperatively. Placing catheters or coil emboli, or intraoperatively injecting methylene blue into supplying mesenteric arteries have all been advocated as helpful procedures [25, 26]. More recently, the development of tiny coaxial catheters, capable of delivering microcoils and particles of varying size, has allowed subselective catheterization and embolization of peripheral mesenteric arteries and gastrointestinal mural vessels.

Retroperitoneal and pelvic congenital AVMs in children share several characteristics: 1) large, high-flow lesions often causing congestive heart failure; 2) the tendency to also involve the mesentery and adjacent organs; and 3) usually multiple, large feeding arteries and an inexhaustible supply of collateral vessels [27]. For these reasons, the prospects for cure are poor [1]. Even with combined embolotherapy and surgery, the recurrence rate has been as high as 67% [28]. After retreatment with both modalities, neither showing an advantage over the other, the recurrence rate was 84% [28].

From our own experience and that reported by others, the following treatment protocol seems reasonable: asymptomatic pelvic and retroperitoneal AVMs should be followed expectantly, documenting size and flow characteristics with ultrasonography or MRI on a 6- to 12-month basis [27, 28]. For symptomatic lesions, a combined approach using preoperative embolization and surgical excision should be followed [28]. Mere ligation or coil embolization of both internal iliac arteries should always be avoided because it prevents future embolization and encourages the formation of collateral supply.

Arteriovenous Fistulae

Arteriovenous fistulae (AVF) are macroscopic arteriovenous connections (Fig. 2-6). In children, these usually represent congenital malformations, although acquired lesions can occur secondary to trauma, cannulation, surgery, or spontaneous rupture in vascular dysplasias, as in neurofibromatosis or Osler-Weber-Rendu syndrome. They may occur in any part of the body but most frequently present in the head or neck area, the spine, and the extremities. Symptomatology depends on the size and location of the fistula and may include congestive heart failure, localized growth disturbances, neurologic deficits due to mass effect of the dilated veins on the spinal cord or intracranial contents, and ischemic changes due to venous hypertension. AVF are frequently diagnosed because of detection of a loud bruit when they are still asymptomatic. Unlike AVMs, which are considered incurable in the majority of patients, AVF can be cured by the endovascular approach. Therefore, because AVF only become larger and more symptomatic with time, those that are curable should be treated when they are

diagnosed or as soon as the risk of the procedure is reasonably low.

The method of occlusion for AVF depends on the size and location of the individual lesions. The goal of treatment is to occlude the fistula and the immediate draining vein and to preserve the feeding artery whenever possible. Suitable devices include detachable balloons, coils, and microcoils, and tissue adhesive especially for fistulae in the central nervous system (Fig. 2-7). Absorbable materials such as Gelfoam should be avoided as should particles. Detachable balloons are ideal for occluding some large fistulae because they can be optimally positioned before being detached and because they conform to the size and shape of the abnormal vessels (Fig. 2-8). Fistulae arising proximally from major branches of the aorta can be occluded with relatively large balloons using a preloaded 4- or 5-French catheter system [29]. For fistulae located more distally in the arterial tree, variable stiffness microcatheters are exceedingly

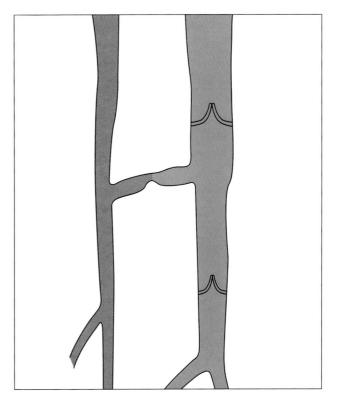

FIGURE 2-6.

An arteriovenous fistula. This condition is a congenital (sometimes acquired) direct connection of variable length between an artery and vein, resulting in high-volume arteriovenous shunting.

useful in catheterizing the fistula and draining vein. Platinum microcoils have several advantages over the larger coils: they can be positioned through the micro-catheters that most readily access the lesion, and they are nonferromagnetic and do not produce a significant artifact on subsequent MRI scanning. However, a disadvantage is their light weight, as they can be dislodged by turbulent arterial flow. They may be used in conjunction with flow-control techniques such as the use of an upstream or downstream balloon

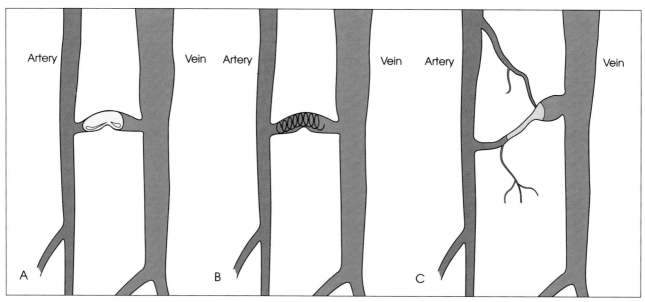

FIGURE 2-7.

Catheter treatment of AVF. **A**, Treatment by detachable balloon.
B, Treatment using coil embolization. **C**, Treatment with tissue adhesive.

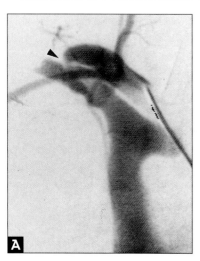
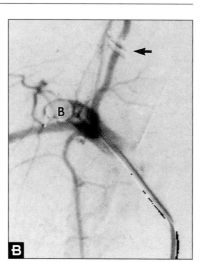
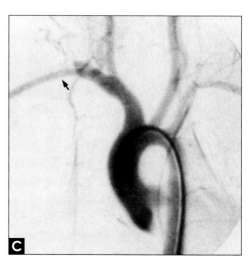

FIGURE 2-8.

Congenital subclavian AVF embolized in a 10-month-old patient using a detachable balloon. **A**, Right subclavian arteriogram prior to embolization shows the fistula (*arrow*) arising from a cervical branch of the right subclavian artery adjacent to the right vertebral artery and connecting directly with the right subclavian vein. **B**, Angiogram performed after inflation but before detachment of the detachable balloon. A second nondetachable balloon has been positioned upstream during balloon inflation to prevent dislodgement during detachment. A Doppler probe (*arrow*) has been placed over the common carotid artery for monitoring during balloon manipulation. **C**, Arch aortogram performed 16 months after the embolization shows the silver clip (*arrow*) at the tip of the balloon, which is now deflated, and continued occlusion of the fistula. (**A** and **B** *From* Burrows *et al.* (29); with permission).

catheter or in the case of extremity lesions, tourniquets, or blood pressure cuffs (Fig. 2-4). A major disadvantage of coils in occluding vascular anomalies is the clot that forms around them may resorb, resulting in recanalization. Therefore, the coils should be packed. Thrombosis may be augmented by previous soaking in topical thrombin, or by injecting a sclerosant around the coils. Tissue adhesive is a powerful agent with many advantages, especially for small fistulae in critical locations such as the central nervous system. Occlusion is permanent and when properly injected it

is possible to precisely cast the fistulae (Fig. 2-9). In lesions where the venous anatomy or short length of the feeding artery does not allow adequate packing of coils, tissue adhesive can be effectively used in combination with microcoils. Coils are placed first to slow the flow and then tissue adhesive is injected to occlude the actual fistula. It must be noted that until the long-term safety of tissue adhesive is ascertained, it is reasonable to restrict their use to those children having lesions that cannot be adequately treated by any other means.

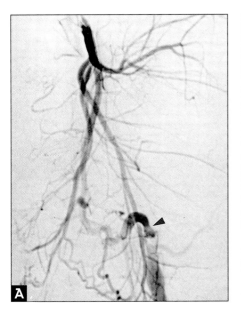

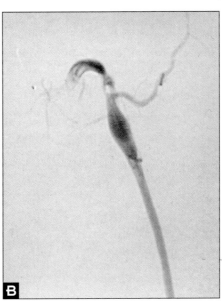

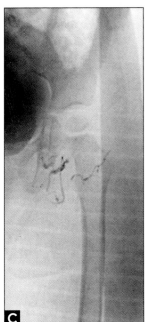

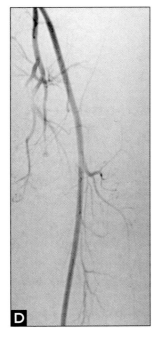

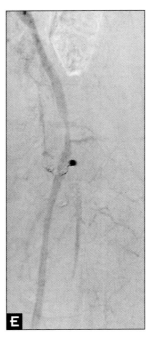

FIGURE 2-9.

Embolization of an AVF at the left groin in a 1 1/2-year-old girl with severe leg swelling and overgrowth. Previous surgery had resulted in ligation of the left common femoral vein above the fistula, aggravating the symptoms. **A**, Left internal iliac arteriogram before embolization shows a direct fistula (*arrowhead*) between a branch of the obturator internus artery and the left superficial femoral vein, with retrograde flow into the lower extremity. **B**, Selective catheterization of the fistula prior to embolization. Injection of tissue adhesive was made using a tourniquet around the thigh to slow flow. **C**, Radiograph showing the tissue adhesive within the feeding artery and immediate draining vein. **D**, Common iliac arteriogram following embolization showing occlusion of the fistula with no evidence of collateral flow. **E**, Venous phase of the postembolization iliac arteriogram showing diversion of flow through the saphenous system.

Venous Malformations

Venous malformations are low-flow vascular malformations. Symptomatic venous malformations are much more common than arteriovenous malformations. The lesions consist of collections of abnormal vascular channels characterized by deficient smooth muscle; on arteriography, these channels opacify in the venous phase or they do not opacify at all (Fig. 2-10). The true size of the lesion is best demonstrated by T_2-weighted MRI and by direct intralesional contrast injection. The number and size of connections with the systemic veins is variable. There are two major forms of venous malformations: one consisting of clusters of interconnecting venous spaces with minimal or no connections to adjacent normal systemic veins, and another in which the clusters of venous channels communicate freely with dysplastic systemic veins [30]. Lesions of the latter type may contain large varicose expansions of major conducting veins. The two forms are frequently found in the same patient.

The clinical symptomatology depends on the location of the malformation. Many are present in the subcutaneous layer or on the skin surface, causing cosmetic deformities. Those in the oral cavity are often responsible for bleeding, airway obstruction, and impaired development of speech and dentition. Intramuscular lesions may cause pain with exertion. Occasionally, relatively small venous malformations can cause severe pain. Venous malformations are the most common vascular malformation found in a number of syndromes, including Klippel-Trenaunay syndrome, Maffucci syndrome, Blue-Rubber Bleb Nevus syndrome, and multiple hereditary venous malformations. Most lesions referred to in the literature as *osseous hemangiomas* are actually venous malformations. The imaging literature is complicated, because many publications refer to the lesions as *cavernous hemangiomas*.

Surgical treatment may be effective in localized lesions, but often involves excision of surrounding normal tissue, and also has a high rate of recurrence [30]. Venous malformations do not respond to arterial embolization [30]. The most effective interventional management is direct intralesional injection of a sclerosant (sclerotherapy) (Fig. 2-11). A variety of materials have been used in the past, including dextrose, sodium morrhuate, sodium tetradecyl, concentrated ethanol, and Ethibloc (Ethicon, Hamburg, Germany). One hundred percent ethanol has been found to have the lowest recurrence rate of the liquid sclerosants. Ethanol can be mixed with metrizamide powder, making it radiopaque. It produces extreme pain on injection and therefore requires general anesthesia. Because of its neurolytic effect, the injection's use is generally associated with relatively minor postprocedural pain. Sodium tetradecyl can be diluted with liquid contrast medium. It has the advantage of causing minor discomfort on injection, so that it can be used without a general anesthetic, and is often administered without fluoroscopic control in the offices of plastic surgeons and dermatologists. Ethibloc consists of a mixture of amino acids, contrast medium, and ethanol, and is frequently used as a sclerosing or fibrosing agent in

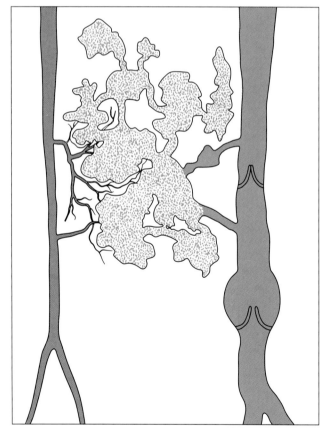

FIGURE 2-10.

Venous malformations appear as a congenital interconnected group of venous channels and spaces at variable sizes that drain to adjacent veins, some of which may contain varicosities or have deficient valves. There often are tiny connecting arteries and occasionally tiny AVF.

Europe but it is not presently approved by the Food and Drug Administration [30, 31]. It can also be used without a general anesthetic.

A direct intralesional injection is performed after clinical evaluation of the patient and MRI of the extent of the lesion. If gradient imaging or MRA is available, arteriography is usually not necessary. However, one of the aforementioned techniques should be performed to rule out associated AVF and other malformations. The skin overlying the lesion is sterilized and draped. The malformation is cannulated, usually through a layer of intact skin and subcutaneous tissue, avoiding the courses of nerves and large blood vessels, with a teflon-sheathed needle (Angiocath 20-gauge, 2-inch; Becton Dickinson Vascular Access, Sandy, UT). After obtaining sufficient blood return, contrast medium is

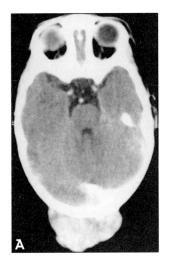
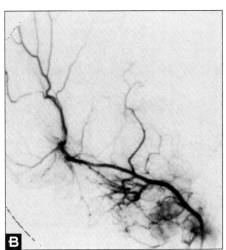
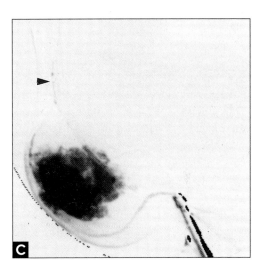
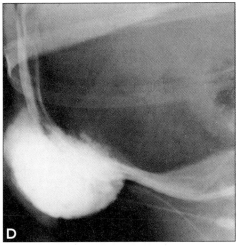
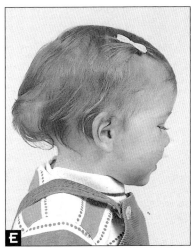
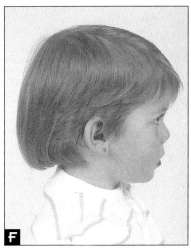

FIGURE 2-11.

Direct intralesional ethanol injection (sclerotherapy) to treat an enlarging venous malformation of the scalp in a 10-month-old girl. **A**, A CT scan after contrast administration shows an inhomogeneously enhancing subcutneous mass. **B**, The right occipital arteriogram, lateral projection, showing no arteriovenous shunting or tumor vascularity. This lesion did not opacify in the venous phase. **C**, The contrast injection (digital subtraction technique) after direct percutaneous cannulation of the lesion, lateral projection, shows filling of typical rounded sinusoidal spaces with opacification of a small subcutaneous vein (*arrow*).

An ethanol injection was made with a tourniquet control to prevent ethanol from entering the intracranial sinuses through emissary veins. **D**, A radiographic image after injection of 100% ethanol made radiopaque with mitrizamide powder, using a tourniquet around the forehead. **E**, A clinical photograph taken after the first ethanol injection procedure. **F**, Another clinical photograph taken 6 weeks after the third intralesional ethanol injection, showing complete resolution of the soft-tissue mass. This result remained stable over the subsequent 3-year follow-up.

injected, with digital-subtraction serial imaging. This confirms the intralesional position of the cannula, and demonstrates the volume of the malformation, and any filling of systemic veins. Maneuvers may then be applied to prevent contrast medium from entering the systemic veins (Fig. 2-12). In the face and trunk, local compression with metal forceps or other devices is usually sufficient. In the extremities, tourniquets, blood pressure cuff, and exsanguination with an Esmark bandage (Critical Specialties, West Chester, PA) may be used to prevent filling of systemic veins, and to prevent refilling of the malformation (which serves to dilute the sclerosant) with blood. An attempt is made to exsanguinate the malformation, either by aspiration or compression, and then a quantity of 100% ethanol less than or equal to the amount of contrast taken to opacify the lesion is slowly injected. The compression or tourniquet is maintained for approximately 10 minutes. By this time, the lesion generally begins to feel firm. Any portions of the malformation not included in the initial injection site can then be cannulated and injected. The total quantity of ethanol used in one session should not exceed 1 mL/kg.

If the injection of ethanol is confined to the malformation without passage of a significant amount into the systemic circulation, the incidence of systemic complications is low. Approximately 50% of children have some hemoglobinuria. To prevent renal toxicity, intravenous fluids are administered at approximately twice the normal rates during the procedure and the recovery period. The most common significant complication of ethanol injection is skin blistering or full-thickness skin necrosis, which usually occurs when the skin surface is involved with the venous malformation. Other complications include neuropathy, thrombophlebitis, and thromboembolism. Yakes and Baker [32] recently reported cardiac arrest in four patients undergoing embolization or sclerotherapy with ethanol. We have not encountered such an effect, but careful monitoring under general anesthesia is mandatory.

The ethanol injection initially produces marked swelling due to a combination of intralesional thrombosis and edema of the adjacent tissues. The edema resolves rapidly in 24 to 48 hours, whereas the thrombus regresses gradually over 2 to 6 months. After 6 months, the lesion can be clinically reassessed for

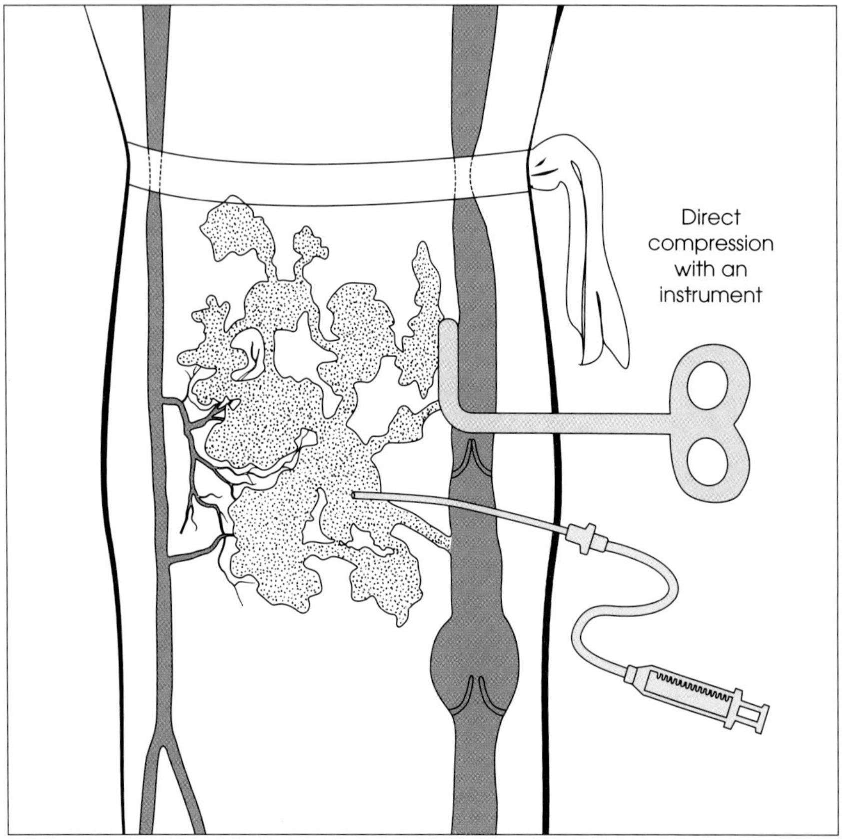

Direct compression with an instrument

FIGURE 2-12.

Direct injection of a sclerosant into the venous malformation, using a tourniquet and direct compression for flow control.

residual refilling of the malformation. The skin blisters or necroses that occur are usually managed conservatively, using antibiotic ointment for small blisters and nonadhesive sterile dressings for more extensive necroses. Patients requiring dressing changes should be followed on a weekly basis in an outpatient clinic to make sure that infection does not develop. If signs of infection appear, they can usually be controlled with oral antibiotics. Simple debridement is often helpful in expediting the healing process.

Most lesions are significantly reduced in size within 2 months after treatment. Some small lesions are "cured" by one injection, but most large lesions require three or four injections 3 to 6 months apart before they reach a stable result. One of the most striking results of sclerotherapy for painful venous malformations is the dramatic, almost immediate relief of pain. In the series by Dubois and colleagues [30], 10 of 23 patients treated with Ethibloc alone appeared to be cured at follow-up

of 6 weeks after sclerotherapy. Most of the cured patients had localized lesions with minimal connections to systemic veins. In our experience, recurrence of the malformation often takes as long as 6 months to manifest; long-term studies using objective methods such as serial MRI to analyze outcome are still required.

Lymphatic Malformations

Lymphatic malformations consist of macro- or microcystic masses containing lymphatic fluid and are usually associated with lymphatic obstruction (Fig. 2-13). They present as local or diffuse soft-tissue masses often associated with a hemovascular malformation of the skin surface (Fig. 2-14). Those lesions with a small number of large cysts sometimes benefit from aspiration and intralesional injection, although the response is less predictable than with venous malformations. A number of chemicals have been used to try to sclerose

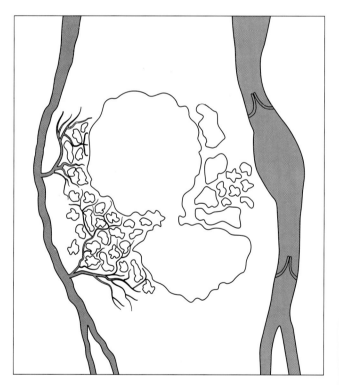

FIGURE 2-13.

A lymphatic malformation appears as a congenital group of micro- and macrocysts filled with lymphatic fluid, often associated with abnormal adjacent veins (varicosities, abnormal valves, tortuosity) and sometimes dilated cutaneous capillaries, causing a blue-purple discoloration.

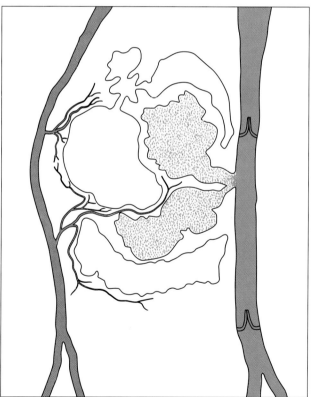

FIGURE 2-14.

A lymphatico-venous malformation. This appears as an association of variably sized vascular spaces, containing either lymphatic third or stagnant venous blood, both draining subtlely and slowly to adjacent veins.

lymphatic malformations, including antibiotics, chemotherapeutic agents, ethanol, Ethibloc, dextrose, sodium tetradecyl, Bleomycin (Nihon, Kayaku, Japan), and most recently OK-432 (Picibanil; Chugai Pharmaceutical, Tokyo, Japan), which is a derivative of group-A *Streptococcus*. Surgical excision is considered the most effective treatment but as with venous malformations, complete removal is often impossible because of the infiltration of the malformation throughout the tissues. Recurrence is frequent after all therapeutic interventions, presumably resulting from the residual lymphatic obstruction and distention of residual cysts. Early experience with OK-432 is promising; lymphatic malformations in 10 of 23 patients injected in one series showed complete or near complete shrinkage with no significant complica-

tions [33•]. However, OK-432 has not been approved by the Food and Drug Administration.

Conclusion

Vascular anomalies in children have long been a misunderstood and mistreated specialty. With increasing understanding of these lesions and the development of better catheter systems, devices, and materials, the treatment of these complex lesions is rapidly improving. Concentration of such investigation and treatment of these complex lesions is best carried out in centers with a multidisciplinary vascular anomalies team where the most current counseling, imaging, and therapy can be offered and where data collection can result in useful outcome analysis.

References and Recommended Reading

Recently published papers of particular interest have been highlighted as:

• Of interest

•• Of outstanding interest

1. Mulliken JB, Young AE: Vascular Birthmarks, Hemangiomas, and Malformations. Philadelphia: WB Saunders; 1988.

2.• Burns AJ, Kaplan LC, Mulliken JB: Is There an Association Between Hemangioma and Syndromes with Dysmorphic Features? *Pediatrics* 1991, 88:1257–1267.
An excellent paper describing the true nature of the cutaneous vascular lesions associated with uncommon syndromes. These lesions have erroneously been referred to as hemangiomas.

3. Jackson IT, Carreno R, Potparre Z, Hussain K: Hemangiomas, Vascular Malformations and Lymphovenous Malformations: Classification and Methods of Treatment. *Plas Reconstr Surg* 1993, 91:1216–1230.

4. Assaf A, Nasr A, Johnson T: Corticosteroids in the Management of Adnexal Hemangiomas in Infancy and Childhood. *Ann Ophthalmol* 1992, 24:12–18.

5. Apfelberg DB, Lane B, Marx MP: Combined (Team) Approach to Hemangioma Management: Arteriography with Superselective Embolization Plus YAG Laser/Sapphire-Tip Resection. *Plas Reconstr Surg* 1991, 88:77–82.

6. Baurmash H, DeChiara S: A Conservative Approach to the Management of Orafacial Vascular Lesions in Infants and Children: Report of Cases. *J Oral Maxillofac Surg* 1991, 49:1222–1225.

7. Enjolras O, Riche MC, Merland JJ, Escande JP: Management of Alarming Hemangiomas in Infancy: A Review of 25 Cases. *Pediatrics* 1990, 85:491–498.

8.•• Ezekowitz RA, Mulliken JB, Folkman J: Interferon Alpha-2a Therapy for Life Threatening Hemangiomas of Infancy. *New Engl J Med* 1992, 326:1456–1463.
This is a scientific report describing the promising results of pharmacologic treatment of serious infantile hemangiomas.

9. Burrows PE, Lasjaunias PL, TerBrugge KG, Flodmark O: Urgent and Emergent Embolization of Lesions of the Head and Neck in Children: Indications and Results. *Pediatrics* 1987, 80:386–394.

10. Argenta LC, Bishop E, Cho KJ, *et al*.: Complete Resolution of Life Threatening Hemangioma by Embolization and Corticosteroids. *Plas Reconstr Surg* 1982, 760:739–742.

11.• Fellows KE, Hoffer FA, Markowitz RI, O'Neill JA: Multiple Collaterals to Hepatic Infantile Hemangioendotheliomas and Arteriovenous Malformations: Effect on Embolization. *Radiology* 1991, 181:813–818.
This manuscript describes the existence of extensive arterial collaterals in infants undergoing embolization of hepatic hemangioendotheliomas for congestive cardiac failure.

12.• McHugh K, Burrows PE: Infantile Hepatic Hemangioendotheliomas: Significance of Portal Venous and Systemic Collateral Arterial Supply. *JVIR* 1992, 3:337–344.
In this manuscript, the significance of portal-vein supply to hepatic hemangioendotheliomas is described and illustrated. The authors emphasize the need to study the portal vein by angiography prior to embolization.

13. Doppman JL, Pevsner P: Embolization of Arteriovenous Malformations by Direct Percutaneous Puncture. *AJR* 1983, 140:773–778.

14. Yakes WF, Haas DK, Parker SH, *et al*.: Symptomatic Vascular Malformations: Ethanol Embolotherapy. *Radiology* 1989, 170:1059–1066.

15.• Gomes AS: Embolization Therapy of Congenital Arteriovenous Malformations: Use of Alternative Approaches. *Radiology* 1994, 190:191–198.
This paper reports long-term results of embolization in the management of symptomatic AVMs of the extremities. The application of new techniques, such as direct intralesional and retrograde embolization, are discussed.

16. Resnick SA, Russel EF, Hanson DH, *et al.*: Embolization of a Life-threatening Mandibular Vascular Malformation by Direct Percutaneous Transmandibular Puncture. *Head Neck* 1992, 14:372–379.

17. Shultz RE, Richardson DD, Kempf KK, *et al.*: Treatment of a Central Arteriovenous Malformation of the Mandible with Cyanoacrylate: A 4-year Follow-up. *Oral Surg Oral Med Oral Pathol* 1988, 65:267–271.

18.• Riles TS, Berenstein A, Fisher FS, *et al.*:Reconstruction of the Ligated External Carotid Artery for Embolization of Cervicofacial Arteriovenous Malformations. *J Vasc Surg* 1993, 17:491–498.

The authors describe the increased difficulty in managing patients with facial AVMs after external carotid artery ligation. Their solution was to reconstruct the ligated vessels with vein grafts, permitting transcatheter embolization in four patients.

19. Komiyama M, Khosla VK, Yamamoto Y, *et al.*:Embolization in High Flow Arteriovenous Malformations of the Face. *Ann Plas Surg* 1992, 28:575–583.

20. Nancarrow PA, Lock JE, Fellows KE: Embolization of an Intra-osseous Arteriovenous Malformation. *AJR* 1986, 146:785–786.

21. Yakes WF, Luethke JM, Merland JJ, *et al.*: Ethanol Embolization of Arteriovenous Fistulas: A Primary Mode of Therapy. *JVIR* 1990, l:89–96.

22. Hartnell GG, Jackson JE, Allison DJ: Coil Embolization of Pulmonary Arteriovenous Malformations. *Cardiovasc Intervent Radiol* 1990, 13:347–350.

23. Papagiannis J, Kantel RJ, Effman EL, *et al.*: Polysplenia with Pulmonary Arteriovenous Malformations. *Pediatr Cardiol* 1993, 14:127–129.

24. Meyerovitz MF, Fellows KE: Angiography in Gastrointestinal Bleeding in Children. *AJR* 1984, 143:837–840.

25. Reed DK, Porter LE, Zajko AB, *et al.*: Pre- and Intraoperative Localization of Small Bowel Arteriovenous Malformation. *J Clin Gastroenterol* 1986, 8:166–170.

26. Kandarpa KW, Fellows KE, Eraklis A, *et al.*: Solitary Ileal Arteriovenous Malformation: Preoperative Localization by Coil Embolization. *AJR* 1986, 146:787–788.

27. Israel PG, Armstrong BE, Effman EL, *et al.*: Retroperitoneal Arteriovenous Malformation, a Rare Cause of Heart Failure in Infancy: Consideration of Therapeutic Approaches. *Pediatr Cardiol* 1993, 14:49–52.

28. Calligaro KD, Sedlacek TV, Savarese RP, *et al.*: Congenital Pelvic Arteriovenous Malformations: Long-term Follow-up in Two Cases and a Review of the Literature. *J Vasc Surg* 1992, 16:100–108.

29. Burrows PE, Lasjaunias P, TerBrugge K: A 4-F Coaxial Catheter for Pediatric Vascular Occlusion with Detachable Balloons. *Radiology* 1989, 170:1091–1094.

30. Dubois JM, Sebag GH, De Prost Y, *et al.*: Soft-Tissue Venous Malformations in Children: Percutaneous Sclerotherapy with Ethibloc. *Radiology* 1991, 180:195–198.

31. Riche MC, Hadjean E, Tran-Ba-Huy P, Merland JJ: The Treatment of Capillary-Venous Malformations Using a New Fibrosing Agent. *Plas Reconstr Surg* 1983, 607–612.

32. Yakes WF, Baker R: Cardiopulmonary Collapse: Sequelae of Ethanol Embolotherapy (abstract). *Radiology* 1993, 189(P):145.

33.• Ogita S, Tsuto T, Deguchi E, *et al.*: OK-432 Therapy for Unresectable Lymphangiomas in Children. *J Pediatr Surg* 1991, 26:263–270.

This is early data on an injection technique using a new agent that is not commercially available in the US.

Select Bibliography

Lasjaunias P, Berenstein A: Technical Aspects of Surgical Neuroangiography. In *Surgical Neuroangiography. Volume 2. Endovascular Treatment of Craniofacial Lesions*. Heidelberg: Springer-Verlag Berlin; 1987.

Lasjaunias P, Berenstein A: Craniofacial Vascular Lesion: General. In *Surgical Neuroangiography. Volume 2. Endovascular Treatment of Craniofacial Lesions*. Heidelberg: Springer-Verlag Berlin; 1987.

Lasjaunias P, Berenstein A: Craniofacial Hemangiomas, Vascular Malformations and Angiomatosis: Specific Aspects. In *Surgical Neuroangiography. Volume 2. Endovascular Treatment of Craniofacial Lesions*. Heidelberg: Springer-Verlag Berlin; 1987.

Mulliken JB, Young AE: Vascular Birthmarks, Hemangiomas, and Malformations. Philadelphia: WB Saunders; 1988.

Radiologic Management of Hemoptysis

Ivan Vujic
Renan Uflacker

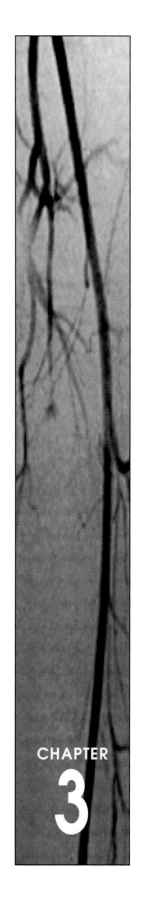

Successful control of hemoptysis remains a continuous challenge in medicine. Bronchial artery embolization (BAE) has proved to be one of the most effective procedures in the field of vascular and interventional radiology. If successful, it results in immediate cessation of bleeding [1,2]. However, it is important to realize that the long-term benefits from the procedure vary depending on the character of the disease and underlying condition of the patient. Hemoptysis in diffuse chronic pulmonary diseases, such as terminal sarcoidosis or cystic fibrosis, complicated by superimposed infection are less likely to be controlled than hemoptysis, which occurs as a result of more localized diseases such as chronic cavitary tuberculosis, empyema, or carcinoma. Therefore, the procedure may initially be successful but recurrent hemoptysis caused by the diffuse nature of the disease may require subsequent intervention [3].

Indications for Bronchial Artery Embolization

Bronchial artery embolization is indicated whenever hemoptysis cannot be controlled by conservative or surgical management. As a rule, hemoptysis exceeding the amount of 300 mL per day is considered life-threatening and is initially treated best by embolization [4]. In patients with episodes of mild hemoptysis occurring over a period of weeks and months, embolization should be the first choice for treatment. However, in recent years the indications for interventional procedures have widened, including patients with very mild bleeding in diffuse lung involvement requiring respiratory therapy such as in cystic fibrosis. This aggressive approach to management is due to the development of safer techniques using digital subtraction angiography and nonionic contrast agents that considerably diminish the risk of neurotoxic damage to the spinal cord [2].

Bronchial Artery Anatomy

It is quite common to have more than one supply source to the area of bleeding. Therefore, a meticulous search is required to identify the target vessel. For a successful procedure, thorough knowledge of the bronchial vascular anatomy is mandatory. The anatomy of the bronchial arteries in cadaver dissections has been described [5]. A more recent study based on angiographic findings in patients with hemoptysis reveals a somewhat different occurrence of anatomic variants. Ten different patterns are described (Fig. 3-1) [2]:

- Pattern 1: An intercostobronchial trunk (ICBT) on the right and a bronchial artery of the left (30.5%)
- Pattern 2: One ICBT on the right and a common trunk with a bronchial artery on the right and left (25%)
- Pattern 3: One ICBT on the right and two bronchial arteries on the left (12.5%)
- Pattern 4: One ICBT on the right and one bronchial artery on the right and left (11.1%)
- Pattern 5: One ICBT on the right, one common bronchial trunk, and one left bronchial artery (8.3%)
- Pattern 6: One ICBT on the right, one bronchial

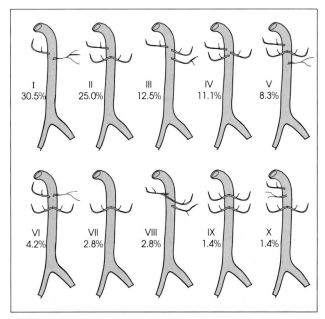

FIGURE 3-1.

Different patterns of bronchial artery variants based on angiographic observation (anterior view). (*From* Uflacker *et al.* (2); with permission).

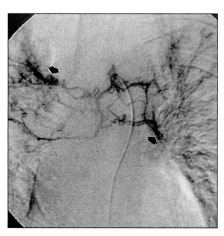

FIGURE 3-2.

Injection into the common bronchial trunk reveals rich collateralization and the opacification of multiple bronchial arteries in cystic fibrosis. Note the bilateral bronchopulmonary artery shunting (*arrows*).

artery on the left, and one common bronchial trunk in caudal position (4.2%)

- Pattern 7: Only one common bronchial trunk (2.8%)
- Pattern 8: One ICBT on the right giving origin to a left bronchial artery and one bronchial artery on the left (2.8%)
- Pattern 9: Two common bronchial trunks giving origin to bronchial arteries on the right and left (1.4%)
- Pattern 10: One ICBT on the right, one bronchial artery on the right, and one common bronchial trunk giving origin to arteries on the right and left (1.4%)

Radicular arteries originating from the ICBT were seen in 58.3% of patients. The most interesting observation of practical value is the frequent occurrence of a common bronchial trunk giving origin to a right and left bronchial artery in more than 45% of patients. The discrepancy between the two observations may be due to the small size of the arteries in normal subjects precluding their identification. A common trunk may be the result of marked hypertrophy of transmediastinal collaterals in response to the increased demand of blood flow to the tumoral or inflammatory lesions. The collateral circulation that develops during the course of the disease between the right and left bronchial arteries and between bronchial arteries and nonbronchial systemic vessels becomes so rich that injection into any of these vessels may opacify multiple arteries within the lung, including the target vessel for embolization (Fig. 3-2) [6,7]. Although a rare occurrence, it must be emphasized that the bronchial arteries may have an unusual origin from the thyrocervical trunk, abdominal aorta, or phrenic arteries (Fig. 3-3)

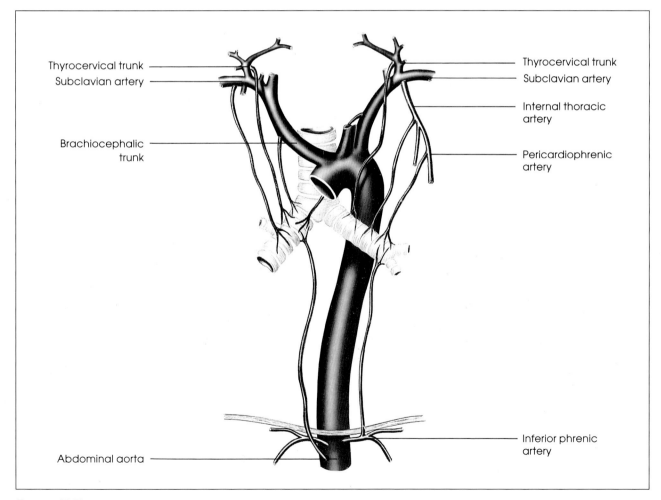

FIGURE 3-3.

Unusual origins of bronchial arteries. (*From* Uflacker R: Atlas of Vascular Anatomy: An Angiographic Approach. Edited by Uflacker R. New York: Thieme Medical Publishers; 1994: in press; with permission).

[7]. Unusual communication between the left bronchial and right coronary artery through the conal branch has recently been reported [8].

PATHOPHYSIOLOGY OF BLEEDING

The normal communication between the systemic bronchial arteries, the pulmonary arterial system, and the pulmonary vein at the capillary pre- and postalveolar level enlarge so much that some degree of systemic-to-pulmonary shunting is always present and may be detected by angiography in approximately half of the patients suffering from hemoptysis (Fig. 3-4). Shunts between the two systems completely change the hemodynamics. Once the shunts are established, the vessels with a thinner wall or with tumoral or inflammatory changes and altered permeability are subject to a much higher pressure regimen; bleeding is a natural consequence of this change. The arteries are most likely not the direct site of the bleeding. Systemic-to-pulmonary shunting may increase pressure, subsequently rupturing pulmonary arteries or veins, which may then bleed into the parenchyma, bronchi, or cavities.

Procedure

The procedure consists of two phases including the diagnostic search for the side and site of bleeding and embolotherapeutic intervention.

DIAGNOSTIC ANGIOGRAPHY

The search for bleeding should begin with a bronchoscopy to identify the side of bleeding [4]. This is

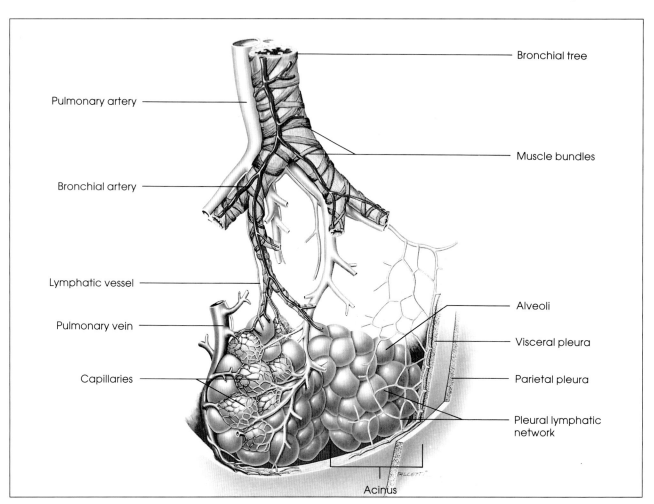

FIGURE 3-4.

The bronchial artery connections with the prealveolar pulmonary artery, as well as fistulas with the postalveolar pulmonary vein at the microcirculation level. (*From*

Uflacker R: Atlas of Vascular Anatomy: An Angiographic Approach. Edited by Uflacker R. New York: Thieme Medical Publishers; 1994: in press; with permission).

particularly important in patients with diffuse lung disease. However, in a large number of patients the findings of the chest studies along with the patient's subjective localization of bleeding point are sufficient enough to obviate a bronchoscopic exam (Fig. 3-5). Occasionally, the condition of patients with massive hemoptysis requires immediate angiography and embolization without a previous assessment.

As a rule, the search for the bleeding area begins by performing a bronchial arteriogram (Fig. 3-6). If the bronchial arteriogram identifies an abnormality, an immediate embolization is carried out and the proce-

dure terminated. However, if the bronchial arteriogram is normal or does not yield a significant abnormality, the angiographic search must be continued in accordance with the changes seen on the chest radiograph or by bronchoscopic location of the bleeding site. The branches of subclavian and axillary arteries, most notably the internal mammary artery, are the most common feeding vessels in the region of upper lobes. The intercostal vessels commonly feed the abnormal lung parenchyma [6]. Occasionally, in the basal segments of the inferior phrenic artery branches, there may be a main supply source (Fig. 3-7). However, it should be noted that any vessel from the neck and lateral chest wall may become a supply source for the blood flow to the abnormal intrathoracic lesion (Fig. 3-8) [9,10•]. Therefore, it is very important to identify these vessels and embolize the most important feeders. Although the thoracic aortogram may be helpful, selective injections are preferred and most likely sufficient.

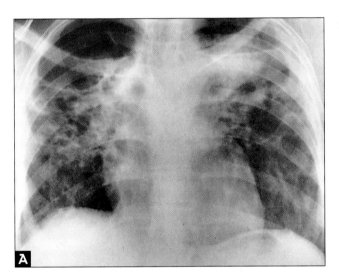

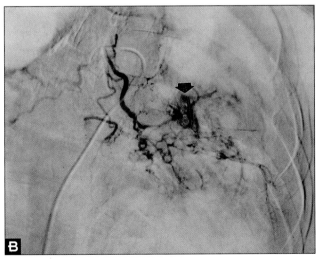

FIGURE 3-5.

A, Massive bleeding in the region of the left upper lobe in a patient suffering from interstitial sarcoidosis. **B,** Left bronchial arteriogram reveals frank extravasation into the bronchial tree (*arrow*).

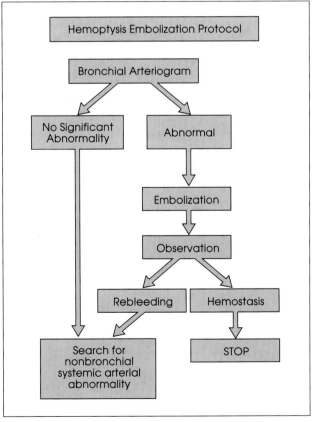

FIGURE 3-6.

Algorithm for the BAE protocol.

The younger the patient, the easier the selective catheterization of intrathoracic vessels. In young patients, simple-curve visceral catheters, such as the RC1, RC2, or RIM are recommended for bronchial arteriography. For intercostal arteries, the renal double-curved catheter is preferred because it is very easy to advance this type of catheter into the intercostal trunk and catheterize the bronchial artery originating from the trunk. Therefore, this catheter should be the first choice used in patients bleeding from the right side. In older patients with a tortuous aorta or moderate-to-advanced arteriosclerosis, sidewinder catheters such as the Mikaelson or Simmons are the best choice for bronchial arteriography; cobra selective catheters are best for use in intercostal trunks. In a great majority of patients, the above described catheters are used for

embolization procedures as well. These catheters are manufactured by Cook, Bloomington, IN; Boston Scientific, Watertown, MA; Mallinckroot, St. Louis, MO; and others. Very rarely, when a more distal embolization is required, coaxial systems are used (Tracker system; Target Therapeutics, Freeport, CA) [11]. This is particularly advantageous when polymerizing agents are used in small peripheral vessels in patients with recurrent hemoptysis.

In rare cases when additional supraortic arteriograms are required, standard cerebral catheters are used; the Head Hunter 1, and the Berenstein catheter are the best choice, at least for initial attempts.

The angiographic findings in hemoptysis that should be sought are listed in Table 3-1. The most common angiographic feature in hemoptysis is the

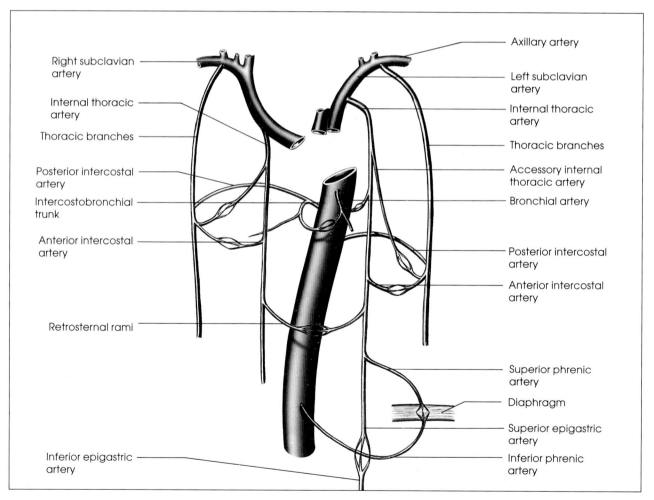

FIGURE 3-7.

The major anatomic connections between bronchial and nonbronchial systemic vessels in the thorax (*From* Uflacker R: Atlas of Vascular Anatomy: An Angiographic Approach. Edited by Uflacker R. New York: Thieme Medical Publishers; 1994: in press; with permission).

enlargement of the systemic vessel supplying the area of abnormality, which is usually associated with increased vascularity of abnormal tissues and systemic-to-pulmonary artery shunting (Fig. 3-8). Angiographic identification of frank extravasation is exceptionally rare, even in patients with massive hemoptysis (Fig. 3-5B). The pseudoaneurysm formation is also uncommon. Nevertheless, it should be noted that the exclusion of this abnormality in pulmonary circulation requires pulmonary angiography in cases of old cavitating tuberculosis resulting in Rasmussen's aneurysm. Patients suspected of having mycotic aneurysms as a consequence of drug abuse should also undergo pulmonary angiography. The lack of normal bronchial vascular architecture, characterized by diffuse parenchymal staining and nonvisualization of bronchial artery branches within the lung parenchyma, is often a sign of an advanced,

usually terminal disease. This pattern is frequently associated with the advanced stages of interstitial sarcoidosis, complicated by systemic aspergillosis (Fig. 3-9). Similar changes in localized form may be encountered in chronic tuberculosis.

EMBOLOTHERAPY

Almost all currently available occlusion devices and materials are useful in the control of hemoptysis, except for absolute ethanol.

It is important to embolize distal branches and preserve the proximal trunk of the vessel. This has a two-fold purpose: 1) the important mediastinal and spinal cord branches remain patent; and 2) access to the area of bleeding is available if a second intervention is required. Particles ranging in size from 0.5 to 2 mm in diameter are the embolic material of choice. Occlusive therapy is usually begun by utilizing the

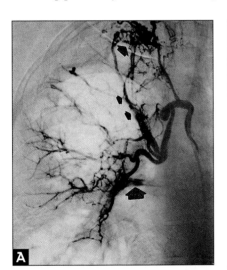
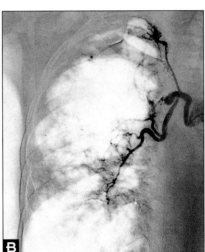
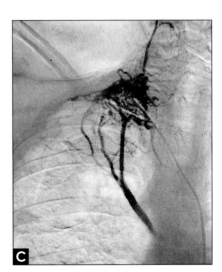
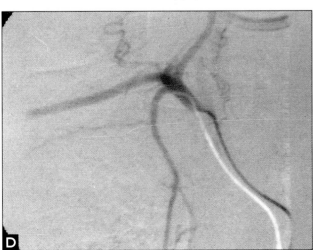

FIGURE 3-8.

An advanced case of cystic fibrosis. **A**, The bronchial arteriogram reveals angiomatous-like lesion in the right apical area (*arrows*) with prompt opacification of the pulmonary artery (*small arrows*). There is also bronchial pulmonary shunting in the right lower lung (*large arrow*). **B**, Satisfactory findings with the lack of shunting following the embolization procedure in the distribution of the right bronchial artery. **C**, Despite successful right bronchial artery embolization, the patient rebled within 24 hours of the procedure. A selective arteriogram of the thyrocervical trunk again reveals an apically-acquired angiomatous lesion with prompt shunting into the pulmonary artery. **D**, A subclavian arteriogram following embolization of the thyrocervical trunk that successfully controlled hemoptysis for several years.

smallest particles and as the flow to the area of interest gradually decreases, larger particles are used to achieve better hemostasis [10•]. Gelfoam (Upjohn, Kalamazoo, MI) is the most commonly used agent. However, if the patient rebleeds from the same source, the use of a permanent occlusive material such as Ivalon (Ivalon, San Diego, CA) is more appropriate. A polymerizing liquid material such as Cyanoacrilate (B Braum, Melsung, Germany) should be reserved for special cases when other methods fail.

Whenever therapeutic embolization is performed, the catheter should be advanced distal to the origin of the mediastinal and spinal cord branches. These small vessels may not be visible in the initial arteriogram, but during embolization, the distal branches gradually occlude and the hemodynamic changes redistribute the blood flow, revealing the proximal branches. It is essential at this point to proceed with extreme care, finalizing the procedure by inserting the occlusive material and pushing it through with a guidewire rather than injecting it. This technique prevents reflux and undesirable embolization of nontarget vessels.

A pseudoaneurysm of the pulmonary artery branches should be embolized with coils or detachable balloons. Detachable balloons are preferred to coils, particularly in patients with hyperdynamic flow, because they comply with both the size and anatomy of the vessel to be embolized.

Absolute ethanol induces coagulation necrosis as it penetrates through the wall of the vessel, causing indiscriminate damage to adjacent tissues. In addition, absolute ethanol may also cause severe spasms when injected into the vessel, causing considerable reflux and inadvertently damaging the small branches supplying the mediastinum and spinal cord. Therefore, it is not recommended for use in patients with BAE [2].

Results

In a series of 64 patients with tuberculosis (TBC) [2], overall immediate control of hemoptysis was achieved in 49 of 64 patients, with 76.6% controlled by BAE. The percentage of immediate control for massive hemoptysis may be as high as 82.8%. Long-term control of massive hemoptysis may be approximately 87%, using all the modalities of treatment including embolization with chemotherapy and surgery whenever possible. Recurrent hemoptysis yields a lower rate of control for both immediate (68.9%) and long-term (76%) results. Rebleeding occurs in approximately 21% of patients, most non-massive, allowing for a nonemergency re-embolization or clinical follow-up.

Patients with chronic diffuse diseases such as interstitial sarcoidosis, cystic fibrosis, bilateral diffuse TBC, aspergillosis, and bleeding bronchial carcinoma tend to have poorer results in bleeding control, because of the progressive course of the disease and gradual deterioration of the patient's condition [12•]. However, BAE still controls acute hemoptysis in this population; the recurrence rate is higher than in TBC, and multiple embolization procedures are often necessary during the life span of these patients [3].

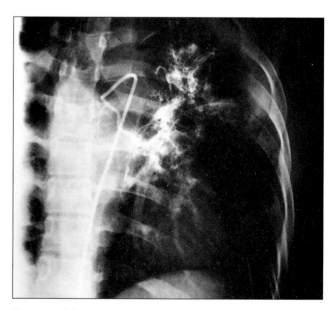

FIGURE 3-9.

Severe form of interstitial sarcoidosis. Total loss of bronchial arterial architecture and irregular dense parenchymal stain. Multiple intercostal angiograms reveal the same features.

Table 3-1. Angiographic Findings in Hemoptysis
Hypertrophy of the feeding vessel with increased vascularity in the area of abnormal intrathoracic tissues
Systemic-to-pulmonary artery shunting
Frank extravasation of contrast
Pseudoaneurysm formation
Total loss of vascular architecture in association with dense staining of diseased tissue

Complications

Following successful embolization procedures, patients may complain of retrosternal pain and dysphagia. These symptoms are related to the ischemia of tissues in the distribution of the embolized vessel and they often subside within a short period of time. Although more serious complications have been occasionally reported (*eg*, bronchoesophageal fistula, necrotic changes in the bronchial wall, and esophagus and spinal cord injury), the technique used at the present time, which utilizes new devices and nonionic contrast agents, is almost risk-free [2]. A more careful approach should be used whenever the subclavian artery branches are embolized. Similarly, occlusive therapy of any intercostal artery should be done gradually with frequent test angiograms obtained by hand injections of diluted, nonionic contrast agents at a slow rate of delivery using digitalized technique [6]. With this method, the possibility of neurotoxic damage or retrograde dislodgement of embolic particles by distant embolization is greatly reduced.

References and Recommended Reading

Recently published papers of particular interest have been highlighted as:
• Of interest
•• Of outstanding interest

1. Remy J, Arnaud A, Fardou H, *et al.*: Treatment of Hemoptysis by Embolization of Bronchial Arteries. *Radiology* 1977, 122:33–37.

2. Uflacker R, Kaemmerer A, Picon P, *et al.*: Bronchial Artery Embolization in the Management of Hemoptysis: Technical Aspects and Long-term Results. *Radiology* 1985, 157:637–644.

3. Fellows K, Khan KT, Schuster S, *et al.*: Bronchial Artery Embolization in Cystic Fibrosis: Technique and Long-term Results. *J Pediatr* 1979, 95:959–963.

4. Uflacker R, Kaemmerer A, Neves C, *et al.*: Management of Massive Hemoptysis by Bronchial Artery Embolization. *Radiology* 1983, 146:627–634.

5. Cauldwell EN, Siekert RG, Liningar RE, *et al.*: The Bronchial Arteries: An Anatomic Study of 150 Human Cadavers. *Surg Gynecol Obstet* 1948, 86:395–412.

6. Vujic I, Pile R, Parker E, *et al.*: Control of Massive Hemoptysis by Embolization of Intercostal Arteries. *Radiology* 1980, 137:617–620.

7. Moore LB, McWey RE, Vujic I: Massive Hemoptysis: Control by Embolization of the Thyrocervical Trunk. *Radiology* 1986, 161:173–174.

8. Nobuaki M, Hiroki I, Akira H, *et al.*: Visualization of Left Bronchial to Coronary Artery Communication After Distal Bronchial Artery Embolization. *Cardiovasc Intervent Radiol* 1994, 17:36–37.

9. Jardin M, Remy J: Control of Hemoptysis: Systemic Angiography and Anastomoses of the Internal Mammary Artery. *Radiology* 1988, 168:377–383.

10.• Cohen AM, Doershuk CF, Stern RC: Bronchial Artery Embolization to Control Hemoptysis Cystic Fibrosis. *Radiology* 1990, 175:401–405.
A study exploring the control of blood flow from source vessels to lesions using small particles to acheive hemostasis.

11. Matsumoto AH, Suhocki PV, Barth CH: Technical Note: Superselective Gelfoam Embolotherapy Using a Highly Visible Small Caliber Catheter. *Cardiovasc Intervent Radiol* 1988, 11:303–306.

12.• Hayakawa K, Tanaka F, Torizuka T, *et al.*: Bronchial Artery Embolization for Hemoptysis: Immediate and Long-term Results. *Cardiovasc Intervent Radiol* 1992, 15:154–159.
In this study, patients with chronic diffuse diseases experienced poorer results in bleeding control, due to the course of the disease and their condition.

Select Bibliography

Keller KS, Rosch J, Loffin TG, *et al.*: Nonbronchial Systemic Collateral Arteries: Significance in Percutaneous Embolotherapy for Hemoptysis. *Radiology* 1987, 164:687–692.

Mauro AM, Jaques PF, Morris S: Bronchial Artery Embolization for Control of Hemoptysis. *Sem Intervent Radiol* 1992, 9:45–51.

Obstetric Embolotherapy

Harold A. Mitty
Keith M. Sterling

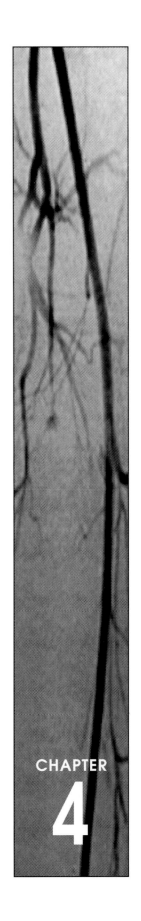

CHAPTER

4

Serious obstetric hemorrhage may become rapidly life-threatening. Traditional methods of control include suture ligation, vaginal or uterine packing, or both. When these local measures fail to control bleeding, obstetricians have resorted to bilateral hypogastric artery ligation. This procedure fails in more than 50% of patients [1,2]. As a result, emergency hysterectomy becomes necessary in many of these patients. This major procedure has the obvious undesirable effect of ending the woman's reproductive ability, as well as the inherent risks associated with emergency surgery.

Transcatheter embolotherapy offers a less-invasive method of controlling postpartum hemorrhage. Despite occasional reports, many obstetricians are not familiar with this form of treatment [3–10].

In an effort to decrease morbidity and the occasional mortality associated with obstetric hemorrhage, two protocols have been established involving interventional radiologists as well as obstetricians at our hospital [11•]. The first protocol involves the interventional radiologic treatment of unexpected obstetric hemorrhage. The second protocol concerns the prophylactic catheterization and possible embolotherapy of patients with known risks for hemorrhage, usually suspected on the basis of antepartum ultrasonograms.

Vascular Anatomy

The normal uterine blood supply is primarily distributed through the uterine arteries. In addition, there are major anastomoses with the ovarian arteries (Fig. 4-1) in the broad ligaments. The uterine arteries arise from the hypogastric artery and have a characteristic medial, often undulating, course in the pelvis (Fig. 4-2). The smaller branches have a corkscrew appearance. It is important to note that the uterine artery and its branches also supply the upper two thirds of the vagina and may be the main source of bleeding from postpartum lacerations in this area.

In the gravid state, the major change is an increase in the amount of uterine vascularity. In addition, the uterine branches rise out of the pelvis to supply the enlarged uterus (Fig. 4-3). The major branches tend to have a tortuous appearance (Fig. 4-4).

The ovarian arteries are an additional supply of uterine blood through the pre-existing anastomoses. These communications occur proximal to the uterus in the broad ligament. As a result, it is rarely necessary to embolize the ovarian vessels because the embolic particles that are introduced into the main uterine arteries find their way to distal branches supplying the bleeding site. For this reason, routine ovarian arteriography is usually not necessary in postpartum hemorrhage.

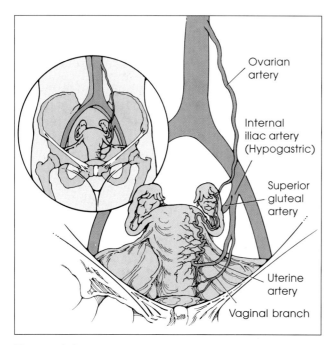

Ovarian artery

Internal iliac artery (Hypogastric)

Superior gluteal artery

Uterine artery

Vaginal branch

FIGURE 4-1.

Normal uterine circulation.

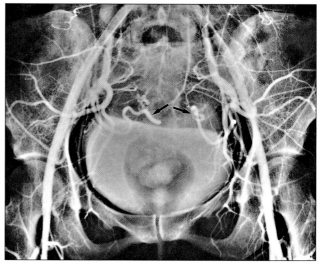

FIGURE 4-2.

An aortogram of pelvic circulation. The uterine arteries arise from the hypogastric arteries and have a medial undulating course (*arrows*).

There are branches described as vaginal and internal pudendal arteries that arise from the hypogastric arteries and supply the lower vagina and perineum. These branches are at risk of laceration during traumatic deliveries. It is important that the angiographic examination include the vulval area, so that extravasation from this area can be recognized. Even very distal vessel disruptions may result in large hematomas that cannot be easily controlled by local surgical techniques. The source of bleeding may be more apparent on the angiogram than by direct inspection in these patients with large hematomas.

Methods and Patients

EMERGENCY PROTOCOL

When unexpected intra- or postpartum hemorrhage occurs, the usual methods of local control are employed. Obstetricians must be warned not to ligate the hypogastric arteries if at all possible, because this eliminates selective catheter access to the uterine circulation. When confronted by serious hemorrhage that does not respond to local measures, the following steps are followed in our hospital: 1) the interventional radiologists are notified. An angiographic room is prepared so that the patient can be catheterized without delay. Syringes containing gelatin-sponge pledgets 1 × 2 mm in size are prepared when awaiting the patient's arrival; 2) the patient is stabilized by a combination of local measures and blood transfusion in the obstetric department; 3) the patient is brought to the interventional suite, accompanied by the obstetrician and the anesthesiologist. This is important because control of the patient's acute medical and surgical status should not be the sole responsibility of the radiologist, who must control the technical aspects of vascular catheterization and embolotherapy; and 4) the femoral artery is catheterized in the standard manner. We use a 5-French cobra C2 to C3 (Medi-Tech, Watertown, MA) to catheterize the contralateral hypogastric artery. This is facilitated by the use of a hydrophilic polymer–coated guidewire (Glidewire; Terumo, Tokyo, Japan). A hypogastric arteriogram is then performed (Fig. 4-5). The most common vessels to show extravasation are the uterine arteries, including the vaginal branch, and the internal pudendal arteries. These are selectively catheterized and embolized to stasis if extravasation is observed.

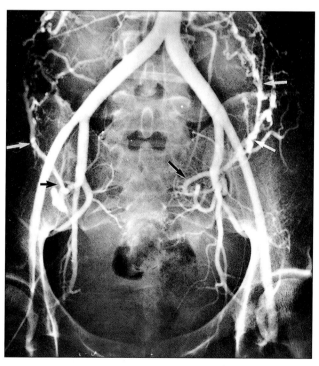

FIGURE 4-4.

An aortogram immediately postpartum. The uterine arteries extend laterally and cephalad to supply the enlarged uterus (*arrows*). Note the increased uterine vasculature that has a tortuous appearance.

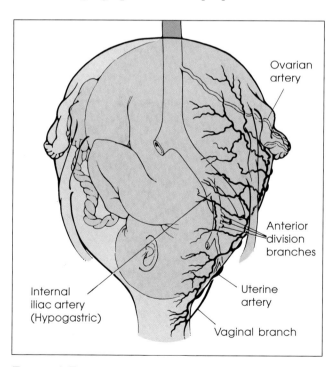

FIGURE 4-3.

The uterine circulation in the gravid state.

The ipsilateral hypogastric artery is catheterized by means of a long, reverse-curve catheter (Bookstein MS-20; Cordis, Miami, FL). This catheter is formed by leaving a guidewire inside the contralateral iliac artery. The catheter is advanced over the wire until the proximal curve is at the aortic bifurcation. The wire is then retracted to the proximal curve and the catheter-guidewire combination pushed cephalad in the aorta. On occasion, it may be necessary to advance the stiff end of the wire to the proximal curve in the catheter to achieve enough rigidity to advance the catheter and form the reverse curve. Once the catheter has formed its curve in the aorta, it is pulled down engaging the ipsilateral hypogastric artery (Fig. 4-6). A second hypogastric angiography and selective uterine or internal pudendal angiography, or both, is then performed. Note that if extravasation from either uterine artery into the uterus occurs, both uterine vessels are embolized because there are normally rich anastomoses between both sides. This reverse-curve catheter is long enough to permit its use in the contralateral hypogastric artery, should the cobra catheter not follow easily over the aortic bifurcation.

PROPHYLACTIC PROTOCOL

Patients with a nonviable fetus and a risk for hemorrhage may be embolized prior to surgery via the femoral route. Patients who have sonographic or clinical evidence of abnormalities (*eg*, placenta accreta or placenta previa) associated with a high risk for bleeding during cesarean section or abdominal surgery are prophylactically catheterized prior to abdominal surgery and embolized in the operating room if necessary.

The patient is brought to an angiography room immediately before surgery. The gravid uterus is shielded in the case of a viable fetus. The left axillary-artery route is used to pass a 5-French H1H head-hunter catheter to a level just above the shielded gravid uterus (Fig. 4-7).

The radiologist, special-procedures nurse, and radiographer go to the operating room with the patient. A procedure tray containing sterile syringes preloaded with gelatin-sponge pledgets is brought to the operating room along with additional catheters and guidewires. Because the H1H catheter is 100-cm long, it is advisable to bring 260-cm exchange wires, should it be necessary to change catheters in the oper-

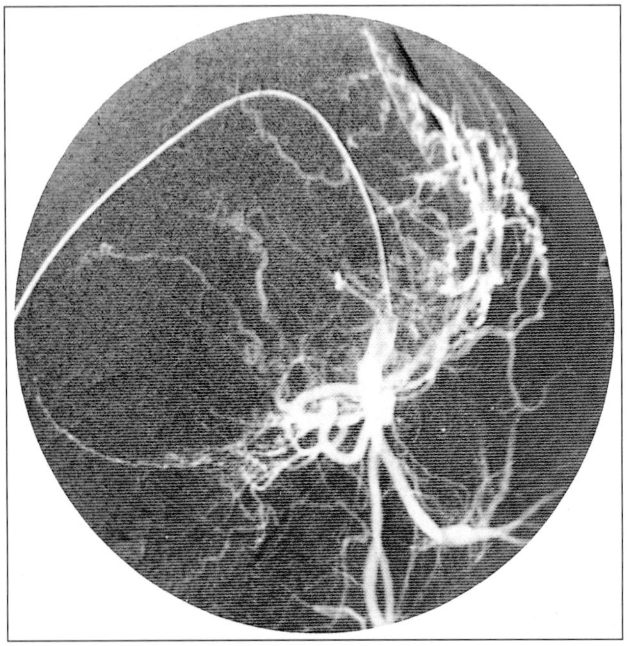

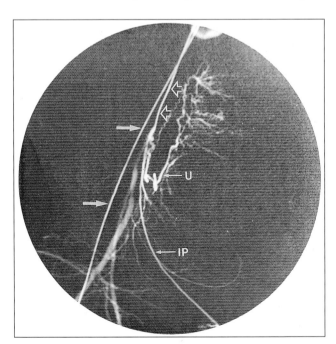

FIGURE 4-5.

Left hypogastric arteriogram via the right femoral approach. Note the course of the cobra catheter. The well-developed uterine circulation extends out of the pelvis to supply the uterine body and fundus.

FIGURE 4-6.

An ipsilateral hypogastric artery catheter with reverse-curve catheter. The ascending shaft (*arrows*) makes a hairpin curve and descends (*open arrows*) to enter the hypogastric artery. U—uterine artery; IP—internal pudendal artery.

ating room. The additional catheters that may be useful are the multipurpose as well as H1H catheters from several different vendors that tend to have variations in their distal curves.

The operating table should be of the type to accept the portable c-arm fluoroscope set in a position to be pushed into place. If the patient develops bleeding uncontrollable by the usual operative methods, the uterus is packed to gain some control. The surgeons then move away from one side of the table and the fluoroscope is pushed into place (Fig. 4-8).

The radiologist should be able to manipulate the catheter from the left axilla without disturbing the sterile abdominal surgical field. The path into the hypogastric artery is basically straight and the uterine vessels are usually easily catheterized. Because the origin of the bleeding has been directly visualized as originating from the uterus, we embolize the uterine arteries without an angiogram showing extravasation. The endpoint is fluoroscopic evidence of stasis in the vessels. The uterine packing is then removed, control of bleeding is visually confirmed, and the abdomen is closed.

Results

THE EMERGENCY CATHETERIZATION GROUP

The indications for arteriography are summarized in Table 4-1. The estimated blood loss for each patient was taken from chart and anesthesia records. The severity of bleeding in these patients was such that all except Patient 6 had disseminated intravascular coagulation at the time of the angiogram. The films demonstrated extravasation in eight patients (Figs. 4-9, 4-10, and 4-11). One of the most interesting radiographic findings was the presence of circumscribed areas of contrast accumulation in two of three patients with placenta accreta. These local collections are consistent with the intervillous spaces related to the adherent placenta (Fig. 4-12). The third patient with placenta accreta had gross accumulation of contrast material in the uterine cavity that was caused by bleeding (Fig. 4-13).

Because there are immediate midline collaterals to the uterus and pelvic vessels, angiography of both uterine and both internal pudendal arteries was performed in patients with lacerations. This was the procedure even when extravasation was initially noted

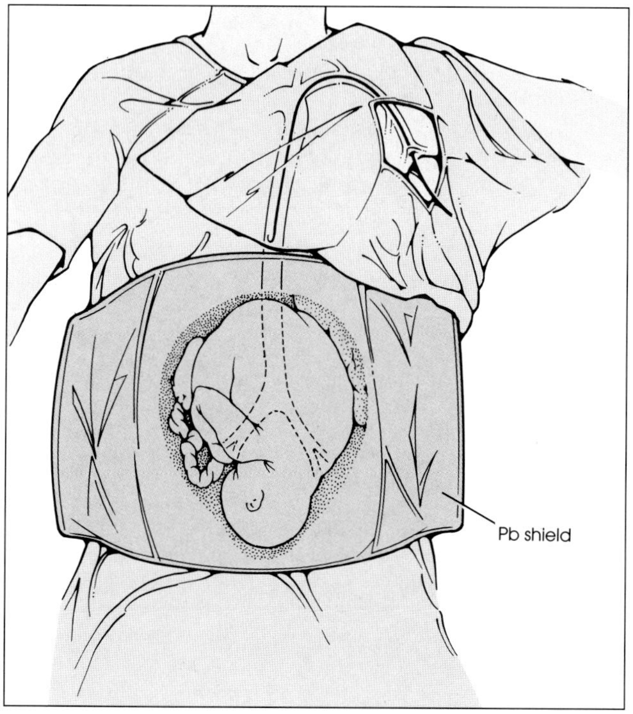

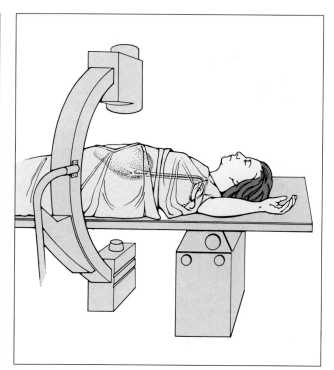

FIGURE 4-7.

Prophylactic catheter placement in patients with risk of intraoperative hemorrhage.

Pb shield

FIGURE 4-8.

The fluoroscopic setup in the operating room.

from one vessel. The endpoint in patients undergoing embolotherapy was clinical evidence of bleeding cessation as well as an angiogram that showed no further extravasation. Patient 4 stopped bleeding during the angiogram and no embolization was performed.

Only one patient in this group (Patient 9) required a hysterectomy. Bleeding was controlled by embolization, but a later-attempted repair of the laceration resulted in new bleeding that led to emergency hysterectomy.

THE PROPHYLACTIC CATHETERIZATION GROUP

Six of these 11 patients did not require embolization because the bleeding during the operation was controlled by the usual surgical measures. Five patients did require embolotherapy—three in the operating room and two in the angiography suite (Table 4-2).

Patient 1 had a nonviable fetus in an interstitial location. Embolization of the right uterine artery was

Table 4-1. Indications for and Results of Transcatheter Embolization in the Emergency Group

Patient	Indications	Estimated blood loss, mL	Arteries embolized*	Results
1	Placenta accreta	4000	Right and left uterine	No further bleeding or blood products
2	Placenta accreta; cervical laceration; uterine atony	4100	Right and left uterine	No further bleeding or blood products; bloodless D & C
3	Abdominal preganancy	8000	Left hypogastric	Bleeding diminished, packing left in place; packing removed, two units of packed erythrocytes given
4	Forceps delivery failure; cesarean section	2500	—	Patient stabilized during angiography
5	Vaginal laceration and enlarging hematoma	4900	Right and left internal pudendal	No further bleeding
6	Placenta accreta	2500	Right and left uterine	No further bleeding; bloodless D & C
7	Retained products of conception	3900	Right and left uterine; right vaginal branch	No further bleeding or blood products; bloodless D & C
8	Transverse tear of cervix and vaginal fornix after forceps delivery	5000	Left uterine; internal pudendal	No further bleeding or blood products
9	Primary uterine atony; cervical and vaginal laceration	6000†	Right and left uterine; right and left internal pudendal	Major bleeding ceased; attempt to repair cervical laceration caused new hemorrhage and led to hysterectomy

*Gelatin-sponge pledgets were used in all patients in whom embolization was performed, except for Patient 1, in whom a coil was used in conjunction with gelatin-sponge pledgets in the left uterine artery.
†Patient 9 was later determined to have acute fatty liver of pregnancy.
D & C—dilation and curettage.

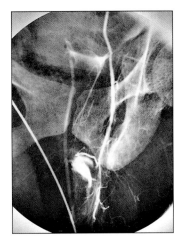

FIGURE 4-9.

A vaginal laceration. Local measures failed to control this patient's bleeding and expanding hematoma. This selective internal pudendal arteriogram demonstrates gross extravasation. This was controlled with gelatin-sponge embolotherapy.

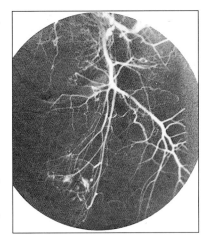

FIGURE 4-10.

Cervical and vaginal lacerations demonstrated by a left hypogastric arteriogram. Several areas of extravasation are demonstrated supplied by vaginal uterine branches and the internal pudendal branches. Gelatin-sponge embolotherapy stopped the bleeding.

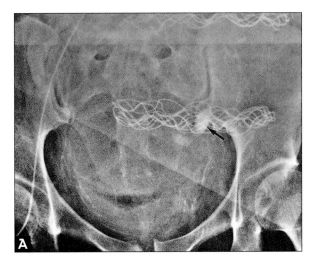

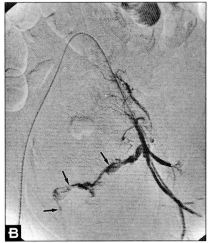

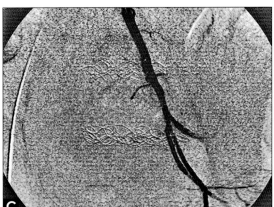

FIGURE 4-11.

Cervical and vaginal lacerations with gross vaginal hemorrhage. **A,** An aortogram. Late film demonstrates an area of extravasation on the left side of the pelvis (*arrow*). Radiopaque markers are in vaginal packing. **B,** A left hypogastric arteriogram. There is gross extravasation from the uterine artery that extends into the vagina (*arrows*). **C,** A left hypogastric arteriogram after embolotherapy with gelatin-sponge pledgets. The uterine artery is occluded, and no further extravasation is present. (**B** and **C** *From* Mitty *et al.* (11•); with permission).

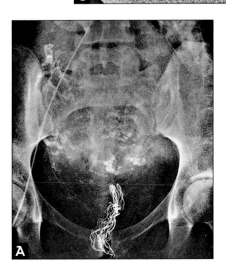

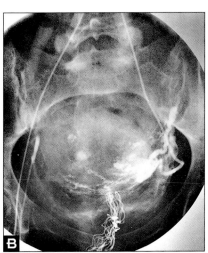

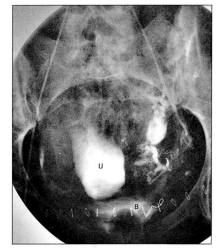

FIGURE 4-12.

Placenta accreta. **A,** An aortogram. The discrete accumulations of contrast material did not change shape during the angiogram and represent the intervillous spaces associated with the adherent placenta. The radiopaque markers are in vaginal packing. **B,** A selective left-uterine arteriogram. Both the intervillous spaces and gross extravasation are seen. Gelatin-sponge embolization was successfully performed. (**A** *From* Mitty *et al.* (11•); with permission).

FIGURE 4-13.

Placenta accreta demonstrated by a selective left-uterine arteriogram. There is accumulation of contrast material in the uterine cavity (*U*). The bladder (*B*) is just inferior to the uterus and is being emptied by a Foley catheter. (*From* Mitty *et al.* (11•); with permission).

performed in the radiology department prior to surgery (Fig. 4-14). The goal was to minimize blood loss and allow removal of the pregnancy and reconstruction of the right side of the uterine wall.

Patient 2 had rapid, 1000-mL blood loss resulting from placenta previa and placenta accreta. The open uterus was packed and both uterine arteries embolized, resulting in cessation of significant bleeding (Fig. 4-15).

Table 4-2. Indications for and Results of Transcatheter Embolization in the Prophylactic Group

Patient	Indication for catheterization	Duration, wk	Indication for embolization	Arteries embolized*	Estimated blood loss, mL	Further results
1	Interstitial pregnancy	12	Nonviable fetus; extrauterine vascular mass	Right uterine	100	—
2	Placenta previa; placenta accreta	39	Hemorrhage during cesarean section	Right and left uterine	1000	Blood loss (at left) before embolization; bleeding ceased after embolization
3	Placenta accreta; dead fetus	24	Bleeding risk before D & C	Right and left uterine	100	Blood loss (at left) during D & C
4	Abdominal pregnancy	17	Nonviable fetus; bleeding risk	Right uterine	1500	Blood loss (at left) from adherence to bowel
5	Placenta accreta	39	Hemorrhage during cesarean section; hypotension	Right and left uterine	1800	Blood loss (at left) before embolization; bleeding ceased after embolization; hysterectomy due to placental depth and adherence
6	Placenta previa; fibroids	34	—	—	850	Patient stabilized
7	Dead twins; fibroids; vaginal bleeding	18	—	—	200	—
8	Placenta previa	33	—	—	1000	—
9	Placenta previa	37	—	—	1500	—
10	Large fibroids	34	—	—	1500	—
11	Placenta accreta	38	—	—	1200	—

*Gelatin-sponge pledgets were used in all patients in whom embolization was performed.
D & C—dilation and curettage.

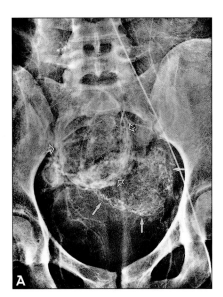
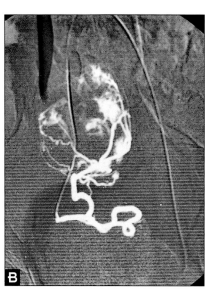

FIGURE 4-14.

An interstitial pregnancy. **A**, An aortogram in late phase. The corkscrew vessels of the uterus are well developed (*arrows*). The interstitial pregnancy involves the right side of the uterus (*open arrows*). **B**, A selective right-uterine arteriogram. This vessel is the primary supply to this pregnancy. Embolization was carried out in this patient. (*From* Mitty *et al.* (11•); with permission).

Patient 3 had placenta accreta and a dead fetus. The patient was judged to be at risk for hemorrhage and embolization of the uterine arteries was performed prior to dilation and curettage (D&C). Patient 4 had prophylactic catheterization of the right uterine artery in the radiology department; in the operating room, significant bleeding associated with mobilization of the abdominal pregnancy led to the embolization of this vessel (Fig. 4-16). This was followed by local applications of gelatin sponge and thrombin at the site that the placenta adhered to the cecum. Patient 5 presented with placenta accreta and significant bleeding, leading to hypotension in the operating room. Embolization of the uterine arteries controlled the bleeding. An attempt to remove the placenta resulted in further bleeding, and a second uterine artery embolization was performed. Once again, bleeding was controlled. Nevertheless, the obstetrician decided to perform a hysterectomy for fear that placental abnormality might lead to further complications.

Discussion

Most bleeding related to normal deliveries and cesarean sections can be controlled with the usual methods of suture ligation, packing, and administration of drugs such as oxytocin. When these methods fail, the traditional preference is to perform a bilateral hypogastric-artery ligation or emergency hysterectomy. Both operations have associated surgical morbidity. In addition, hysterectomy precludes further child-bearing. A review of 123 cases of emergency peripartum hysterectomies revealed an incidence of 1.3 per 1000 births [12•]. Indications for surgery were placenta accreta (*n*=61), uterine atony (*n*=25), unspecified uterine bleeding (*n*=19), and uterine rupture (*n*=14). The high incidence of placenta accreta and anterior placenta previa appears to be related to the rising rate of cesarean section and the scarring of these previously operated uteri [13].

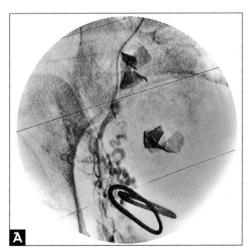

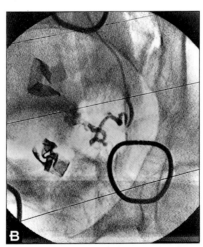

FIGURE 4-15.

Placenta previa and placenta accreta. This patient was embolized in the operating room with packing in the open uterus. **A**, A right hypogastric arteriogram demonstrating uterine vessels. **B**, A left-uterine arteriogram following embolization. There was stasis in this vessel. (*From* Mitty *et al.* (11•); with permission).

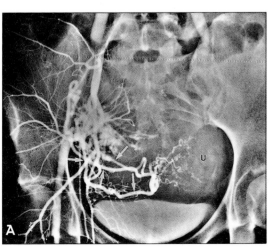

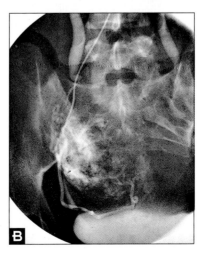

FIGURE 4-16.

An abdominal pregnancy. **A**, A right hypogastric arteriogram demonstrating normal uterine vessels (*U*) and the right uterine supply to the abdominal pregnancy (*arrows*). **B**, Selective right-uterine artery injection. Note the intense stain in the placenta that was attached to the right pelvic sidewall as well as the cecum. The uterine artery was embolized with gelatin-sponge pledgets in the operating room. (*From* Mitty *et al.* (11•); with permission).

Bilateral hypogastric-artery ligation is a poor method of controlling uterine or other forms of pelvic hemorrhage. Clark and colleagues [1] report 15 patients with uterine atony, three with low-transverse cesarean section incisions, and one with placenta accreta. Hypogastricartery ligation controlled bleeding in eight of 19 patients (42%). Eleven patients (58%) required emergency hysterectomies. A similar experience is reported by Evans and McShane [2], involving 18 patients treated with bilateral hypogastric-artery ligation. They reported an overall failure rate of 57% (10 patients). The failures included three of six patients with placenta accreta and all five patients with uterine lacerations.

Transcatheter embolotherapy is a useful method of treating pelvic bleeding associated with trauma, tumors, and vascular malformations [14–18]. There has been a gradual acceptance of this form of treatment for obstetric hemorrhage. An early report by Heaston and colleagues [19] describes a patient who continued to bleed after bilateral hypogastric ligation and hysterectomy. Bleeding was controlled by means of embolizing the medial circumflex artery that was providing anastomic flow to a bleeding site from the internal pudendal artery. This report was also of importance because the authors describe six additional patients who became pregnant after ligation of both hypogastric and ovarian arteries. This experience supports the concept that the rich collateral supply of the pelvis protects the uterus from ischemic damage, so that future pregnancies may be possible. Rosenthal and Colapinto [5] report experience in using embolotherapy in six patients with nonobstetric pelvic hemorrhage and two patients with postcesarean section hemorrhage. The treatment was successful in one of these patients, although the other required hysterectomy to control the bleeding. It is also important to rule out underlying coagulation diseases as causes of postpartum hemorrhage. Postpartum bleeding caused by unrecognized von Willebrand's disease or the prophylactic administration of aspirin or anticoagulants has been described [17,20]. Embolotherapy has also been reported to be valuable in patients with cervical pregnancy, abdominal pregnancy, and gestational trophoblastic disease (Fig. 4-16) [21,22,23•]. Greenwood and colleagues [24] report the efficacy of embolotherapy in postpartum and postabortal hemorrhage in eight patients.

Gilbert and colleagues [25•] recently reported successful embolization of bleeding sites in 10 patients with pregnancy-related hemorrhage. These included three postcesarean section patients, two cervical pregnancies, four vaginal hematomas, and one case of postpartum bleeding associated with uterine myomas. Yamashita and colleagues [26] describe five patients with uncontrollable postpartum hemorrhage caused by cervical and vaginal lacerations, and one patient with uterine rupture. Bleeding was controlled with gelatinsponge embolotherapy in all six patients. Two of these patients were treated successfully after emergency hysterectomy failed to control the bleeding. Normal menses resumed in the patients who did not have a hysterectomy. Our patients who retained their uteri have also had a return of normal menses.

The patients in our emergency catheterization group (Table 4-1) all experienced serious bleeding prior to catheterization. Estimated blood loss ranged between 2500 mL and 8000 mL. Eight of nine patients also had disseminated intravascular coagulation (DIC) at the time of the angiogram. DIC is believed to result from release of thromboplastin from a dead fetus or damaged muscle. This leads to hypofibrinoginemia and delayed clotting. Fresh-frozen plasma should be administered to these patients to correct the coagulation disorder, and packed erythrocytes used to replace blood loss.

One of our nine patients in the emergency group stopped bleeding during the diagnostic arteriogram and no embolization was performed. Bleeding in the remaining eight patients was controlled by means of gelatin-sponge embolotherapy in the angiography suite. No hypogastric-artery ligations were performed. It is unfortunate that one patient did require a hysterectomy. This occurred as a result of surgical repair of a laceration, which led to renewed bleeding and emergency hysterectomy. This patient was later found to have acute fatty liver of pregnancy, an entity associated with an increased risk for hemorrhage [27,28]. Our high rate of success in controlling postpartum bleeding with no mortality or significant morbidity is related to the team approach our protocol has established. The active involvement of the obstetricians and anesthesiologists in patient management during the angiographic procedure ensures adequate blood replacement and ventilation. This gives the interventional radiologist the opportunity to perform an efficient and successful procedure.

Prophylactic arterial catheterization is a new approach in the management of threatened intraoperative obstetric hemorrhage. Many of these patients have abnormal placental implantations or ectopic pregnancies that are detected by antenatal ultrasound examination. As an example, placenta previa is reported to occur in one per every 200 to 250 live births and leads to a perinatal mortality of 81 per 1000 births when it is a factor. Placenta accreta is less common and is the result of deficient decidua in the placental bed so that trophoblastic invasion of the myometrium can take place [29]. There is good evidence that the sites of previous curettage or scarring related to cesarean section are more prone to this pathology. When the myometrium is deeply invaded, the abnormality is described as placenta increta. When the serosal surface is involved, the condition is described as placenta percreta [30].

Patients with increased risk for hemorrhage and with a nonviable fetus may receive an angiogram and embolization in the radiology department prior to surgery. This was the case in two of our patients—one with an interstitial pregnancy and one with a dead fetus and placenta accreta (Table 4-2). We performed intraoperative embolotherapy in three patients. Patient 2 had hemorrhage following cesarean section as a result of placenta accreta and placenta previa. Bleeding was controlled by gelatin-sponge embolotherapy. This patient has had a subsequent normal pregnancy. Patient 5 also had placenta accreta; the intraoperative bleeding was controlled by means of bilateral uterine-

artery embolization. The obstetrician elected to remove the uterus because of the adherence and depth of the placenta. Patient 4 had prophylactic catheterization of the right uterine artery that was supplying an abdominal pregnancy. This branch was embolized in the operating room to diminish blood loss during removal of this pregnancy. Six additional patients had prophylactic axillary-artery catheterization, but did not require embolization because bleeding was either insignificant or was controlled by the usual surgical means. With more experience, we hope to be able to reduce the number of prophylactic catheterizations that do not require embolization.

Conclusion

Our experience is additional evidence of the usefulness of arterial catheterization and embolotherapy in obstetric patients with hemorrhage-associated conditions. The radiologist must educate the obstetrician as to the indications and availability of this form of treatment. Moreover, it is important that ligation of the hypogastric arteries be avoided as a form of treatment because it virtually prohibits access to the uterine arteries for transcatheter therapy. Joint efforts between radiologists and obstetricians can reduce the need for emergency hysterectomy.

References and Recommended Reading

Recently published papers of particular interest have been highlighted as:
• Of interest
•• Of outstanding interest

1. Clark SL, Phelan JP, Yeh SY, et al.: Hypogastric Artery Ligation for Obstetric Hemorrhage. Obstet Gynecol 1985, 66:353–356.

2. Evans S, McShane P: The Efficacy of Internal Iliac Artery Ligation in Obstetric Hemorrhage. Surg Gynecol Obstet 1985, 160:250–253.

3. Pais SO, Glickman M, Schwartz P, et al.: Embolization of Pelvic Arteries for Control of Postpartum Hemorrhage. Obstet Gynecol 1980, 55:754–758.

4. Haseltine FP, Glickman MG, Marchesi S, et al.: Uterine Embolization in a Patient with Postabortal Hemorrhage. Obstet Gynecol 1984, 63(suppl):78S–80S.

5. Rosenthal DM, Colapinto R: Angiographic Arterial Embolization in the Management of Postoperative Vaginal Hemorrhage. Am J Obstet Gynecol 1985, 151:227–231.

6. Heffner LJ, Mennuti MT, Rudoff JC, McLean GK: Primary Management of Postpartum Vulvovaginal Hematomas by Angiographic Embolization. Am J Perinatol 1985, 2:204–207.

7. Kivikoski A, Martin C, Weyman P, et al.: Angiographic Arterial Embolization to Control Hemorrhage in Abdominal Pregnancy; A Case Report. Obstet Gynecol 1988, 71:456–459.

8. Chin HG, Scott DR, Resnik R, et al.: Angiographic Embolization of Intractable Puerperal Hematomas. Am J Obstet Gynecol 1989, 160:434–438.

9. Martin JIV, Ridgway LE, Conners JJ, et al.: Angiographic Arterial Embolizations and Computed Tomography-Directed Drainage in the Management of Hemorrhage and Infection with Abdominal Pregnancy. Obstet Gynecol 1990, 76:941–943.

10. Lobel SM, Meyerovitz MF, Benson CC, et al.: Preoperative Angiographic Uterine Artery Embolization in the Management of Cervical Pregnancy. Obstet Gynecol 1990, 76:938–941.

11.• Mitty HA, Sterling KM, Alvarez M, Gendler R: Obstetric Hemorrhage; Prophylactic and Emergency Arterial Catheterization and Embolotherapy. Radiology 1993, 188:183–187.
This article describes the protocols we have been using in clinical practice.

12.• Stanco LM, Schrimmer DB, Paul RH, Mishell DR Jr: Emergency Peripartum Hysterectomy and Associated Risk Factors. *Am J Obstet Gynecol* 1993, 168:879–883.

The clinical background for increased incidence of these obstetric complications is presented in this study.

13. Manyonda IT, Varma TR: Massive Obstetric Hemorrhage Due to Placenta Previa/Accreta with Prior Cesarean Section. *Int J Gynaecol Obstet* 1991, 34:183–186.

14. Jander HP, Russinovich AE: Transcatheter Gelfoam Embolization in Abdominal Retroperitoneal and Pelvic Hemorrhage. *Radiology* 1980, 136:337–344.

15. Matalon TS, Athanasoulis CA, Margolies MN, *et al.*: Hemorrhage with Pelvic Fractures: Efficacy of Transcatheter Embolization. *AJR* 1979, 133:859–864.

16. Lang EK: Transcatheter Embolization of Pelvic Vessels for Control of Intractable Hemorrhage. *Radiology* 1981, 140:331–339.

17. Bakri YN, Linjawi T: Angiographic Embolization for Control of Pelvic Genital Tract Hemorrhage. Report of 14 Cases. *Acta Obstet Gynecol Scand* 1992, 71:17–21.

18. Vogelzang RL, Nemcek AA Jr, Skrtic Z, *et al.*: Uterine Arteriovenous Malformations: Primary Treatment with Therapeutic Embolization. *JVIR* 1991, 2:517–522.

19. Heaston DK, Mineau DE, Brown BJ, Miller FJ: Transcatheter Arterial Embolization for Control of Persistent Massive Puerperal Hemorrhage After Bilateral Surgical Hypogastric Artery Ligation. *AJR* 1979, 133:152–154.

20. Reubinoff BE, Eldor A, Laufer N, Sadovsky E: Maternal Hemorrhagic Complications Following Prophylactic Low-dose Aspirin and Dipyridamole Therapy. *Gynecol Obstet Invest* 1992, 33:241–243.

21. Sepulveda WH, Vinals F, Donetch G, *et al.*: Cervical Pregnancy. A Case Report. *Arch Gynecol Obstet* 1993, 252:155–157.

22. Simon P, Donner C, Delcour C, *et al.*: Selective Uterine Artery Embolization in the Treatment of Cervical Pregnancy: Two Case Reports. *Euro J Obstet Gynecol Reprod Biol* 1991, 40:159–161.

23.• Kerr A, Trambert J, Mikhail M, Hodges L, Runowicz C: Preoperative Transcatheter Embolization of Abdominal Pregnancy: Report of Three Cases. *JVIR* 1993, 4:733–735.

A current report of the efficacy of this procedure in the potentially serious condition of abdominal pregnancy.

24. Greenwood LH, Glickman MG, Schwartz PE, *et al.*: Obstetric and Nonmalignant Gynecologic Bleeding: Treatment with Angiographic Embolization. *Radiology* 1987, 164:155–159.

25.• Gilbert WM, Moore TR, Resnik R, *et al.*: Angiographic Embolization in the Management of Hemorrhagic Complications of Pregnancy. *Am J Obstet Gynecol* 1992, 166:493–497.

This article describes one of the larger series of patients treated by transcatheter embolization.

26. Yamashita Y, Takahashi M, Ito M, Okamura H: Transcatheter Arterial Embolization in the Management of Postpartum Hemorrhage Due to Genital Tract Injury. *Obstet Gynecol* 1991, 77:160–163.

27. Kaplan MM: Acute Fatty Liver of Pregnancy. *N Engl J Med* 1985, 313:367–370.

28. Riely CA, Latham PS, Romero R, Duffy TP: Acute Fatty Liver of Pregnancy. *Ann Intern Med* 1987, 106:703–706.

29. Barron SI: Antepartum Hemorrhage. In *Obstetrics*. Edited by Turnbull A, Chamberlain G. Edinburgh, Scotland: Churchill Livingston; 1989:469–477.

30. Dunnihoo DR: *Gynecology and Obstetrics*. Philadelphia: JB Lippincott; 1992:292–297.

Select Bibliography

Bakri YN, Linjawi T: Angiographic Embolization for Control of Pelvic Genital Tract Hemorrhage. Report of 14 Cases. *Acta Obstet Gynecol Scand* 1992, 71:17–21.

Gilbert WM, Moore TR, Resnick R, *et al.*: Angiographic Embolization in the Management of Hemorrhagic Complications of Pregnancy. *Am J Obstet Gynecol* 1992, 166:493–497.

Mitty HA, Sterling KM, Alvarez M, Gendler R: Obstetric Hemorrhage; Prophylactic and Emergency Arterial Catheterization and Embolotherapy. *Radiology* 1993, 188:183–187.

Diagnosis and Ablation of Parathyroid Adenomas

Barry A. Sacks

Johanna Pallotta

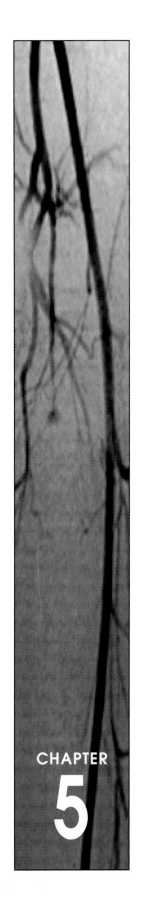

CHAPTER

5

In the vast majority of patients, primary hyperparathyroidism is caused by a single adenoma (85% in most reported series, but > 90% in our experience), with the remainder caused by hyperplasia (5% to 10%), double adenomas (< 5%), or carcinomas (< 1%) [1••,2–5]. There are two major reasons for radiologic interest in this disease: 1) radiographic findings that help to establish the diagnosis (*eg*, bone changes, renal calculi, and soft-tissue calcification); and 2) location of the lesion causing the disease. The anatomic location of parathyroid glands (Fig. 5-1), and as a consequence the adenomas (Fig. 5-2) (though usually related to the posterior thyroid), is inconsistent and unpredictable, often requiring radiographic localization.

Experts debate the necessity for preoperative localization of parathyroid lesions in patients who present with primary hyperparathyroidism [6–12,13••,14–17]. Many skilled parathyroid surgeons believe they can successfully locate the lesion in greater than 95% of patients without localization assistance. Others believe

that even though preoperative localization may be helpful, it is not cost-effective, particularly if they belong to the school that recommends bilateral neck exploration in all patients to visualize or perform a biopsy in all four glands.

There is a significant problem with the above philosophy. The vast majority of primary parathyroid patients are treated in a community hospital setting by general surgeons. Regardless of skill level, this is not equivalent to a specialized parathyroid surgeon, and success rates are very unlikely to mirror the rates found in published surgical series. As a consequence, other investigators including ourselves believe that the localization is not only helpful in reducing the number of failed operations, but can also limit the surgical approach to a unilateral neck dissection. If the lesion is confidently identified, the surgeon will remove the abnormal gland and examine the ipsilateral parathyroid. If the gland appears normal, the opposite side is not explored because there is such an

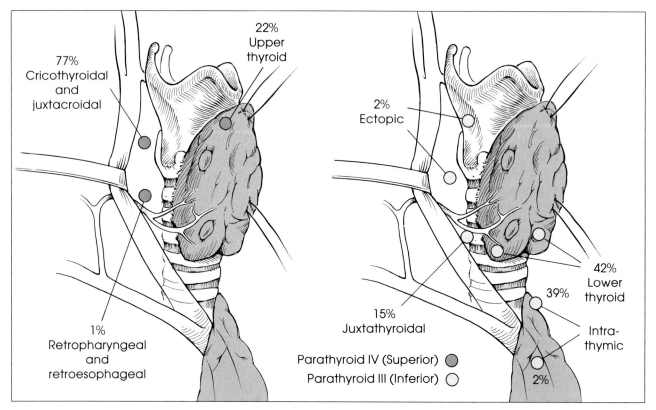

FIGURE 5-1.

Normal and ectopic location of parathyroid glands. Parathyroid III represents the inferior gland and may be detected from the angle of the mandible to the anterior mediastinum. The parathyroid IV or superior gland can lie

from high in the neck to the posteromedial neck (even the tracheoesophageal groove) to the posterior mediastinum. (Adapted from Wang CA: The Anatomic Basis of Parathyroid Surgery. *Ann Surg* 1976, 183:271, with permission.)

overwhelming incidence of single adenomas, the chance of finding an abnormality on the opposite side is extremely remote, particularly if the imaging study showed only a single lesion.

Diagnostic Work-up

Noninvasive modalities used to image parathyroids include ultrasound, computed tomography (CT),

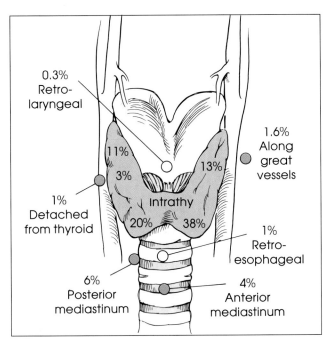

FIGURE 5-2.

The location of detected adenomas in a large surgical series. (*Adapted from* Sacks BA, *et al.*: Parathyroid Adenomas: Cinearteriography. *AJR* 1980, 135:535, with permission.)

nuclear medicine, and magnetic resonance imaging (MRI). The method preferred depends largely on the expertise at the particular institution. The reported accuracies of each method are summarized in Table 5-1. Localization information using these modalities is based on finding a mass in the proper location and demonstrating specific ultrasound, CT, or MRI characteristics. Absolute differentiation from other masses, particularly thyroid nodules, is often impossible on morphologic grounds alone. Often, the imager uses a number of criteria to make a diagnosis.

Despite our strong belief about the value of preoperative localization, we do limit our initial search to one radiologic study (usually a small-parts ultrasound of the neck), unless there are extenuating circumstances. When the results show a lesion with a classical appearance, the ultrasound has been extremely reliable. When results are negative, no further radiographic work-up is undertaken and the patient is usually sent directly to surgery. Although arguments have been made to pursue noninvasive tests such as CT, thallium-technetium subtraction, or MRI to reduce or eliminate the 5% miss rate, we have elected not to follow this procedure. Multiple exams are often diffcult to justify because of the high costs of these tests and because the surgical community often questions the value of any imaging studies.

However, once patients have had failed exploration exams, the situation is completely different. Preoperative localization becomes imperative, as surgery is much more difficult and there is greater likelihood of an ectopic lesion [18,19,20–22,23••,24,25]. The major causes of failed surgery are missed glands (62%), ectopic glands

Table 5-1. Localization of Parathyroid Lesions					
Modality	Accuracy unexplored, %	Accuracy explored, %	Ectopic local, %	False positive, %	Single vs multiple
Ultrasound	71–80	40–50	40–50	—	Fair
Thallium-technetium	75	27–49	75	18–27	Fair
Computed tomography	78	44–47	78	2–12	Fair
Magnetic resonance imaging	56–81	50–75	50–75	10–18	Fair
Arteriography	—	85–88	85–88	1–2	Good
Arteriography and vein catheterization	—	91–95	91–95	—	Excellent
Computed tomography and thallium-technetium	88	59	—	—	—
Computed tomography and ultrasound	—	71	—	—	—
Computed tomography, ultrasound, and thallium-technetium	—	78	—	—	—

(15%), supernumery glands (15%), and malignancy or autotransplantation (8%). In this group, the differentiation between adenoma and hyperplasia (single vs multigland disease) as the cause of hyperparathyroidism was established at the time of the initial operation. After localization, only the abnormal gland must be excised. At this stage, sequential radiographic localization studies including CT scanning, MRI, thallium-technetium subtraction (the order in which tests are performed will vary by institution and case), and angiography (if other tests are inconclusive) may be necessary. In failed previous exploration, the detection rates of noninvasive tests are inconsistent and substantially lower than usually quoted for the virgin neck (Table 5-1). Despite low detection rates, noninvasive tests should be attempted first. If these tests are positive with a reasonable degree of certainty, a second surgery can be undertaken. Angiography is pursued only if these localization studies are either negative or inconclusive. In these difficult situations, our suggested approach is to perform an extensive venous sampling to localize the site of parathyroid hormone (PTH) step-up. Directed angiography should then be performed to specifically demonstrate the lesions. If work-up requires this sequence of studies to culminate in arteriography, angiographic ablation can be a reasonable therapeutic alternative.

Ultrasound

In our experience, a small-parts ultrasound is approximately 75% accurate in detecting parathyroid adenomas. If the 4% to 6% incidence of mediastinal adenomas is subtracted, this would leave 19% to 21% of adenomas that occur in the neck but are not detected sonographically. The reason many parathyroid lesions cannot be demonstrated ultrasonically is both unclear and frus-

trating. Unusual ectopic location may be a factor, but not for all cases. Perhaps in some lesions the textural changes are such that they are indistinguishable, and blend in with the juxtathyroidal tissue.

On ultrasound, a parathyroid adenoma classically appears as a round, oblong teardrop or cigar-shaped hypoechoic lesion posterior to the thyroid (Fig. 5-3). Its position may vary, but the ultrasound features are relatively consistent. Although the glands may lie close to one another toward the midportion of the posterior thyroid, the lower gland is often found at or below the lower pole of the thyroid lobe. When not in its usual location, the upper gland lies posteromedial, and may lie often as far as the tracheoesophageal groove. If the glands are not detected immediately, the more common ectopic locations must be examined. This includes scanning from the angle of the mandible, along the carotid vessels, and past the thyroid to the thoracic inlet. It is also important to scan at the thoracic inlet and direct the patient to swallow. This may reveal a lesion that moves cephalad with the thyroid and can only be seen using this maneuver.

One of the confusing issues with ultrasound is the common presence of incidental thyroid nodules. Although diagnosis of parathyroid adenomas is based on position or textural characteristics, it is often difficult to differentiate the lesions. Thyroid nodules are often multiple, can appear in the posterior portion of the gland, and have similar texture to that of parathyroid adenomas. To complicate matters, parathyroid adenomas may also be intrathyroidal (Fig. 5-4). A newer aspect of ultrasound, color-flow imaging, adds specificity to the examination. Parathyroid adenomas are reported to demonstrate hypervascularity within the lesions, whereas thyroid lesions show more circumferential hypervascularity.

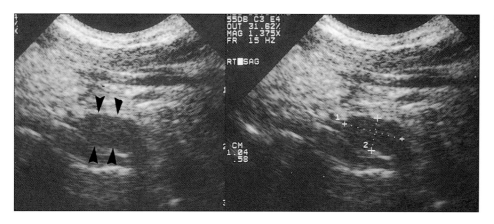

FIGURE 5-3.

Ultrasound demonstrates the classical appearance of a parathyroid adenoma (*arrows*). The lesion is smooth, well demarcated, oblong, and hypoechoic in comparison with the thyroid tissue texture.

We have improved the specificity of ultrasound diagnosis by performing needle aspiration of suspicious lesions to measure PTH, particularly in the patients mentioned above (Fig. 5-5). [26•,27,28••,29, 30•,31,32]. We recently reviewed our series of needle aspiration in 80 lesions in 66 patients (Sacks, unpublished data). Elevated levels of PTH in the aspirate indicated a positive result and confirmed the diagnosis and location of the abnormal gland. Most negative results were truly negative, with all lesions representing thyroid nodules. There were six false-negative aspirates caused by the needle missing the lesion. The technique is simple and extremely helpful in clinical decision-making. A number of publications have indicated the value of cytology in specifically confirming parathyroid adenomas [1••]. However, this is not a reliable technique at our institution, even with special stains. The technique was attempted in 10 patients, was not helpful, and was subsequently abandoned.

Nuclear Medicine

A variety of nuclear medicine localization techniques have been used to treat parathyroid adenomas [20,33–35,36••,37–46]. The most popular is the thallium-technetium subtraction, in which a focal area of isotope concentration is demonstrated, corresponding to the adenoma (Fig. 5-6). Using this approach, the technetium injection results in visualization of the thyroid gland; the thallium helps to visualize both the thyroid and parathyroid glands. When the two images are photographically subtracted, a localized area of increased activity usually corresponds to the parathyroid adenoma. A variation of this approach uses tech-

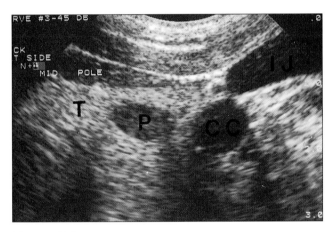

FIGURE 5-4.

An intrathyroidal parathyroid adenoma. Ultrasound demonstrated the hypoechoic lesion within the substance of the thyroid.

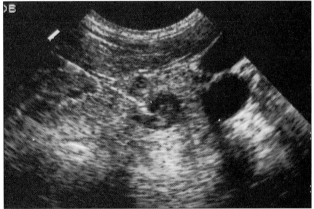

FIGURE 5-5.

Diagnostic aspiration under ultrasound guidance. The needle tip is demonstrated within the parathyroid adenoma. Two tenths of a mL is injected, and the needle agitated in and out a few millimeters during continuous aspiration.

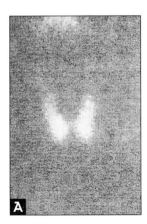

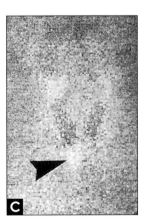

FIGURE 5-6.

Right lower-pole adenoma shown on a thallium-technetium subtraction. **A**, The technetium study showing only the thyroid. **B**, Both the thyroid and parathyroid perfusion on the thallium examination. **C**, Following subtraction of **A** from **B**, only the parathyroid is seen (*arrow*).

netium sestamibi instead of the thallium and is reported to be superior [40,42]. Other investigators have used the technetium sestamibi alone.

As can be expected with this technique, adenomas that lie either within or immediately behind the thyroid gland will be difficult, if not impossible, to see. The technique relies on the lesion being partially or completely separate from the thyroid; this technique should theoretically be ideal for detecting cervical ectopic lesions. Lesions in the mediastinum are not usually seen because the isotope is attenuated by the sternum. We have found the cine-loop to be helpful in this situation. This implies a collection of images sequentially during injections of the isotopes and is the equivalent of a flow study. Playing the loop over and over can sometimes be very useful in detecting subtle abnormalities.

Computed Tomography

The standard CT approach, to obtain thin sections through the lower neck and mediastinum with or without intravenous contrast, has had mixed results and is very much dependent on the expertise of the interpreting radiologist and the quality of the study. If the thyroid is situated low in the neck or the patient has a short neck, attempting to image through the shoulders can degrade the results.

One of the major functions of CT and MRI is to exclude a mediastinal adenoma. As an indirect approach, exclusion of a mediastinal adenoma is helpful because it suggests that the adenoma is cervical.

The interpretation of CT findings is usually very difficult and demands meticulous sequential examination of each thin slice (Fig. 5-7). When a physician is

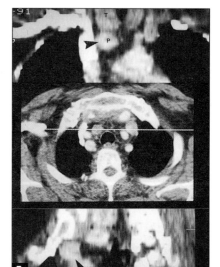

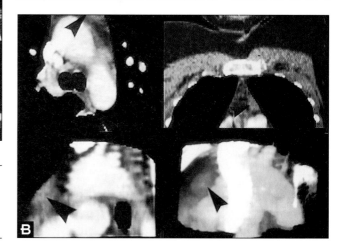

FIGURE 5-8.

Computed tomography reconstruction. Thin, contiguous-slice CT as well as spiral CT allows examination of the neck and mediastinum in more than the axial projection. **A**, A sagittal and coronal view of a right lower-pole adenoma. **B**, Sagittal, coronal, and three-dimensional reconstruction of a mediastinal adenoma following spiral CT.

FIGURE 5-7.

Computed tomography demonstrates the need for careful examination of a sequence of slices to compare the right side with the left side and look for a soft-tissue abnormality that could correspond to the parathyroid adenoma (*arrows*).

looking for a small enhancing nodule, comparison of the two sides of the neck for any asymmetry is the key. Sometimes the lesion is very obvious; mostly the findings are subtle, particularly if the lesion is in contiguity with the thyroid gland. All that may be seen is an asymmetry or a bulbous region posteriorly. In the mediastinum, the physician is usually looking for a lesion that does not correspond to a normally expected structure.

The advent of spiral CT will certainly have a substantial impact on the detection ability of this technique [5]. Using this approach, rapid sequential scans can be obtained at the peak of contrast enhancement. Not only will the axial scans be superior to those obtained with conventional CT, but also the ability to perform sagittal, coronal (Fig. 5-8A), or three-dimensional reconstructions (Fig. 5-8B) demonstrates the exact location of the lesion and enables the entire tissue volume to be rotated in any desired position. This also improves mediastinal detection. Unfortunately, no randomized studies on the overall accuracy of this method have been reported.

Magnetic Resonance Imaging

The MRI-enhanced features of a parathyroid adenoma that show a significant increase in T_2 signals are unfortunately undependable. Often the findings are a soft-tissue mass similar to the thyroid that is slightly higher in signal to the vascular flow void, but is in a location consistent with the parathyroid. The T_1 images are often more useful because the resolution is superior (Fig. 5-9). Sometimes in T_2, the lesion may even be more difficult to see because it may become isosignal with the surrounding tissue. However, when the T_2 appearances are classical, the lesions are easy to see (Fig. 5-10). Gadolinium enhancement seems to be an appropriate approach in an attempt to improve lesion

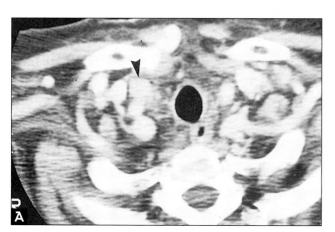

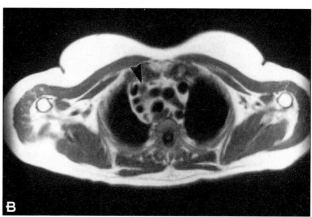

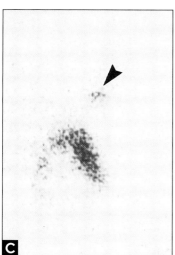

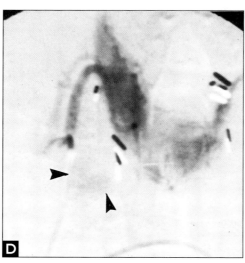

FIGURE 5-9.

Four studies of the same patient showing a right lower-pole lesion (*arrows*). **A**, Computed tomography. **B**, Magnetic resonance imaging. **C**, Nuclear medicine. **D**, An arteriogram.

detection with MRI, but this has not been adequately assessed [5,34,36••,38,47–49].

One major advantage of MRI is the ability to obtain high-resolution studies in both sagittal and coronal planes (Fig. 5-11).

Venous Sampling and Arteriography

Angiography is reserved only for patients with hyperparathyroidism who have been previously explored and have had inconclusive noninvasive localization studies [5,50–52]. Initially, we perform an extensive venous catheterization and use that data to proceed with a limited arteriogram directed by the results. However, this approach is not universally accepted. Some angiographers would prefer to go directly to the arteriogram and adopt one of two approaches: 1)

confining the study to examination of the mediastinum (selective internal mammary artery injections); or 2) a complete study involving bilateral internal mammary, inferior, and superior thyroid arteries. The limited approach is based on the idea that if the mediastinum results are negative, the surgeon can be advised to re-explore the neck. In our opinion, this leaves too much uncertainty because the lesion has still not been specifically identified.

The venous sampling procedure is safe but tedious. Although it has previously required 3 to 4 hours to perform, an experienced radiologist can complete the procedure within 1.5 hours. Our major aim in this proceudre is to determine two points: 1) if the lesion is in the chest or the neck; and 2) if it is on the right or left side. We sample what is left of the thyroid venous plexus (the middle thyroid veins are always tied off if

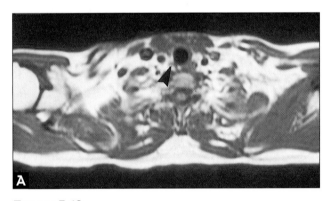

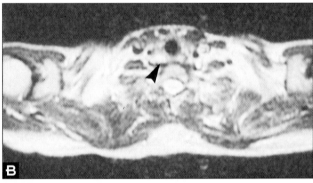

FIGURE 5-10.

Magnetic resonance imaging of a right-sided neck lesion. **A,** Using T_1, a small soft-tissue mass is seen in the tracheoesophageal groove (*arrow*). **B,** Using T_2, the lesion shows the classical bright signal (*arrow*).

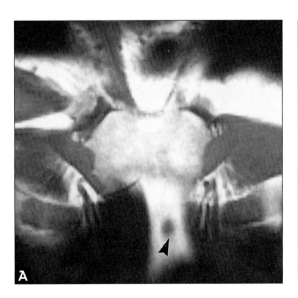

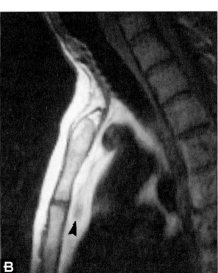

FIGURE 5-11.

A and **B,** Magnetic resonance imaging in sagittal and coronal planes demonstrates a small adenoma shown as a low-density lesion within the bright fat of the mediastinum using T_1.

the patient has had surgery), the thymic vein, the vertebral veins (a collateral after surgery), and the large neck veins (*ie*, the jugular, innominate, and superior vena cava) (Fig. 5-12). Often additional small veins are found in the lower neck and chest. Although the specific names of these veins are ignored, the important factor is the region these veins drain (*ie*, low right neck or left chest). Many institutions attempt to quickly sample the large veins in the neck that are easily catheterized. The data from this type of procedure are usually unsatisfactory and often more confusing than helpful; it is necessary to be more selective.

It is impossible to perform a venous study with standard-size catheters. Each vein sampled requires a different shape and the number of catheters changes required would make the procedure intolerable. As a result, an unconventional approach must be used. Doppman and colleagues [32] use an externally directable system that permits changing the shape of the catheter *in vivo*. We have used the Cope/Eisenberg coaxial system. This requires a 7-French, straight, 80- to 90-cm thin-walled catheter that acts as a long sheath. Through this catheter, a 5-French teflon catheter is directed by an inner torquable parathyroid wire. The wire can be one of two shapes: a very gentle distal curve, or a 3-cm C curve. By advancing or retracting the two catheters and the wire, the shapes can be continuously varied as needed. The samples are difficult to draw and the wire helps in this regard. By

advancing the bulbous-ended wire 1 or 2 mm out of the catheter tip, the vein wall is kept away, permitting easy flow of venous blood.

Choosing to begin a lesion search with a complete arteriogram in previously explored patients presents a different set of problems. Although the vascular parathyroid lesion is usually quite easy to identify, the areas of blush are often not as clear cut, intimately related to the thyroid, and difficult to interpret with confidence. It is in this situation that venous data helps the most. The venous data are functional information and invaluable in interpreting the arteriographic findings. Viewing a lesion on the side of the step-up of PTH adds confidence that it is the adenoma. Additionally, vein catheterization allows tailoring of the arteriographic examination which significantly shortens the procedure and renders it safer.

Although arteriography is normally done in a standard fashion with a groin puncture to simplify selective catheterization, the catheter is introduced into the brachial artery on the side of the step-up. This is performed in patients who are older, hypertensive, or have tortuous vessels, making selective catheterization of the internal mammary and inferior thyroid arteries from the groin extremely difficult and subselective catheterization impossible. Because both superior and inferior parathyroid glands can be visualized by injecting the inferior thyroid artery, the brachial approach is the logical choice in many patients. However, there can be a problem when no lesions are immediately seen; this will require a contralateral arteriography or injection of the superior thyroid vessels. By using a Simmons I or II catheter (Cook, Bloomington, IN and Cordis, Miami Lakes, FL), bilateral, nonselective subclavian and common carotid injections from either brachial approach can be achieved. This will demonstrate the lesion but usually rules out ablation via this catheter because superselective catheterization of the feeding vessel is necessary. If the lesion is identified, either a second appropriate puncture for selective catheterization is performed or ablation is canceled in favor of surgery. Attempted ablation from the superior thyroid artery is much more dangerous; we have only performed this procedure once (Fig. 5-4).

Conventional catheters are used, usually 4-French in size. For catheterization from the groin, an H1 catheter (Cook, Bloomington, IN and Cordis, Miami Lakes, FL) is the first choice and for the arm, a cobra catheter

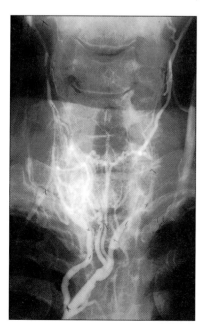

FIGURE 5-12.

Vein catheterization. During venous sampling of the thyroid plexus for the parathyroid hormone, venography is performed to show the anatomy. This provides a road map of the vein to be sampled as well as sites of drainage.

(Cook, Bloomington, IN and Cordis, Miami Lakes, FL) is preferred. The shapes may be modified as needed, depending on the specific anatomy. Although we previously performed subclavian arteriograms as an initial step, we now proceed directly to selective catheterization. If all vessels fail to reveal the lesion, bilateral subclavian arteriograms will be performed to rule out an unusual vessel supplying the lesion. All studies are performed with digital subtraction angiography (DSA) using nonionic contrast. This procedure has improved safety by significantly expediting the examination and allowing the use of safer and more dilute contrast mediums. Often, many projections are necessary. If the lesion is not visualized on injection of the expected arterial supply, we proceed to inject the ipsilateral internal mammary and superior thyroid and then proceed to the opposite side.

The classical appearance of a parathyroid adenoma is a blushing hypervascular lesion, staining more prominently than the thyroid tissue and persisting for a longer period of time. When the lesion is identified (Fig. 5-13A), the diagnosis is relatively obvious. If the lesion protrudes beyond the outline of the thyroid, diagnosis becomes even easier (Fig. 5-13B). However, when the lesion is projected over the thyroid or shows nontypical staining, diagnosis may be very difficult. It is in these cases that the venous data improve the diagnostic confidence level. Occasionally, the lesion may be completely avascular and not detectable with arteriography.

ARTERIAL ABLATION

The accepted treatment of parathyroid adenomas is surgical excision of the abnormal gland or glands. However, surgery may sometimes be risky because of a patient's significant medical problems or technically difficult because of a scarred previously explored neck. In these patients, it is valuable to have an alternative

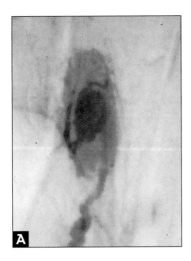
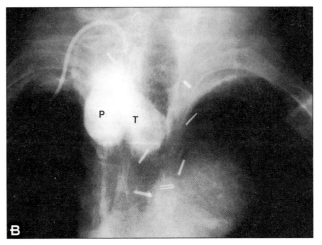

FIGURE 5-13.

A, Arteriography shows the small parathyroid adenoma superimposed over the thyroid. The adenoma is identified because the blush is more prominent than the thyroid and persists for a longer period of time. **B**, An adenoma (*P*) separate from the thyroid (*T*) that is much easier to identify.

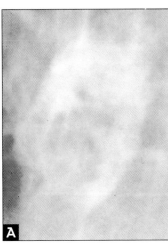
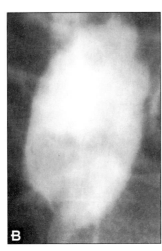

FIGURE 5-14.

Ablation. **A**, The appearance of the adenoma during the regular arteriogram. There is a prominent blush with an avascular area in the lower aspect, caused by some necrosis or cystic degeneration. **B**, Following the ablation, the marked difference in stain can be seen. Not only is the stain much more intense, but it is also almost homogeneously bright. This is a result of the highly concentrated ionic contrast forced into the interstitium.

therapeutic option. Two forms of alternative nonsurgical therapy have been used: 1) percutaneous ablation using direct absolute alcohol injection into the adenoma; and 2) angiographic ablation using a variety of agents injected via the arterial supply [53–61,62••, 63••,64–66].

In the past, consideration for an angiographic ablation procedure was restricted to those patients who had very complicated prior clinical courses. This group included multiple or difficult surgical procedures or significant medical problems that rendered patients high-risk surgical candidates. Now, if the patient has reached the stage where noninvasive studies are inconclusive and angiographic localization is necessary, we obtain informed consent for ablation at the time of diagnostic arteriography. We explain to the patient that a final decision about ablation can only be made once the lesion has been identified, the arterial supply superselectively catheterized, and the procedure considered safe. Ablation does not add significant extra risk to the diagnostic arteriogram and a successful ablation also negates further surgery. Ablation failure necessitates a second surgery but following the arteriographic examination, the lesion has been well localized and beautifully demonstrated, making the surgery routine.

Technique

Once the lesion has been identified arteriographically, the specific blood supply is assessed and subselective catheterization performed. The catheter is advanced as distal as possible and wedged into the supplying vessel. Five- to 10-mL boluses of 60% to 76% regular ionic contrast are then injected until a dense homogeneous stain is attained within the lesion (Fig. 5-14). Usually a total volume of 40 to 60 mL of contrast is necessary. The contrast has two major effects: 1) direct cytotoxicity; and 2) hyperosmolarity. As the contrast is forced into the interstitium, it will result in fluid being drawn out of the cells, causing cellular dehydration and subsequent destruction of the lesion.

When a satisfactorily persistent dense stain is achieved, the supplying vessel is occluded with Gelfoam (Cook, Bloomington, IN and Target Therapeutics, Freemont, CA) or small coils (Fig. 5-15). Coils used are usually 0.018- to 0.025-inch, 5- to 10-mm, straight microcoils; occasionally in a large vessel, the S coil (Target Therapeutics, Freemont, CA) or the 2 × 3 mm coil (Cook, Bloomington, IN) are used. This final maneuver achieves two important functions: 1) it perpetuates the stain by preventing contrast washout, allowing maximal time for the contrast ablative effects;

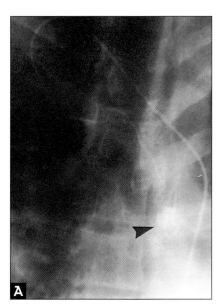
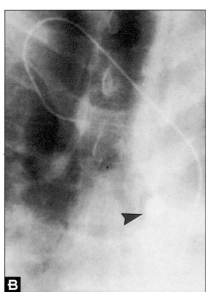
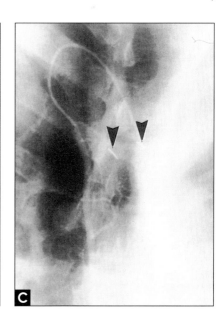

FIGURE 5-15.

Ablation. **A**, A mediastinal lesion is seen, supplied by a branch of the left internal mamary artery (*arrow*). **B**, The lesion following subselective catherization and dense staining (*arrow*). **C**, At the end of the ablation, the arterial supply was occluded with two straight mini 5-mm coils (*arrows*).

and 2) it results in ischemia that aids in the ablative process. Another use of coils is to redistribute blood flow for the contrast staining. For example, if the adenoma is supplied by a branch of the inferior artery but cannot be selectively catheterized, the radiologist can occlude the vessel to the thyroid allowing subsequent injections of contrast to flow directly into the adenoma. When it is impossible to subselectively catheterize the vessel to the adenoma in neck lesions, we have successfully ablated such lesions from the main inferior thyroid trunk. No thyroid complications occurred, indicating a rich collateral vascular supply and intrinsic resistance of thyroid tissue to the contrast.

However, some unanswered questions remain. There is no objective way to determine when enough contrast material has been injected into the lesion or when the stain becomes adequately dense. The surgeon must rely on experience and a ball park contrast volume in the to 40- to 60-mL range. No biochemical tests are quick enough to give meaningful information. The endpoint is empirical and the surgeon can only wait and follow the clinical course to assess the procedure's success. If the stain remains a few hours after the procedure, the chances of success are increased (Fig. 5-16).

In our series of approximately 30 patients (Sacks, unpublished data), we were able to achieve long-term success in approximately 60% of patients with cervical lesions (18 patients). These patients are definitely the most difficult because of the extensive collateral vascular supply of the thyroid. On the other hand, the success rate is much higher in the mediastinum (five of six patients). This is because the lesion is usually at the end of a pedicle (an end organ)

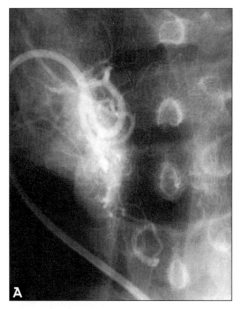

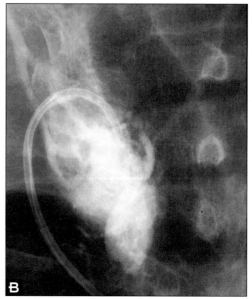

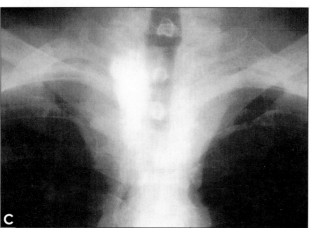

FIGURE 5-16.

Ablation of a cervical adenoma. **A,** Arterial and **B** tissue phases of the right inferior artery injection. The lesion is demonstrated posteromedial to the lower pole of the thyroid lobe. This was injected with 50 to 60 mL of Renografin-60 and the arterial supply occluded. **C,** A chest radiograph obtained 3 hours after the procedure shows persistence of the stain within the lesion.

and if selective catheterization is possible, staining and embolization are more effective. Additionally, in the chest, other ablative agents can be used that would not be safe in the cervical region, specifically absolute alcohol. Using these agents, the likelihood of success is also much greater (Fig. 5-17). It is usually possible to assess the success of the procedure within 24 to 48 hours. The serum calcium levels drop rapidly, often requiring temporary calcium supplementation. If the ablation fails, the calcium levels rapidly return to the elevated state. In most patients, the levels did so within 48 hours, although one or two took 2 to 8 weeks. If the calcium and PTH levels remain normal for longer than 2 months, the patients continue to remain normocalcemic and are considered cured.

Complications

In our study, no major complications were encountered. Two patients complained of temporary hoarseness that resolved after a few hours. The hoarseness may have been a result of either direct staining of the vocal cords or involvement of a supplying nerve with minor neuropraxia. Despite the high incidence of branchial artery catheterizations (usually using a 5-French catheter), no problems were encountered. All patients complained of pain during the contrast injections; this pain is mainly caused by the contrast effect on cervical muscle supplied by small branches from the thyroid arteries. It is for this reason that ablation with absolute alcohol may be dangerous and contraindicated intra-arterially. Some small branches may also supply important nerves in the region.

Other ablative agents such as heated contrast and Yb-90 microspheres (causing radiation necrosis) have also been used, but experience with these agents is too limited to draw any meaningful conclusions.

DIRECT ALCOHOL ABLATION

Attempts have also been made to inject absolute alcohol directly into the lesion, with promising results. This approach does have exciting possibilities. Solbiati [28••] has the largest clinical experience and has attempted treatment of both adenomas and hyperplastic glands. As would be expected, results with adenomas are much better than those with the hyperplastic glands. The amount of alcohol necessary was

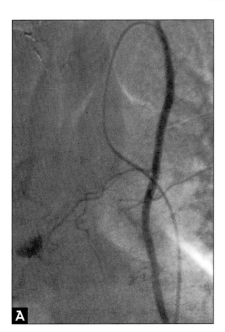 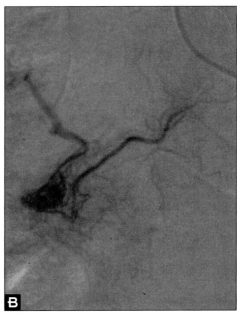 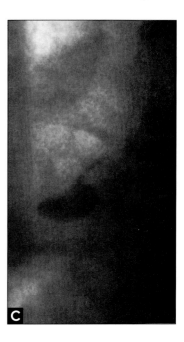

FIGURE 5-17.

Ablation. Three films during ablation of a mediastinal adenoma in a patient who had a significant thymic-vein elevation of PTH. **A**, The adenoma during injection of the left internal mamary artery. **B**, Subselective catheterization of the feeding vessel shows the lesion as well as the thymic-vein drainage. **C**, Following ablation with 40 mL of Renografin-60, absolute alcohol, and micro-coil occlusion of the supplying artery, the lesion shows a persistent stain, stasis in the artery, and swelling.

calculated as the volume of the lesion and approximately 10% was added. All procedures were performed under ultrasound guidance on an outpatient basis. The alcohol was injected until the lesion completely changes its texture. In many cases, the technique was repeated days to weeks later until adequate ablation was achieved. Reported complications included pain from alcohol leaking into the surrounding tissue which led to temporary dysphonia; this was believed to be related to a temporary effect on the recurrent laryngeal nerve. Because a new needle specifically designed for ethanol injection (with an occluded end and multiple sideholes) was developed, problems with dysphonia have been eliminated.

Conclusion

Although surgery remains the treatment of choice for hyperparathyroidism, arteriographic ablation of parathyroid adenomas is a definite alternative therapeutic consideration in some patients. Our experience has been with both neck and mediastinal lesions and Doppman and colleagues [58] and Miller and colleagues [62••] have had experience with adenomas in the mediastinum. There is no doubt that arteriographic ablation of mediastinal lesions offers a tremendous advantage. Not only is major thoracotomy avoided, but there is also a high success rate

with these lesions. Miller and colleagues [62••] report a success rate in excess of 70% with the mediastinal lesions; our success has been slightly higher, but in a smaller series. We have elected to use intra-arterial absolute alcohol in the mediastinal adenomas whenever possible, and we believe this will significantly improve ablation success rates without adding significant risk.

Treatment of neck lesions is more controversial and likely to be questioned by our colleagues, especially those with expertise in this field. They can rightly argue that a second neck surgery by an experienced surgeon once the lesion has been identified is simple and absolutely curative. However, if work-up requires proceeding to arteriography and the lesion is identified during that study, it makes perfect sense to consider ablation. Every patient undergoing arteriography who has been offered angiographic ablation with the possibility of avoiding a second surgery, unanimously elects to give this approach a try. Patients are tremendously disappointed if this approach is either impossible or unsuccessful. The success rate with cervical lesions is approximately 60%, which is reasonably acceptable for using only contrast and embolization. We do not advise the use of absolute alcohol for neck lesions. Certainly, we have had enough experience to determine that the procedure is successful if the calcium and PTH remain normal for up to 3 months.

References and Recommended Reading

Recently published papers of particular interest have been highlighted as:
•Of interest
••Of outstanding interest

1.•• Wang CA: Surgical Management of Primary Hyperparathyroidism. In *Endocrinology*, vol 2. Edited by Degroot L. New York: Grune and Stratton; 1979:735–737.
The author has extensive experimental and clinical experience with both anatomy and surgical treatment of parathyroid disease. These writings give an excellent overall approach to management.

2. Obara T: Diagnosis and Treatment of Primary Hyperparathyroidism (in Japanese). *Nippon Naibunpi Gakkai Zasshi* 1992, 68:1167–1176.

3. Duh QY, Uden P, Clark OH: Unilateral Neck Exploration for Primary Hyperparathyroidism: Analysis of a Controversy Using a Mathematical Model. *World J Surg* 1992, 16:654–661.

4. Salti G, Fedorak I, Yashiro T, *et al.*: Continuing Evolution in the Operative Management of Primary Hyperparathyroidism. *Arch Surg* 1992; 127:831–836.

5. Eisenberg H, Pallotta JA: Special Localizing Techniques for Parathyroid Disease. In *Endocrinology*, vol 2. Edited by Degroot LJ. New York: Grunne and Stratton; 1979:717–724.

6. Deftos LJ, Parthemore JG, Stabile BE: Management of Primary Hyperparathyroidism. *Ann Rev Med* 1993, 44:19–26.

7. Shaha AR, Jaffe BM: Cervical Exploration for Primary Hyperparathyroidism. *J Surg Oncol* 1993, 52:14–17.

8. Barbier J, Kraimps JL, Denizot A, Henry JF: Primary Hyperparathyroidism. Results of a French Multicenter Study. *Bull Acad Natl Med* 1992, 176:1033–1047.

9. Sarfati E, DeAngelis P, D'Acremont B, *et al.*: Minerva Anatomic Localization of Parathyroid Adenomas. Experience with 1200 Cases of Primary Hyperparathyroidism. *Minerva Chir* 1992, 47:89–94.

10. Kaplan EL, Yashiro T, Salti G: Primary Hyperparathyroidism in the 1990s. Choice of Surgical Procedures for This Disease. *Ann Surg* 1992, 215:300–317.

11. Morioka WT: Trends in Primary Hyperparathyroidism Surgery. *Laryngoscope* 1992, 102:422–425.

12. Lesser T, Bartel M: Primary Hyperparathyroidism. Pathogenesis–Diagnosis–Therapy. *Zentralbl Chir* 1992, 117:41–49.

13.•• Clark OH, Duh QY: Primary Hyperparathyroidism. A Surgical Perspective. *Endo Metab Clin North Am* 1989, 18:701–714.
This chapter reviews the disease, clinical approach, and surgical management. Indications for particular imaging studies and when the studies are required are covered.

14. Hasselgren PO, Fidler JP: Further Evidence Against the Routine Use of Parathyroid Ultrasonography Prior to Initial Neck Exploration for Hyperparathyroidism. *Am J Surg* 1989, 164:337–340.

15. Zhang J: Re-evaluation of Ultrasonographic Localization in Primary Hyperparathyroidism. Report of 55 Cases (in Chinese). *Chung Kuo I Hsueh Ko Hsueh Yuan Hseuh Pao* 1992, 14:408–412.

16. Kairaluoma MI, Makarainen H, Salo-Zetterman E, *et al*: Cost Effectiveness of Ultrasound in Primary Parathyroid Surgery. *Br J Surg* 1989, 76:596–597.

17. Murchison J, McIntosh C, Aitken AGF, *et al*.: Ultrasound Detection of Parathyroid Adenomas. *Br J Radiol* 1991, 64:679–682.

18. Brennan MF, Norton JA: Reoperation for Persistent and Recurrent Hyperparathyroidism. *Ann Surg* 1984, 201:40–44.

19. Wang CA: Parathyroid Re-exploration: A Clinical and Pathological Study of 112 Patients. *Ann Surg* 1977, 186:140.

20. Carter WB, Carter DL, Cohn HE: Cause and Current Management of Reoperative Hyperparathyroidism. *Am Surg* 1993, 59:120–124.

21. Silver CE, Velez FJ: Parathyroid Re-exploration. *Am J Surg* 1992, 164:606–609.

22. Wei JP, Burke GJ, Mansberger AR Jr: Cause and Current Management of Reoperative Hyperparathyroidism. *Surgery* 1992, 112:1111–1116.

23.•• Brennan MF, Norton JA: Reoperation for Persistent and Recurrent Hyperparathyroidism. *Ann Surg* 1984, 201:40–44.
A paper by authors who have treated a large number of patients. They follow the belief that advocates extensive bilateral neck exploration in initial primary hyperparathyroidism without primary imaging. The authors also agree to imaging in the previously explored patient.

24. Palmer JA, Rosen IB: Reoperative Surgery for Hyperparathyroidism. *Am J Surg* 1982, 144:406–410.

25. Flickinger FW, Sathyanayana, White JE, McWhirt EB: MRI in Hyperparathyroidism Requiring Reoperation. *Clin Imaging* 1991, 15:210–212.

26.• Sardi A, Bolton JS, Mitchell WT Jr, Merritt CR: Immunoperoxidase Confirmation of Ultrasonically Guided Fine Needle Aspirates in Patients with Recurrent Hyperparathyroidism. *Surg Gynecol Obstet* 1992, 175:563–568.
This paper discusses evaluation of the aspiration technique in establishing the diagnosis. Invariably, this is used to establish whether an imaged mass actually represents parathyroid tissue. Most of the cases were treated by cytology; with special stains, a few cases were treated with PTH estimation from the aspirate. See Solbiati *et al*. [28••] and Verbanck *et al*. [30•] for further reading.

27. Karstrup S, Glenthoj A, Torp-Pedersen S, *et al*.: Ultrasonically Guided Fine Needle Aspiration of Suggested Enlarged Parathyroid Glands. *Acta Radiol* 1988, 29:213–216.

28.•• Solbiati L, Montali G, Croce F, *et al*.: Parathyroid Tumors Detected by Fine-Needle Aspiration Biopsy Under Ultrasonic Guidance. *Radiology* 1983, 148:793–797.
This paper relates to the information presented in Sardi *et al*. [26•] by discussing the use of the aspiration technique in establishing parathyroid diagnosis.

29. Gooding GA, Clark OH, Stark DD, *et al*.: Parathyroid Aspiration Biopsy Under Ultrasound Guidance in the Postoperative Hyperparathyroid Patient. *Radiology* 1985, 155:193–196.

30.• Verbanck J, Clarysse J, Loncke R, *et al*.: Parathyroid Aspiration Biopsy Under Ultrasound Guidance. *Arch Otolaryngol Head Neck Surg* 1986, 112:1069–1073.
Another paper relating to Sardi *et al*. [26•] and Solbiati *et al*. [28••] that reports on the aspiration technique for parathyroid diagnosis.

31. Winkler B, Gooding GA, Montgomery CK, *et al*.: Immunoperoxidase Confirmation of Parathyroid Origin of Ultrasound Guided Fine Needle Aspirates of the Parathyroid Glands. *Acta Cytol* 1987, 31:40–44.

32. Doppman JL, Krudy AG, Marx SJ, *et al*.: Aspiration of Enlarged Parathyroid Glands for Parathyroid Hormone Assay. *Radiology* 1983, 148:31–35.

33. Thompson CT, Bowers J, Broadie TA: Preoperative Ultrasound and Thallium-Technetium Subtraction Scintigraphy in Localizing Parathyroid Lesions in Patients with Hyperparathyroidism. *Am Surg* 1993, 59:509–511.

34. Kohri K, Ishikawa Y, Kodama M, *et al*.: Comparison of Imaging Methods for Localization of Parathyroid Tumors. *Am J Surg* 1992, 164:140–145.

35. Krausz Y, Horne T, Hain D, *et al*.: Scintigraphic Techniques in Preoperative Localization of Parathyroid Adenoma. *Isr J Med Sci* 1992, 28:217–220.

36.•• Eisenberg H, Pallotta J, Sacks BA, Brickman AS: Parathyroid Localization, Three Dimensional Modeling and Percutaneous Ablation Techniques. Endocrine and 31. *Metab Clin North Am* 1989, 18:659–700.
This article discusses all the various modalities in detail and numerous excellent examples are given. In particular, examples of three-dimensional CT reconstructions are shown.

37. Summers GW, Dodge DL, Kammer H: Accuracy and Cost-Effectiveness of Preoperative Isotope and Ultrasound Imaging in Primary Hyperparathyroidism. *Otolaryngol Head Neck Surg* 1989, 100:210–217.

38. Kohri K, Ishikawa Y, Kodama M, *et al*.: Comparison of Imaging Methods for Localization of Parathyroid Tumors. *Am J Surg* 1992, 164:140–145.

39. Simon I, Simo R, Mesa J, *et al*.: Subtraction Scintigraphy with Thallium-201 Chloride and Technetium-99m Pertechnetate Versus High Resolution Ultrasonography in the Localization of the Parathyroid Glands in Primary Hyperparathyroidism. *Med Clin Barc* 1992, 99:774–777.

40. Taillefer R, Boucher Y, Potvin C, Lambert R: Detection and Localization of Parathyroid Adenomas in Patients with Hyperparathyroidism Using a Single Radionuclide Imaging Procedure with Technetium-99m Sestamibi. *J Nucl Med* 1992, 33:1801–1807.

41. Suehiro M, Fukuchi M: Localization of Hyperfunctioning Parathyroid Glands by Means of Thallium-201 and Iodine-131 Subtraction Scintigraphy in Patients with Primary and Secondary Hyperparathyroidism. *Ann Nucl Med* 1992, 6:185–190.

42. O'Doherty MJ, Kettle AG, Wells P, *et al.*: Parathyroid Imaging with Technetium-99m Sestamibi: Preoperative Localization and Tissue Uptake Studies. *J Nucl Med* 1992, 33:313–318.

43. Bergenfelz A, Tennvall J, Ahern B: Thallium-Technetium of Enlarged Parathyroid Glands After Calcitonin Stimulation of Parathyroid Hormone Secretion. *Acta Radiol* 1992, 33:319–322.

44. Kao CH, Lin WY, Wang SJ: Comparison Between Thallium-Technetium Subtraction Scan and Other Imaging Modalities in the Preoperative Localization of Abnormal Parathyroid Glands. *Kao Hsiung I Hsueh Ko Hsueh Tsa Chih* 1992, 8:272–276.

45. Goris ML, Basso LV, Keeling C: Parathyroid Imaging. *J Nucl Med* 1991, 32:887–889.

46. Basso LV, Keeling C, Goris ML: Parathyroid Imaging. Use of Dual Isotope Scintigraphy for the Localization of Adenomas Before Surgery. *Clin Nucl Med* 1992, 17:380–383.

47. Noyek AM, Bain J, Chapnik JS, *et al.*: Decision Making in Thyroid and Parathyroid Surgery: The Influence of Imaging. *Isr J Med Sci* 1992, 28:221–224.

48. Yao M, Jamieson C, Blend R: Magnetic Resonance Imaging in Preoperative Localization of Diseased Parathyroid Glands: A Comparison with Isotope Scanning and Ultrasonography. *Can J Surg* 1993, 36:241–244.

49. Wright AR, Goddard PR, Nicholson S, *et al.*: Fat-Suppression Magnetic Resonance Imaging in the Preoperative Localization of Parathyroid Adenomas. *Clin Radiol* 1992, 46:324–328.

50. Bergenfeltz A, Lundstedt C, Stribeck H, Ahern B: Large Vein Sampling for Intact Parathyroid Hormone in Preoperative Localization of Enlarged Parathyroid Glands. *Acta Radiol* 1992, 33:528–531.

51. Eisenberg H, Pallotta J, Sherwood LM: Selective Arteriography, Venography and Venous Hormone Assay in Diagnosis and Localization of Parathyroid Lesions. *Am J Med* 1974, 56:810–820.

52. Krudy AG, Doppman JL, Miller DL, *et al.*: Work in Progress: Abnormal Parathyroid Glands. Comparison of Nonselective Arterial Digital Arteriography, Selective Parathyroid Arteriography, and Venous Digital Arteriography as Methods of Detection. *Radiology* 1983, 148:23–29.

53. Reading CC: Percutaneous Biopsy of Neck Masses and Percutaneous Ablation of Parathyroid Glands. In *Current Practice of Interventional Radiology*. Edited by Kadir S. Philadelphia: BC Decker; 1991.

54. Futh U, Hofereiter F, Frohling PT: Method and Initial Results of Percutaneous Ultrasound-Controlled Sclerotherapy of Parathyroid Adenoma in Secondary or Tertiary Hyperparathyroidism (in German). *Z Urol Nephrol* 1989, 82:437–441.

55. Charboneau JW: Persistent Primary Hyperparathyroidism: Successful Ultrasound-Guided Percutaneous Ethanol Ablation of an Occult Adenoma. *Mayo Clin Proc* 1988, 63:913–917.

56. Karstrup S, Holm HH, Glenthoj A, Hegedus L: Nonsurgical Treatment of Primary Hyperparathyroidism with Sonographically Guided Percutaneous Injection of Ethanol: Results in a Selected Series of Patients. *AJR* 1990, 154:1087–1090.

57. Geelhoed GW, Doppman JL: Embolization of Ectopic Parathyroid Adenomas. A Percutaneous Treatment of Hyperparathyroidism. *Am J Surg* 1978, 44:71–80.

58. Doppman JL, Brown EM, Brennan MF, *et al.*: Angiographic Ablation of Parathyroid Adenomas. *Radiology* 1979, 130:577–582.

59. Doppman JL, Popovsky M, Girton M: The Use of Iodinated Contrast Agents to Ablate Organs: Experimental Studies and Histopathology. *Radiology* 1981, 138:333–340.

60. Geelhoed GW, Krudy AG, Doppman JL: Long-Term Follow-Up of Patients with Hyperparathyroidism Treated by Transcatheter Staining With Contrast Agent. *Surgery* 1983, 94:849–862.

61. Gunther R, Beyer J, Hesch H, Reinwein D: Percutaneous Transcatheter Ablation of Parathyroid Gland Tumors by Alcohol Injection and Contrast Media Infusion (in German). *ROFO* 1984, 140:27–30.

62.•• Miller DL, Doppman JL, Chang R, *et al.*: Angiographic Ablation of Parathyroid Adenomas: Lessons From a 10-Year Experience. *Radiology* 1987, 165:601–607.

These authors (Doppman) pioneered angiographic ablation of parathyroid adenomas. This study represents a 10-year follow-up of patients treated with this technique. As opposed to our own experience involving cervical adenomas, their experience involves the treatment of mediastinal adenomas.

63.• Sacks BA, Pallotta J: Angiographic Ablation of Parathyroid Adenomas. In *Current Practice of Interventional Radiology*. Edited by Kadir S. Philadelphia: DC Becker; 1991.

This chapter discusses our technique and approach to ablation of parathyroid adenomas.

64. Reidy JF, Ryan PJ, Fogelman I, Lewis JL: Ablation of Mediastinal Parathyroid Adenomas by Superselective Embolization of the Internal Mammary Artery with Alcohol. *Clin Radiol* 1993, 47:170–173.

65. Leight GS Jr: Angiographic Ablation of Mediastinal Parathyroid Adenoma (editorial, comment). *Ann Surg* 1992, 215:99–100.

66. Doherty GM, Doppman JL, Miller DL, *et al* .: Results of a Multidisciplinary Strategy for Management of Mediastinal Parathyroid Adenomas as a Cause of Persistent Primary Hyperparathyroidism. *Ann Surg* 1992, 215:101–106.

Select Bibliography

Calliada F, Sala G, Conti MP, *et al.*: Clinical Applications of Color Doppler: The Parathyroid Glands. *Radiol Med Torino* 1993, 85(suppl 1):114–119.

Falke THM, Schipper J, Patton JA, Sandler MP: Parathyroid Glands. In *Endocrine Imaging*. Edited by Sandler MP, Patton JA, Gross MD, Shapiro B, Falke THM. Norwalk: Appleton and Lange; 1991:149–174.

Heath DA: Primary Hyperparathyroidism: Clinical Presentations and Factors Influencing Clinical Management. *Endo Metab Clin North Am* 1989, 18:631–646.

Miller DL, Doppman JL, Shawker TH, *et al.*: Localization of Parathyroid Adenomas in Patients Who Have Undergone Surgery. Part I. Noninvasive Imaging Methods. *Radiology* 1987, 162:133–137.

Miller DL, Doppman JL, Krudy AG, *et al.*: Localization of Parathyroid Adenomas in Patients Who Have Undergone Surgery. Part II. Invasive Procedures. *Radiology* 1987, 162:138–141.

Pallotta JA, Sacks BA, Moller DE, Eisenberg H: Arteriographic Ablation of Cervical Parathyroid Adenomas. *J Clin Endocrinol Metab* 1989, 69:1249–1255.

Winkelbauer F, Ammann ME, Langle F, Niederle B: Diagnosis of Hyperparathyroidism with Ultrasonography After Autotransplantation Results of a Prospective Study. *Radiology* 1993, 186:255–257.

Uses of Intravascular Ultrasound in Vascular Intervention

Gerald E. Grubbs
Barry T. Katzen

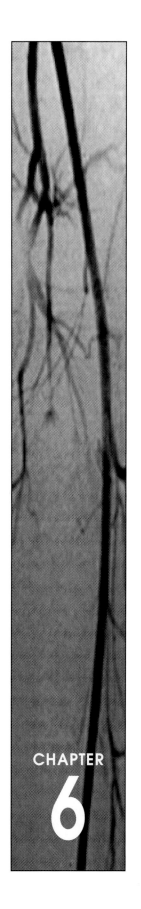

CHAPTER
6

During the past several decades, angiography has been well established as the gold standard for detailed assessment of arterial structures. Detailed evaluation of diverse portions of the circulation can be obtained over large areas of the vascular system. Angiography provides a two-dimensional detailed evaluation of vessels, including branches and collateral circulation in patients with occlusive disease. By definition, angiography provides images of the luminal surfaces showing irregularities, stenosis, and occlusions, but it provides no information about the vessel wall. The two-dimensional images obtained with angiography often provide a deficient or misleading representation of the vessels. Lesion morphology and percent of stenosis are not well quantified. Detailed visualization of intimal irregularities such as intimal flaps is sometimes difficult because overlying tissue can reduce contrast. The known harmful effects of ionizing radiation and concerns about the osmotic effects of radiographic dyes restrict the imaging time available. In addition, intra- and inter-observer variability limits the quantitative assessment of disease and therapeutic interventions [1,2]. Quantitation of lumen diameter and cross-sectional area has important hemodynamic and prognostic value; the arteriogram cannot be used to accurately assess plaque composition and associated thrombus. It is becoming apparent that atherosclerotic plaque instability may be a strong predictor of its future development of fissures, ulcerations, and thrombosis [3,4••,5,6].

Although intraluminal ultrasonographic imaging was attempted in the vascular system via the intravenous route as early as 1960 by Omoto [7] and further developed in the early 1970s by Bom and colleagues [8], the main interest was in obtaining more detailed evaluation of cardiac chambers because of the limitations of external ultrasonography at the time. The rapid progress in interventional radiology and more particularly the introduction of new therapeutic techniques such as atherectomy and endovascular stents, has stimulated the development of an imaging method to characterize vessel wall pathology and monitor plaque ablation procedures in real time, to provide operator feedback on the efficacy of intervention. With the recent development of clinically useful intravascular ultrasonography (IVUS), the interventionalist can now obtain unique and additional information about the vessel wall in comparison with that obtained through angiography. The continued miniaturization

of ultrasound technology and concomitant effects in catheter technology have facilitated this growth. At the same time, significant advances in percutaneous intervention for vascular disease have made the information obtained by IVUS more directly relevant to intervention. The number of catheter-based therapeutic interventions is rapidly increasing. The unique information provided by IVUS will be of major help before, during, and after the newer therapeutic techniques for the removal of atherosclerotic plaques and for determining the endpoint of the intervention.

Technical Considerations in Intravascular Ultrasonography

Successful acquisition of IVUS images involves a combination of both ultrasound and catheter technologies. Because of the invasive nature of IVUS, the examination is limited to adjunctive use during diagnostic and therapeutic angiography procedures. Characteristics such as flexibility, trackability over a guidewire, radiopacity, and durability are as important as the technologic aspects of the ultrasound transducers and imaging consoles. If the IVUS catheter cannot be placed in the area of interest, a failure of acquisition occurs as surely as if the ultrasound imaging device had failed. Cooperative efforts with catheter manufacturers have led to investigations that have evaluated both phased-array and mechanical transducers for use in IVUS, with each type of probe having characteristic advantages and limitations.

Phased-array catheters have multiple small transducers in the catheter tip. There are normally 64 multiple crystals arranged circumferentially around the tip, which simulate and reconstruct a cross-sectional two-dimensional image. Due to the mechanical simplicity of the transducer assembly, it is possible to incorporate this imaging component into multifunction catheters. Currently, a combination of imaging and angioplasty catheters is undergoing clinical trials. The transducer assembly is located just proximal to the dilatation balloon. This allows the deflated balloon profile to be low enough for routine use in dilating severely stenotic lesions. The coaxial guidewire then allows the catheter to be advanced slightly to bring the imaging element into the stenosis. The simplicity of the imaging element allows this catheter to behave similarly to contemporary balloon angioplasty catheters with respect to flexibility, trackability, and axial control. Limitations of a phased-array system include the need for more computer power to handle data, the secondary increase in cost, and difficulty in imaging of larger vessels in the peripheral circulation. High-quality images have been obtained in the coronary circulation, but the limitations described have led to the abandonment of this technology.

Mechanical transducers employ a rotating transducer driven by an externally supplied motor drive (Diasonics; Boston Scientific, Watertown, MA and Cardiovascular Imaging Systems, Sunnyvale, CA). Frequently, internal mirrors are used to reduce the imaging window of the transducer and to further enhance image quality. Catheters used with these types of systems are somewhat larger (4.8- to 8-French) and employ monorail or over-the-wire introduction using small (0.014- to 0.025-inch) guides. Traversing the aortic bifurcation or delivering the IVUS catheter selectively to visceral vessels is somewhat difficult without the use of a guiding catheter.

Intravascular ultrasound catheters have been evaluated in a variety of frequencies ranging from 20 to 40 MHz. These frequencies are considerably higher than those used with conventional external vascular ultrasonography (5 MHz), and give improved resolution. The 20-MHz probes that are most widely used in the peripheral circulation and provide tissue penetration of 1.5 to 2.0 cm have produced images of consistently high quality with axial resolution in the order of 0.1 mm.

The use of IVUS catheters requires an introducing sheath and guidewires of smaller size than usual for their exchange (0.014- to 0.025-inch). With experience, the extra time required for IVUS catheters can take 5 minutes or less. To justify the increase in procedure time and the cost of ultrasound equipment, this imaging modality must provide unique information that enhances the understanding of the interventional procedure and affects therapeutic decision-making. Initial studies performed in patients suggest that an IVUS is feasible, safe, and provides useful clinical information [9–12].

Unique Information Provided by Intravascular Ultrasonography

Angiography provides detailed two-dimensional longitudinal information about vessels but is limited in its ability to assess the vessel wall anatomy. IVUS permits two-dimensional axial imaging of the vessels and by providing information about the luminal surfaces, luminal morphology, vessel wall architecture, extent of atheroma, and other pathology, it offers unique advantages for the diagnosis and treatment of arterial disease (Fig. 6-1). This unique capability is not possible with angioscopy or any external imaging modality. There is excellent correlation between ultrasound-derived vascular dimensions and those obtained by angiography *in vivo* and histology *in vitro*

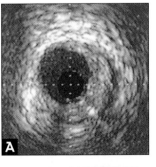
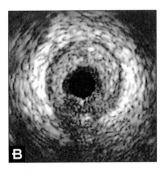
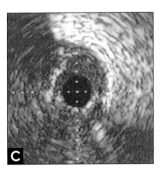
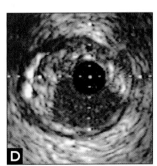
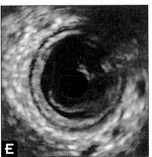
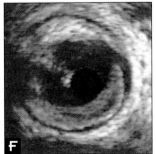

FIGURE 6-1.

Representative images acquired with an IVUS catheter.
A, Eccentric plaque. **B**, Concentric plaque. **C**, Plaque with superficial calcification (9 o'clock to 10 o'clock positions) and distal shadowing. **D**, Deep calcification (9 o'clock to 10 o'clock positions) with eccentric plaque. **E**, Intimal dissections (5 o'clock to 7 o'clock positions). The intimal flap is separated from the normal intima by a thin dark band representing flowing blood. **F**, Medial dissection. The tear through intima and media at the 3 o'clock position with a dark band of dissecting blood is seen deep to the media from the 3 o'clock to 6 o'clock positions.

[13–15]. The ability to determine vessel diameter and cross-sectional area accurately affects diagnostic decisions and therapeutic interventions (Fig. 6-2).

Intravascular ultrasound has provided us with a better understanding of the compensatory arterial dilation that occurs with the development of atherosclerosis [16]. When approximately 40% of the cross-sectional area is filled with atheroma, the artery does not dilate further but new atheroma encroaches upon the lumen. The implication of this pathology study is that a truly normal artery segment may be indistinguishable by angiogram from one that has up to 40% of its cross-sectional area filled with atheroma. These results from autopsy series have now been confirmed in *in vivo* by IVUS.

Postprocessing of the two-dimensional axial images permits three-dimensional reconstruction of image segments, further enhancing the quality of information. Because IVUS does not require ionizing radiation or injection of fluids, there is no inherent time limit on imaging. The information provided is digitized and therefore suitable for quantitative analysis such as diameter, area, and percent stenosis calculations.

Investigations of ultrasound applied to vessels *in vivo* and *in vitro* have demonstrated similar findings. Basically, there are two types of arteries: elastic and muscular. The two types are not sharply divided because elastic arteries gradually merge into muscular arteries. The aorta, pulmonary, and proximal segments of the brachiocephalic, carotid, subclavian, and common iliac arteries are of the elastic type. All other arteries such as femoral, coronary, and renal are of the muscular type.

Several histologic layers of the arterial wall can be identified clearly by IVUS. The intima is hypoechoic with a varying course and a smooth echogenic pattern. In normal arteries, it is quite thin but can increase significantly if intimal hyperplasia develops after percutaneous intervention. The adventitia is hypoechoic with an indistinct outer margin where the outer wall of the artery blends with surrounding soft tissue. The presence of circularly arranged elastin fibers in the media of an elastic artery results in a significant amount of acoustic back scatter, causing the media to appear as echogenic as the intima and adventitia. Conversely, muscular arteries have a typical three-layered wall. The media, bounded internally and externally by the elastic membranes, is a distinctive thin hypoechoic layer amidst the hyperechoic intima and adventitial layers. The ability to identify the echolucent media is important because it allows measurement of the circumferential intimal plaque thickness separately from the total

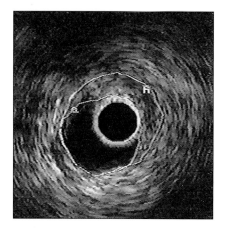

FIGURE 6-2.

Intravascular ultrasound is used to measure percent stenosis and cross-sectional area. The central anechoic circle with a bright ring is the IVUS catheter, the darker hypoechoic region is the residual lumen containing flowing blood. Note the echogenic eccentric plaque extending from the 9 o'clock to 5 o'clock positions. Sixty-seven percent stenosis was recorded by cross-sectional area measurement.

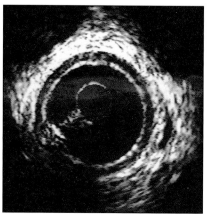

FIGURE 6-3.

A good example of the typical three-layered appearance of a muscular artery. The thin echogenic inner ring is the intima. The next hypoechoic ring is the media. The outer echogenic region is the adventitia. A superficial calcified plaque is seen at the 8 o'clock position.

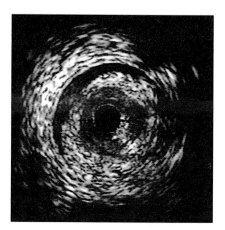

FIGURE 6-4.

Postangioplasty medial dissection. The anechoic IVUS catheter is seen centrally with faint echoes formed by flowing blood within the vessel lumen. At the 10 o'clock position, a dissection plane through the intima and media is seen with faint echoes representing the jet of flowing blood. The hyperechoic rim of blood dissecting beneath the media extends from the 8 o'clock to 4 o'clock position.

wall thickness and thus permits determination of the atherosclerotic plaque cross-sectional area (Fig. 6-3).

Calcium within the wall of the vessel produces acoustic shadowing, a typical sonographic characteristic (Figs. 6-1C, 6-1D and 6-3). Generally, this calcium is deep to the intima and does not result in degradation of the image. Simple atheromas are echogenic because of the deposition of lipids within the tunica intima. Plaque is hyperechoic, but may have a mixed pattern with hypoechoic areas. This is compatible with the known histologic complexity of a plaque, including predominantly fibrous materials mixed with lipid components. Thrombus is hyperechoic but frequently has a distinctive fine bright-speckled pattern recognizable to experienced observers. Flowing blood is easily identified during real-time evaluations with pulsations of the cardiac cycle. Vessel wall elasticity can be evaluated subjectively during imaging, and wall dynamics can be assessed so that the dilation of atherosclerotic segments by vasodilating drugs can be studied.

Variables in the ultrasonic appearance of vessels occur due to differences in manufacturing parameters, gain settings during examination, frequency of transducer, and the vessel size. Nonetheless, the characteristics previously described are reproducible, predictable, and clinically useful. More recently, investigators have begun to assess the potential of ultrasonography to distinguish plaque types in smaller (coronary) muscular arteries. *In vitro* studies have demonstrated the possibility of differentiating between noncalcified, fibromuscular atheroma with fibrosis and lipid deposits, more advanced calcified atheroma, thrombus, plaque rupture, and dissections [17–25]. Potkin and colleagues [26] compared ultrasonographic images with corresponding histologic images of excised coronary arteries. They were able to correctly predict the presence of fibrous and calcified plaque with an accuracy of 77% and 83%, respectively. Both types of plaques are highly echogenic, with calcification producing typical acoustic shadowing [21]. It was considerably harder to determine the presence of lipid-containing or mixed plaque with 23% and 43% success, respectively. Because lipid-filled areas are hyperechoic, they may be obscured by areas of calcification or surrounding tissue. Nonetheless, improved technology and further investigations may increase ultrasonography potential for tissue specificity.

The ability to identify thrombus by ultrasound is important because thrombus is frequently associated with atherosclerotic plaque. A more homogeneous reflective pattern is a possible identifying feature [27]. Fresh thrombus appears as a bright, sparkling, speckled pattern.

A limitation of all currently available IVUS devices is that the device designs allow only for side viewing. Because forward viewing is impossible, IVUS cannot be currently employed to determine the composition (*eg*, thrombus vs plaque) of a total occlusion prior to recanalization.

Clinical Applications

The unique information provided by IVUS has its greatest value during vascular disease treatment by percutaneous methods. The angiographic appearance of the postintervention region is often suboptimal for interpretation of the result and does not allow prediction of acute and chronic complications (Fig. 6-4). Using IVUS, the presence and severity of wall dissection may be directly visualized and could be used to develop criteria for stent implantation (Fig. 6-5).

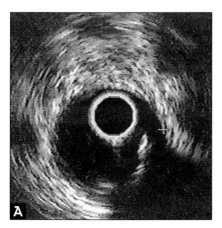
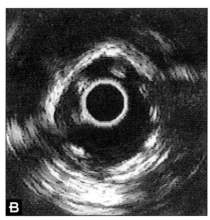

FIGURE 6-5.

Postangioplasty intimal flap. **A**, The echogenic intimal flap extends vertically into the vessel lumen from the 5 o'clock position. This necessitated placement of a sent. **B**, Echogenic struts of the stent surround the IVUS catheter. This is a good example of incomplete stent deployment. A larger balloon was placed within the stent and inflated to abut the struts against the intima.

Morphologic criteria may be established that predict acute or chronic restenosis, the major problem of balloon angioplasty, because it occurs in up to 30% of patients.

VESSEL MEASUREMENT

Although digital subtraction angiography has provided significant clinical benefit in performing diagnostic and therapeutic vascular procedures, one of the limitations has been the difficulty in determining accurate cross-sectional diameter. As previously mentioned, recent pathologic studies have further elucidated the atherosclerotic disease process. In the earlier stages of the disease, arteries enlarge as a result of a remodeling process of normal segments in relation to plaque area, and functionally important luminal stenosis will not develop until a lesion occupies 40% of the circumference of the internal elastic lamina [16]. Thus serious wall disease may be present, despite a nearly normal luminal cross-sectional area by arteriography. The usual evaluation of an angiogram is based on a measurement of the diameter of the presumed normal vessel and the diameter of the arterial lesion judged most severe in multiple views. This percent diameter stenosis measurement must therefore assume that the adjacent wall is truly normal, but this is often not the case [28,29]. The IVUS findings of luminal narrowing at sites devoid of stenosis underscore the fact that angiographic assessment of luminal narrowing may be compromised by diffusely distributed intimal disease allowing determination of any focal stenosis only as a relative function of adjacent disease, albeit less-narrowed site. The IVUS imaging catheter provides a reproducible method for measuring the arterial lumen area *in vitro* with excellent intra- and interobserver correlation [30]. The benefits of IVUS are the ability to accurately measure not only vessel diameter, but also cross-sectional area and percent stenosis. Another benefit is the potential for evaluating vessel compliance. These measurements can be done on-line without significant procedural delay. Such measurements have proved valuable in determining balloon size for percutaneous transluminal angioplasty, atherectomy device size, and for measuring postprocedure accurate residual stenosis. The measurements have also been of value in obtaining accurate sizing before stent deployment [31].

Intravascular Ultrasound Use During Transluminal Angioplasty

Intravascular ultrasound provides definitive information about lesion location, percent stenosis, lesion length, and extent of calcification. Therefore, it is useful as an adjunct during angioplasty of peripheral lesions. During the percutaneous transluminal angioplasty (PTA) procedure, detailed information about the arterial wall (luminal diameter) can be evaluated, allowing correct balloon size to be selected. IVUS offers particular advantages in patients with decreased renal function with or without diabetes, by reducing contrast injections used for localization. Following balloon dilatation, characteristic findings in ultrasound images are the presence of a tear in the plaque with separation of the torn ends and subsequent enlargement of the arterial lumen cross-sectional area.

Of primary importance to the interventionalist is the IVUS description of the morphology of the arterial wall following balloon angioplasty. Ultrasound imaging reveals six morphologic patterns following balloon dilatation. In most cases, the plaque fractures, usually at the thinnest section. The tear may extend to the media and create a dissection of varying extent around the circumference of the plaque (Fig. 6-4). In some cases, the plaque appears to be torn completely away from the media, as if a force of torsion has twisted the base of the plaque away from its mooring to the media. The mechanism of this type of circumferential dissection is caused by tortional forces that rotate and shear the plaque relative to the underlying media; the atheroma is pulled off of its base but remains still attached to the media, which holds it in place at a short distance proximal or distal to the circumferential dissection. IVUS imaging may also clearly demonstrate that blood is flowing within the dissection plane (Fig. 6-4). The final pattern consists of a plaque that does not demonstrate any evidence of tear or dissection. In this case, balloon dilatation stretches the plaque or free wall without tearing the atheroma. This tends to occur in concentric diffuse atheroma where the balloon apparently stretches the plaque uniformly but does not crack it.

The IVUS images demonstrate not only that the lumen area is increased after the balloon tears the plaque and separates the torn ends, but also the external dimensions of the arterial wall and adventitia. This suggests the fibrous band that prevents arterial distention also acts as a scar to bind the artery and prevent distensibility. Other investigators have reported that inflation of an angioplasty balloon produces complex alterations in the ultrasound cross-sectional profile of the artery [32]. Because of the differences between ultrasound and angiography observed in eccentric plaques, it is hypothesized that distortion of the vessel lumen by balloon dilatation might significantly impair the accuracy of angiography. Luminal dimensions compared by using angiography and IVUS have been examined in vessels immediately following angioplasty. These studies demonstrate a poor correlation between minimum luminal dimensions by angiography and IVUS. A spectrum of morphologic findings including complex cracks or splits in the vessel walls was observed in patients following balloon angioplasty. Measurements of luminal cross-sectional areas following angioplasty are generally smaller with ultrasound than with angiography. This difference may represent an enhancement of the apparent angiographic diameter of the vessel produced by extraluminal contrast within cracks or splits in the intima or media of the vessel. It is likely that a tomographic technique such as IVUS is more accurate in determining the actual cross-sectional area following an angioplasty [33•]. Therefore, IVUS offers great promise in increasing the *in vivo* understanding of the angioplasty process, perhaps leading to improved outcomes in therapy and decreased rates of restenosis.

Early prototypes of balloon catheters integrated with central transducers are currently being evaluated and may contribute to a better understanding of the angioplasty process. On-line ultrasound monitoring of balloon inflation facilitates the identification of plaque fracture initiation. On-line analysis of pressure volume curves has been previously investigated as a means of characterizing the mechanism responsible for vascular

dilatation *in vivo* [34]. Cracking, identified as sudden yielding of the balloon at a given inflation pressure, was less commonly observed than patterns indicative of either stretching or compacting. The results of on-line ultrasound analysis of balloon inflation suggests that plaque fracture is proportionately more common than indicated by pressure volume analysis and this is further supported by post hoc ultrasound analysis [33•,35–38] and previously reported necropsy studies [39]. As suggested by Kleinman and colleagues [40], any technique (whether it be pressure volume or ultrasound analysis) that permits immediate on-line recognition of plaque fracture might theoretically be employed to modify the remainder of the dilatation procedure to prevent the development of a flow-limiting dissection.

Observations made during PTA have documented that IVUS shows excellent sensitivity for calcium and a high accuracy for demonstrating the degree of luminal narrowing. Clinical experience at the Miami Vascular Institute confirms the observations made by Tobis and colleagues [41] in coronary arteries: residual atheroma of significance is still present (average residual stenosis, 73% by area), suggesting a possible cause of inherent restenosis or early failures. Maximal plaque ablation could result in a lower restenosis rate and too much thinning of the arterial wall with risk of aneurysm formation could also be avoided.

DETECTION OF INTIMAL DISSECTIONS

Both spontaneous and iatrogenic intimal dissections are well visualized by two-dimensional, cross-sectional ultrasonographic imaging. Although spontaneous dissections are generally detected by other means, IVUS has been shown to be useful in detection of aortic dissections [42,43•,44•] (Fig. 6-6). More conventional

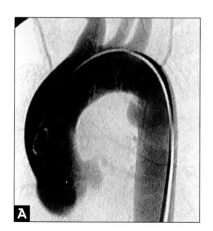
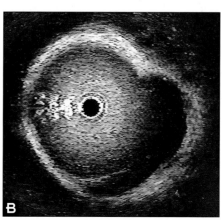

FIGURE 6-6.

Aortic dissection performed on a patient suffering injuries from a motor vehicle accident. **A,** Left anterior oblique arch aortogram showing aortic dissection with pseudoaneurysm at ductus attachment. **B,** IVUS imaging precisely shows the site of intimal disruption at the 2 o'clock position. This image also demonstrates a good example of an elastic artery. The elastin within the media increases the echogenicity of this layer, causing all three layers to appear echogenic.

methods such as CT or angiography can establish this diagnosis more simply, but IVUS may be of assistance during angiography in detecting the precise point of re-entry or termination of dissection.

Increasing experience with IVUS during intervention has shown it to be more sensitive than angiography in detecting both the presence and extent of post-PTA dissections (Fig. 6-5). This superiority is to be expected because dissections are longitudinal and IVUS images are perpendicular to the plane of dissection. In many instances, fully appreciating the extent of the dissection will influence therapeutic decision-making (*eg*, placing an intravascular stent, prolonging balloon inflation, or atherectomy).

Dissections have been noted to be of two predominant types: localized longitudinal and spiral. Either type may extend to compromise the lumen, but spiral dissections are generally a cause for immediate luminal compromise and will generally lead to intravascular stent placement.

Intravascular Ultrasound Use During Atherectomy

Percutaneous atherectomy is emerging as a major new therapeutic modality in the treatment of atherosclerotic vascular disease. This technique relies on the removal of plaque to restore luminal patency rather than the controlled injury of plaque dissection associated with balloon angioplasty. Early experience with various atherectomy catheters suggests that plaque extraction produces a more predictable result than balloon angioplasty and with a lower incidence of acute complications such as abrupt reclosure. Some investigators

believe that this method may be superior to PTA, but this has not been well established at present in the scientific literature [45,46].

As experience with atherectomy is accumulating, it is becoming increasingly clear that conventional angiography may not be precise enough to guarantee maximally safe and effective procedures because it is not capable of judging the amount, location, and plaque accumulation relative to the lumen [47]. Previous pathologic studies have demonstrated that atherosclerotic disease is frequently present in segments of vessels that appear angiographically normal. Even more important from the standpoint of atherectomy is the fact that it is often difficult to appreciate the asymmetric nature of plaque accumulation from an angiogram (Fig. 6-7). Pathologic studies have shown that approximately three quarters of coronary artery segments that have severe stenosis will have an arch of the normal wall on one side of the vessel—a much higher percentage of truly eccentric lesions than is revealed by angiography.

Ultrasound imaging is well-suited to provide imaging guidance for atherectomy because detailed information about vessel wall composition can be obtained well below the intimal surface and thus, images acquired can be used to determine the most strategic positioning of cuts (Fig. 6-8). The imaging plane of current ultrasound catheters, which is perpendicular to the catheter tip, is also favorable for the application of percutaneous atherectomy. The operator can develop a detailed three-dimensional sense of the distribution of atheroma by actually moving the catheter back and forth through the region of interest. This information allows the oper-

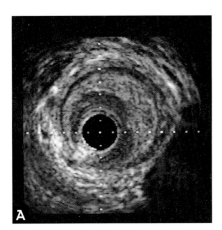 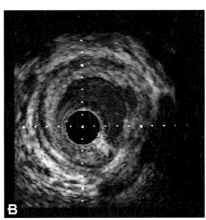

FIGURE 6-7.

A, Intravascular ultrasound used to direct atherectomy. Image shows eccentric plaque extending from the 9 o'clock to 5 o'clock positions. **B**, Postatherectomy image shows that the atherectomy cuts were concentrated to the region of the eccentric plaque with significant decrease in lumen stenosis.

ator to position the interventional device accurately with respect to actual position in the vessel, as well as directing the device radially to the appropriate segment of the wall (Fig. 6-9).

A recent study of the coronary arteries has confirmed previously reported observations that angiography provides a gross underestimation of residual plaque in comparison with IVUS [48,49]. Although the mean percent area stenosis by angiography was only 29% (17% diameter stenosis) following atherectomy, ultrasound scanning showed that an average of 43% of the lumen area was still occupied by plaque [50]. This finding supports previous work performed by Yock and colleagues [51]. In patients who were found to have an adequate result (stenosis less than 10%), 68% of lesions were found to have residual stenosis greater than 30%, the traditional endpoint of intervention. Several factors contribute to the discrepancy between the angiographic and ultrasonic measurements of residual plaque burden. The most important of these is the failure of angiography to detect the plaque accumulation in the proximal segments chosen as normal reference areas for the determination of percent stenosis. Experiences at the Miami Vascular Institute parallel with those of Tobis and colleagues [32] and Nissen and colleagues [52] in that these adjacent normal segments have an average of 25% to 30% of the lumen occupied

by plaque. When the lumen diameter of this segment is used as a reference to compare with the diseased segment on angiography, the plaque burden at the more stenotic site is underestimated.

In addition to the concern for vessel perforation, there is evidence that suggests subintimal injury may accelerate the restenosis rate after atherectomy. Early animal models of balloon angioplasty demonstrate that when media was exposed by deep dissection, there was enhanced platelet deposition acutely and long-term higher restenosis rates [53]. More recent clinical pathologic studies by Nobuyoshi and colleagues [54] and Waller and colleagues [55] have confirmed that the areas of myointimal proliferation are markedly increased when media or adventitia are involved in a deep dissection compared with a tear that is confined to the diseased intimal layer alone. In the series of Backa and colleagues [56], restenosis in peripheral vessels was 80% when subintimal tissue was present within the atherectomy specimens compared with 35% when no media or adventitia was excised. In the Mayo Clinic Coronary Study by Garratt and colleagues [57], restenosis rates were 42% when intima alone was sampled; 50% for media; and 63% for adventitia.

Studies by Kuntz and colleagues [58] and others have suggested that for any interventional device, the rates of restenosis measured by conventional angio-

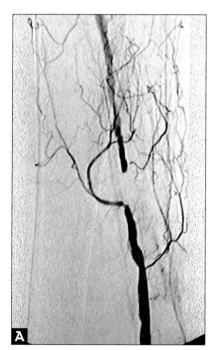

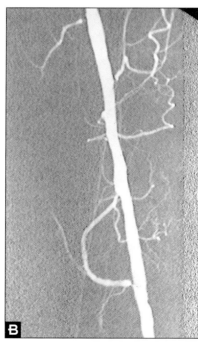

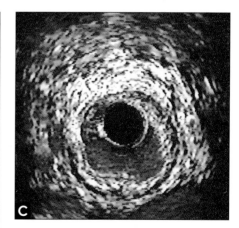

FIGURE 6-8.

Superficial femoral artery occlusion treated by atherectomy. **A,** Angiography shows occlusion of left superficial femoral artery. **B,** Postatherectomy angiogram shows good morphologic result. **C,** IVUS image shows residual plaque despite the apparent patent lumen on angiogram.

graphic criteria are lower for cases in which the post-procedural lumen is relatively large. One interpretation of these findings is that the larger lumen can tolerate a certain degree of intimal hyperplasia without narrowing the lumen sufficiently to trigger the angiographic definition of restenosis. These limited data appear to support the concept that the optimal result from an atherectomy device would be to remove the maximum amount of plaque, leaving the largest post-procedural lumen without violating the normal layers of the vessel wall. One would assume that assessment of the efficacy of atherectomy has been limited by these significant observations and that continued studies should be performed to re-evaluate outcomes. It seems intuitive that a procedure to remove plaque would depend on an adequate method of determining a therapeutic endpoint. Restenosis rates could be significantly lower with atherectomy than for balloon angioplasty, depending on how completely atheromas are removed. Aggressive debulking of a vessel increases the risk of weakening the vessel wall and aneurysm formation or actual perforation of the vessel acutely thus emphasizing another benefit of IVUS in monitoring atherectomy procedures.

Recently, investigators have considered the integration of IVUS into atherectomy devices [59]. Although stand-alone imaging catheters are proving to be useful in monitoring atherectomy, a combined imaging and atherectomy device could enhance the convenience and precision of graded atherectomy. This combination will be particularly useful with the directional atherectomy device, where both the rotational and axial positioning of the device could be facilitated by means of the images. A prototype has been developed by Yock and colleagues [51] based on the Simpson Atherocath (Devices for Vascular Intervention, Redwood City, CA). A transducer is mounted immediately behind the cutting element of the catheter so that a single cable is used to provide rotation for both the imaging and cutting elements. The basic elements of atherectomy are not altered by imaging. The catheter is delivered with the cutter in the protected forward position. When the housing is placed within a segment of interest, images are created perpendicular to the catheter tip through the open window of the housing, corresponding to the portion of the vessel wall that will be exposed to the cutter. This will permit on-line assessment of the efficacy of plaque removal and reduced procedure time.

Use of Intravascular Ultrasound During Stent Placement

Balloon-expandable, implantable, intra-arterial stents have been developed in an effort to improve safety, efficacy, and patency during angioplasty procedures. Indications for their use include a significant intima dissection compromising flow, complex lesions, and total occlusions. Intravascular prosthetic devices have been developed to serve as scaffolds to provide optimal acute patency opposing recoil of elastic vascular stenosis and to help reduce the frequency of restenosis. Preliminary reports indicate that the stents show promise in reducing complications and improving short- and long-term efficacy compared with balloon angioplasty [60–62].

As previously reported by Palmaz [63], ideal stent placements result in incorporation of the endovascular device into the arterial wall by endothelialization of the

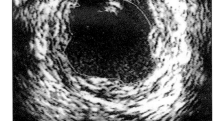

FIGURE 6-9.

Postatherectomy IVUS image. The typical appearance of multiple semicircular troughs from the atherectomy catheter are seen circumferentially.

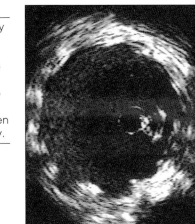

FIGURE 6-10.

Intravascular ultrasound imaging after stent placement. The echogenic stent struts are evenly spaced circumferentially around the vessel lumen.

stent surface. Recently, it has become apparent that an incomplete deployment of the stent will result in delayed or incomplete endothelial covering. Because of the highly reflective nature of stent surfaces by IVUS, the resultant arterial wall structural changes alterations in stent geometry, and stent sites can be more accurately evaluated [21,26,64,65].

In several clinical trials, including a recent trial at the Miami Vascular Institute, IVUS was used to assess the degree of stent inflation (abutment) against the arterial wall after deployment with satisfactory end results based on angiography [42]. In 20% of patients, stents were noted to be incompletely deployed, requiring additional intervention with a larger balloon to achieve complete deployment (Fig. 6-5B). Stent struts are clearly identified by their regularly spaced, highly echogenic appearance (Fig. 6-10). IVUS may also be useful in evaluating the extent of intimal dissection and in particular, the effectiveness of stenting in eliminating the adverse effects of dissections. Following recanalization in total occlusions, IVUS can determine whether subintimal passage has occurred. Ultrasonography is also a sensitive detector of intimal hyperplasia that may develop within the stent.

Stents can also be evaluated for circumferential and axial strut expansion. Stent-vessel wall contact in the circumferential and axial planes can also be evaluated, as can lumen dimensions within the stent at proximal, middle, and distal locations. Stent struts are detected as bright, highly reflective hyperechoic dots or dashes within small subjacent acoustic shadows behind each strut. Struts can usually be observed over a complete circumference in most patients, although the interstrut distance is variable. The typical morphologic appearance of a stented artery consists of an internal layer of highly reflective stent struts surrounded by an echolucent zone that probably includes compressed and displaced atheroma in the media, obscured in part by acoustic shadowing. A third outer layer that corresponds to the adventitia can also be seen in most patients. Previous animal studies have demonstrated an orderly sequence of vessel wall adaptation to the presence of an implanted metallic tubular slotted stent [60,66–70]. There is early multicentric endothelialization that should be completed in several weeks, followed by the formation of a homogenous neointima and late thinning and atrophy of the media. The use of IVUS permits enhanced visual capacity of the transmural vessel wall changes after stent implantation. In addition, physical properties and geometry of the stent can be clearly determined as a result of the hyperechoic nature of the stent itself (Fig. 6-11).

Over time, stents adapt to the vessel wall and subsequent lumen compromise occurs as a complex multifactorial process. In many patients, a thin relatively echolucent zone of intimal hyperplasia on the luminal surface of the stent can be observed. This accounts for a portion of lumen diameter narrowing noted during follow-up angiography. However, there also appears to be evidence of progressive narrowing of the stent itself with further reduction measured in strut diameters by IVUS techniques. Importantly, contrast angiography is unable to determine intimal hyperplasia above the stent and intrastent narrowing as a cause of lumen compromise and restenosis. This late recoil of the stent may be caused by a constant stress associated with vessel motion or vessel tortuousity, mechanical fatigue of the stent strut scaffold, or intimal hyperplasia resulting in compression of the stent from the outer vessel wall.

Future Directions

Intravascular ultrasound will continue to improve as more investigators consider its importance. Technologies are currently being explored to integrate IVUS capabil-

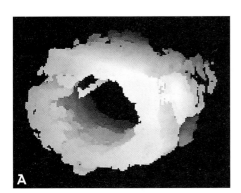 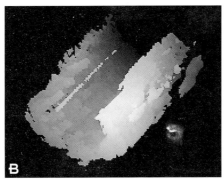

FIGURE 6-11.

Three-dimensional reconstruction of IVUS image enhances the appearance of diagnostic information in this patient with polypoid plaque protruding through stent struts. **A**, End three-dimensional view.
B, Cutaway view looking into lumen (same patient as shown in Fig. 6-10).

ities within interventional devices including PTA balloons and atherectomy devices, with several concepts being presented [71]. Additional emphasis will be placed on image quality and processing, including three-dimensional reconstructions in real time. It is anticipated that future studies using a combination of therapeutic and imaging devices will improve initial results as well as further our understanding of the pathophysiology of vascular intervention and subsequent restenosis. In theory, the ability to characterize and quantitate plaque before, during, and after intervention should allow selection of lesion-specific therapy designed to maximize the initial result and minimize restenosis. The practical result of these effects will be a more accurate assessment and control of intervention, perhaps resulting in improved initial long-term outcome.

Conclusion

Significant advances have been made in IVUS technologies from its first clinical application. Smaller, more flexible catheters in conjunction with improved image quality have greatly reduced catheter time, making IVUS less cumbersome and more practical during intervention. Unique information obtained includes: 1) tissue-specific data about the vessel wall deep to the lumen; 2) more sensitive and accurate demonstration of the extent of plaque as well as the

extent of calcification; and 3) accurate measurements of luminal diameter and percent stenosis. Ultrasonography also has the potential for specific tissue characterization in detecting fibrous, calcific, or lipid-laden plaque as well as the presence of thrombus. This information may be valuable in determining which type of intervention might be best suited for a particular lesion. In fact, a fundamental hypothesis of this technology is that IVUS images will provide predictive information about the likelihood of restenosis, which maybe helpful in selecting the most appropriate therapeutic option. Additionally, early prototypes of devices including PTA balloons, atherectomy devices, and lasers in which IVUS has been integrated, offer hope for more precise localization and on-line assessment of therapy efficacy. Three-dimensional reconstructions can be formed in or near real time, providing the additional perspectives about the extent of disease and effects of therapy. The established increase in sensitivity of IVUS versus angiography makes ultrasonography a suitable method for the comparison of various types of interventional devices. In the current environment of critical cost-effective analysis, IVUS contributes significantly to the efficacy of intervention, which will hopefully lead to improved long-term results. Studies are underway to evaluate the effect of this increased accuracy on long-term outcome. Based on current clinical experience, IVUS is a useful imaging tool for the interventionalist.

References and Recommended Reading

Recently published papers of particular interest have been highlighted as:
• Of interest
•• Of outstanding interest

1. Fisher LD, Judkins MP, Lesperance J, *et al.*: Reproducibility of Coronary Arteriographic Reading in the Coronary Artery Surgery Study (CASS). *Cathet Cardiovasc Diagn* 1982, 8:565–575.

2. Arnett EN, Isner JM, Redwood DR, *et al.*: Coronary Artery Narrowing in Coronary Artery Disease: Comparison of Cineangiographic and Necropsy Findings. *Ann Intern Med* 1979, 91:350.

3. Falk E: Morphologic Features of Unstable Atherothrombotic Plaques Underlying Acute Coronary Syndromes. *Am J Cardiol* 1989, 63:114E.

4.•• Levin DC, Fallon JT: Significance of the Angiographic Morphology of Localized Coronary Stenoses: Histopathologic Correlations. *Circulation* 1982, 66:316.
This paper is a detailed discussion of the histopathologic changes in atherosclerotic lesions and the correlation with angiographic appearance. It is a good primer for understanding the basis for IVUS findings.

5. Beeuwkes R III, Barger AC, Silverman KJ, Lainey LL: Cinemicrographic Studies of the Vasa Vasorum of Human Coronary Arteries. In *Pathobiology of the Human Atherosclerotic Plaque*. Edited by Glagov S, Newman KWP, Schaffer SA. New York: Springer-Verlag; 1990:425.

6. Ambrose JA, Winters SL, Arora RR, *et al.*: Angiographic Evolution of Coronary Artery Morphology in Unstable Angina. *J Am Coll Cardiol* 1986, 7:472.

7. Omoto R: Intracardiac Scanning of the Heart with Aid of Ultrasonic Intravenous Probe. *Jpn Heart J* 1967, 8:569–581.

8. Bom N, Lancee CT, Van Egmond FC: An Ultrasonic Intracardiac Scanner. *Ultrasonics* 1972, 10:72–76; and US Patent No. 1, 402,192, filed February 22, 1973.

9. Yock PG, Linker DT, Seather D, *et al.*: Intravascular Two-Dimensional Catheter Ultrasound: Initial Clinical Studies. *Circulation* 1988, 78:II–21.

10. Meyer CR, Chiang EH, Fechner KP, *et al.*: Feasibility of High Resolution Intravascular Ultrasound Imaging Catheter. *Radiology* 1988, 168:113–116.

11. Pandian N, Kreis A, Desnoyer M, *et al.*: *In-Vivo* Ultrasound Angioscopy in Humans and Animals: Intraluminal Imaging of Blood Vessels Using a New Catheter-Based High Resolution Ultrasound Probe. *Circulation* 1988, 78:II.

12. Hodgson JMcB, Graham SP, Savakos A: Percutaneous Intravascular Ultrasound Imaging in Humans: Initial Peripheral and Coronary Studies. Proceedings of the 4th International Congress on Cardiac Doppler; Anaheim, 1989.

13. Hodgson JMcB, Graham SP, Sheehan H, *et al.*: Percutaneous Intracoronary Ultrasound Imaging: Initial Application in Patients. *Echocardiography* 1990, 7:403.

14. Hodgson JMcB, Graham SP, Sheehan, *et al.*: Percutaneous Intravascular Ultrasound Imaging: Validation of Real Time Synthetic Aperture Array Catheter. *Am J Cardiac Imaging* 1991, 5:65.

15. Nissen SE, Grines CL, Gurley JC, *et al.*: Application of a New Phased-Array Ultrasound Imaging Catheter in the Assessment of Vascular Dimensions: *In-Vivo* Comparison to Cineangiography. *Circulation* 1990, 81:660.

16. Glagor S, Weinserberg E, Zarins CK, *et al.*: Compensatory Enlargement of Human Atherosclerotic Arteries. *N Engl J Med* 1987, 316:1371–1375.

17. Pandian N, Kreis A, O'Donnell T, *et al.*: Intraluminal Two-Dimensional Ultrasound Angioscopic Quantitation of Arterial Stenosis: Comparison with External High Frequency Ultrasound Imaging and Anatomy. *J Am Coll Cardiol* 1989, 13:5A.

18. Pandian N, Kreis A, Brockway BS, *et al.*: Detection of Intravascular Thrombus by High Frequency Intraluminal Ultrasound Angioscopy: *In-Vitro* and *In-Vivo* Studies. *J Am Coll Cardiol* 1989, 13:5A.

19. Roelandt JR, Serruys PW, Bom N, *et al.*: Intravascular Real Time High Resolution Two-Dimensional Echocardiography. *J Am Coll Cardiol* 1989, 13:4A.

20. Bartonelli AL, Potkin BN, Almagor Y, *et al.*: Intravascular Ultrasound Imaging of Atherosclerotic Coronary Arteries: An *In-Vitro* Validation Study (abstract). *J Am Coll Cardiol* 1989, 13:4A.

21. Gussenhoven EJ, Essed CE, Lancee CT, *et al.*: Arterial Wall Characteristics Determined by Intravascular Ultrasound Imaging: An *In-Vitro* Study. *J Am Coll Cardiol* 1989, 14:957–962.

22. Pandian N, Kreis A, Brockway BS, *et al.*: Intraluminal Ultrasound Angioscopic Detection of Arterial Dissection and Intimal Flaps; *In-Vitro* and *Vivo* Studies. *Circulation* 1988, 78:II–21.

23. Mallery JA, Tobis JM, Gessert J, *et al.*: Evaluation of an Intravascular Ultrasound Imaging Catheter in Porcine Peripheral and Coronary Arteries *In-Vivo*. *Circulation* 1988, 78:II–21.

24. Yock PG, Johnson EL, Linker DT: Intravascular Ultrasound: Development and Clinical Potential. *Am J Card Imaging* 1988, 2:185–193.

25. Mallery JA, Tobis JM, Gessert J, *et al.*: Identification of Tissue Components in Human Atheroma by an Intravascular Ultrasound Imaging Catheter. *Catheter* 1988, 78:II–22.

26. Potkin BN, Bartorelli AL, Gessert JM, *et al.*: Coronary Artery Imaging with Intravascular High Frequency Ultrasound. *Circulation* 1990, 81:1575.

27. Pandian N, Kreis A, Brockway BS, *et al.*: Detection of Intra-arterial Thrombosis by Intravascular High Frequency Two-Dimensional Ultrasound Imaging *In-Vitro* and *In-Vivo* Studies. *Am J Cardiol* 1990, 65:1280.

28. McPherson DD, Hiratzka LF, *et al.*: Delineation of the Extent of Coronary Atherosclerosis by High Frequency Epicardial Echocardiography. *New Engl J Med* 1987, 316:304–305.

29. Harrison DG, White CW, *et al.*: The Value of Lesion Cross-Sectional Area Determined by Quantitative Coronary Angiography in Assessing the Physiologic Significance of Proximal Left Anterior Descending Coronary Arterial Stenosis. *Circulation* 1984, 69:1111–1119.

30. Moriuchi M, *et al.*: Validation of Intravascular Ultrasound Images. In *Intravascular Ultrasound Imaging*. Edited by Tobis JM, Yock PG. New York: Churchill Livingstone; 1992:58.

31. Katzen BT: Current Status of Intravascular Ultrasonography. The Radiologic Clinics of North America: Ultrasonography of Small Parts. 30:895–905.

32. Tobis JM, Mallery JA, Mahon D, *et al.*: Intravascular Ultrasound Imaging of Human Coronary Arteries *In-Vivo*. *Circulation* 1991, 83:913.

33.• Gurley JC, Nissen SE, Grines CL, *et al.*: Comparison of Intravascular Ultrasound and Angiography Following Percutaneous Transluminal Angioplasty. *Circulation* 1990, 82:III–72.

This paper is an interesting comparison of IVUS and angiography in determining the outcome of PTA. Examples are shown of the limitations of angiography in detecting the extent of dissection.

34. Jain A, Demer LL, Raizner AE, *et al.*: *In-Vivo* Assessment of Vascular Dilatation During Percutaneous Transluminal Coronary Angioplasty. *Am J Cardiol* 1987, 60:988.

35. Isner JM, Rosenfield K, Losordo DW, *et al.*: Percutaneous Intravascular US as Adjunct to Catheter-Based Interventions: Preliminary Experience in Patients with Peripheral Vascular Disease. *Radiology* 1990, 175:61.

36. Isner JM, Rosenfield K, Losordo DW, *et al.*: How Reliable are Images Obtained by Intravascular Ultrasound for Making Decisions During Percutaneous Interventions? Experience with Intravascular Ultrasound Employed in Lieu of Contrast Angiography to Guide Peripheral Balloon Angioplasty in 16 Patients (abstract). *Circulation* 1990, 82:III–440.

37. Tobis JM, Mallery JA, Gessert J, *et al.*: Intravascular Ultrasound Cross-Section Arterial Imaging Before and After Balloon Angioplasty *In-Vitro*. *Circulation* 1989, 80:873.

38. Losordo DW, Rosenfield K, Ramaswarry K, *et al.*: How Does Angioplasty Work? Intravascular Ultrasound Assessment of 30 Consecutive Patients Demonstrating that Angiographic Evidence of Luminal Patency is the Consistent Result of Plaque Fractures and Dissections (abstract). *Circulation* 1990, 82:III–338.

39. Waller BF: Pathology of New Interventions Used in the Treatment of Coronary Heart Disease. *Curr Prob Cardiol* 1986, 11:666.

40. Kleinman NS, Raizner AE, Roberts R: Percutaneous Transluminal Coronary Angioplasty: Is What We See What We Get? *J Am Coll Cardiol* 1990, 16:576.

41. Tobis JM, Mahon D, Lehmann K, *et al.*:Intracoronary Ultrasound Imaging After Balloon Angioplasty. *Circulation* 1990, 82:III–676.

42. Cavaye DM, French WJ, White RA, *et al.*: Intravascular Ultrasound Imaging of an Acute Dissecting Aortic Aneurysm: A Case Report. *J Vasc Surg* 1991, 13:510–512.

43.• Pande A, Meier B, Fleisch M, *et al.*: Intravascular Ultrasound for Diagnosis of Aortic Dissection. *Am J Cardiol* 1991, 67:662–663.

This article along with Williams, *et al.* [44•], demonstrates an important use of IVUS in the diagnoses of traumatic injuries to the aorta and large vessels. We have found this to be of increasing importance, particularly in the treatment of aneurysmal disease by endovascular techniques.

44.• Williams DM, Simon HJ, Marx MV, *et al.*: Acute Traumatic Aortic Rupture: Intravascular Ultrasound Findings. *Radiology* 1992, 182:247–249.

This article discusses important uses of IVUS in diagnosing traumatic injury to the aorta and large vessels. Refer to Pande, *et al.* [43•] for additional information.

45. Selmon M, Robertson G, Hinohara T, *et al.*: Factors Associated with Restenosis Following Successful Peripheral Atherectomy (abstract). *J Am Coll Cardiol* 1989, 13:108A.

46. Simpson JB, Selmon MR, Robertson GC, *et al.*: Transluminal Atherectomy for Occlusive Peripheral Vascular Disease. *Am J Cardiol* 1988, 61:96G–101G.

47. Yock PG, Linker DT, *et al.*: Clinical Applications of Intravascular Ultrasound Imaging in Atherectomy. *Int J Card Imaging* 1989, 4:117–125.

48. Katzen BT, Benenati JF, Becker GJ, *et al.*: Role of Intravascular Ultrasound in Peripheral Atherectomy and Stent Placement (abstract). *Circulation* 1991, 84:II–542.

49. Ehrlich S, Honye J, Mahon D, *et al.*: Unrecognized Stenosis by Angiography Documented by Intravascular Ultrasound. *Cathet Cardiovasc Diagn* 1991, 3:198–201.

50. White NW, Webb JG, Roue MH, Simpson JB: Atherectomy Guidance Using Intravascular Ultrasound: Quantitation of Plaque Burden (abstract). *Circulation* 1989, 80(suppl):II–374.

51. Yock PG, Fitzgerald PJ, Linker DT, *et al.*: Intravascular Ultrasound Guidance for Catheter-Based Coronary Interventions. *J Am Coll Cardiol* 1991, 17(suppl):39B–45B.

52. Nissen SE, Grines CL, Gurley JC, *et al.*: Comparison of Intravascular Ultrasound and Angiography in Quantitation of Coronary Dimensions and Stenosis in Man: Impact of Lumen Eccentricity (abstract). *Circulation* 1990, 82:III–440.

53. Steele PM, Cresebro JGH, Stanson AW, *et al.*: Balloon Angioplasty: Natural History of the Pathophysiological Response to Injury in Pig Model. *Circ Res* 1985, 57:105.

54. Nobuyoshi M, Kimura T, Ohishi H, *et al.*: Restenosis After Percutaneous Transluminal Coronary Angioplasty: Pathologic Observations in 20 Patients. *J Am Coll Cardiol* 1991, 17:433.

55. Waller BF, Pinkerton CA, Orr CM, *et al.*: Morphological Observations Late (>30 Days) After Clinically Successful Coronary Balloon Angioplasty. *Circulation* 1991, 83:28.

56. Backa D, Polnitz AV, Nerlich A, Hofling B: Histologic Comparison of Atherectomy Biopsies from Coronary and Peripheral Arteries (abstract). *Circulation* 1990, 82(suppl):III–34.

57. Garratt KN, Holmes DR, Bell MR, *et al.*: Restenosis After Directional Coronary Atherectomy: Differences Between Primary Atheromatous and Restenosis Lesions and Influence of Subintimal Tissue Resection. *J Am Coll Cardiol* 1992, 16:1665.

58. Kuntz RE, Safian RD, Schmidt DA, *et al.*: Restenosis Following New Coronary Devices: The Influence of Post-Procedure Luminal Diameter (abstract). *J Am Coll Cardiol* 1991, 17:2A.

59. Yock PG: Catheter Apparatus. European Patent No. 0234951, 1987.

60. Palmaz JC: Balloon Expandable Intravascular Stents. *Cardiol Clin* 1988, 6:357.

61. Schatz RA: Introduction to Intravascular Stents. *Cardiol Clin* 1988, 6:357.

62. Ellis SG, Savage M, Baim DS, *et al.*: Intracoronary Stenting to Prevent Restenosis: Preliminary Results of a Multicenter Study Using the Palmaz-Schatz Stent Suggest Benefit in Selected High Risk Patients. *J Am Coll Cardiol* 1990, 15:118A.

63. Palmaz JC: Intravascular Stents. Syllabus: A Categorical Course in Interventional Radiology. In *Programs and Abstracts of the RSNA*. 1991:185–192.

64. Nishimura RA, Edwards WD, Warnes CA, *et al.*: Intravascular Ultrasound Imaging: *In-Vitro* Validation and Pathologic Correlation. *J Am Coll Cardiol* 1990, 16:145.

65. Siegel RJ, Fishbein MC, Chae JS, *et al.*: Comparative Studies of Angioscopy and Ultrasound for the Evaluation of Arterial Disease. *Echocardiography* 1990, 7:495.

66. Schatz RA, Palmaz JC, Tio FO, *et al.*: Balloon Expandable Intracoronary Stents in the Adult Dog. *Circulation* 1987, 76:450.

67. Schatz RA: A View of Vascular Stents. *Circulation* 1989, 79:445.

68. Palmaz JC, Windeler SA, Garcia F, *et al.*: Atherosclerotic Rabbit Aortas: Expandable Intraluminal Grafting. *Radiology* 1986, 160:723.

69. Robinson KA, Roubin GS, Siegel RJ, *et al.*: Intra-arterial Stenting in the Atherosclerotic Rabbit. *Circulation* 1988, 78:646.

70. Bartonelli AL, Neville RF, Almagor Y, *et al.*: Intravascular Catheter-Based Ultrasound: *In-Vivo* Imaging of Artery Wall and Stents. *Circulation* 1989, 80:II–580.

71. Crowley RJ, Hamm MA, Joshi CD, *et al.*: Ultrasound Guided Therapeutic Catheters: Recent Developments and Clinical Results. *Int J Card Imaging* 1991, 6:145–146.

Select Bibliography

Bresnahan DR, Davis JL, Holmes DR, Smith HC: Angiographic Occurrence and Clinical Correlates of Intraluminal Coronary Artery Thrombus: Role of Unstable Angina. *J Am Coll Cardiol* 1985, 6:285.

Eusterman JH, Achor RWP, Kincaid OW, Brown AL Jr: Atherosclerotic Disease of the Coronary Arteries: A Pathologic-Radiologic Correlative Study. *Circulation* 1962, 26:1288.

Garratt KN, Kaufman OP, Edwards WD, *et al.*: Safety of Percutaneous Coronary Atherectomy with Deep Arterial Resection. *Am J Cardiol* 1989, 64:538.

Johnson DE, Alderman EL, Schroeder JS, *et al.*: Transplant Coronary Artery Disease: Histopathologic Correlation with Angiographic Morphology. *J Am Coll Cardiol* 1991, 17:449.

Seigel RJ, Swan K, Edwards G, *et al.*: Limitations of Post-mortem Assessment of Human Coronary Artery Size and Luminal Narrowing: Differential Effects of Tissue Fixation and Processing on Vessels with Different Degrees of Atherosclerosis. *J Am Coll Cardiol* 1985, 5:342–346.

Puncture Site Hemostasis

Kenneth R. Kensey

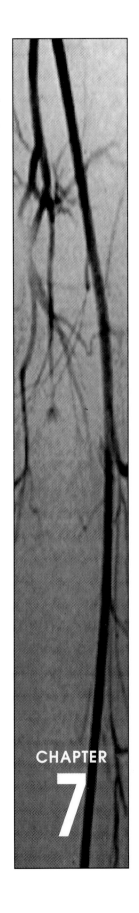

The achievement of sustained puncture site hemostasis has been a difficult, complication-ridden, and time-consuming task following the inception of percutaneous diagnostic and therapeutic procedures. The use of large-bore introducers and the more aggressive use of anticoagulants during interventional percutaneous procedures has made postprocedure hemostasis even more difficult to achieve without complications [1•]. Historically, direct manual pressure has been the gold standard for puncture hemostasis; however, this method causes discomfort and inconvenience for the patient, reduces blood flow to the distal extremity, and can be excessively time-consuming for hospital staff, as well as increasing the staff's exposure to patient blood. The patient usually remains immobile for at least 6 hours postcatheterization and is often required to stay overnight in the hospital for observation [2]. In addition, serious complications can occur as a result of persistent bleeding or hematoma formation [3].

In 1986, a personal experience led to a new idea and the subsequent development of a new method for producing hemostasis. Having successfully recanalized a 50-cm chronically occluded femoral artery, I was ecstatic to palpate a bounding popliteal pulse. However, after a few minutes the pulse suddenly disappeared. I immediately believed the artery had acutely occluded, but then observed that the assistant resident was pressing far too forcefully on the puncture site. I requested that less pressure be applied in the hope that the pulse might return. Fortunately, once groin pressure was reduced, the popliteal pulse did return. This event emphasized the need for a method to control bleeding at the puncture site without compromising distal blood flow.

Materials and Methods

Following that experience, Kensey Nash investigated and researched this problem with a team of engineers and as a result, developed the Angio-Seal (American Home Products, Madison, NJ) Hemostatic Puncture Closure Device (HPCD). The Angio-Seal is an absorbable hemostatic plug, both simple and easy to use, that produces almost immediate hemostasis after a percutaneous vascular procedure (Fig. 7-1). Upon removal of the introducer and carrier, the HPCD is activated and the arteriotomy is sealed automatically, generally without the need for any manual pressure.

The Angio-Seal is made of three bioresorbable components: 1) a polymer anchor; 2) a collagen plug; and 3) a resorbable suture (Fig. 7-2). These three parts are deployed from a carrier system as described in Figure 7-3. The anchor is molded from a resorbable copolymer, polyglycolic or polylactic acid (the same materials found in most resorbable sutures). The anchor is designed to seat itself on the intraluminal artery wall upon retraction of the device. Once seated on the artery wall, the anchor acts as a pulley system with the resorb-

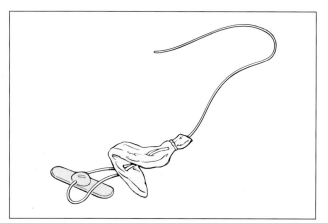

FIGURE 7-1.

The Angio-Seal device. The device, containing an absorbable hemostatic plug, is placed to control bleeding at the puncture site following a percutaneous vascular procedure.

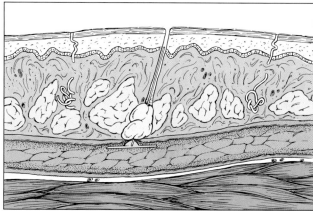

FIGURE 7-2.

Components of the Angio-Seal device are a polymer anchor molded from polyglycolic or polyactic acid, a collagen plug, and a resorbable suture.

able suture passing through a hole in the anchor. One end of the suture is tied to a collagen plug and the other end is attached to the removable carrier. As the device and introducer are withdrawn, the pulley mechanism pulls the collagen plug down and attaches onto the outside of the artery, causing mechanical hemostasis within seconds. Within minutes, in a nonanticoagulated patient, the collagen initiates platelet aggregation, causing a secondary chemical hemostasis [4]. The resorbable suture secures the collagen and anchor together, sandwiching the arterial wall between them. In a highly anticoagulated patient (as in a stent place-

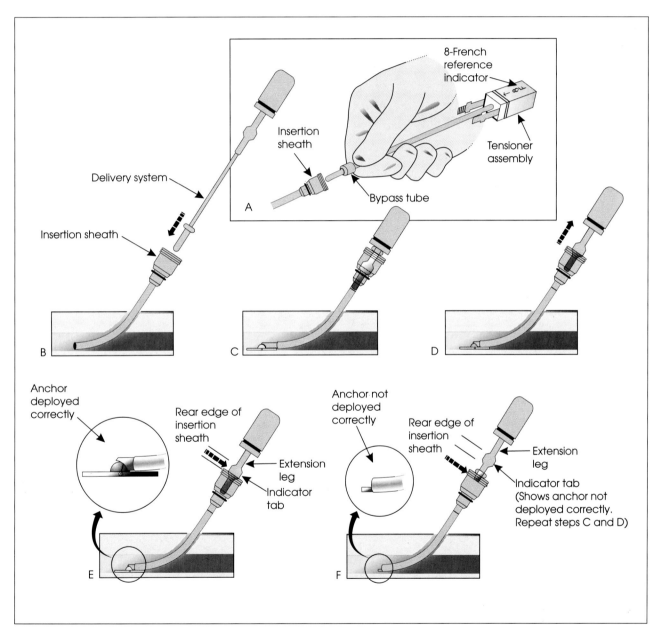

FIGURE 7-3.

The Angio-Seal insertion sequence is performed as follows: **A** and **B**, The bypass tube delivery system is placed into the insertion sheath. **C**, Once fully inserted, **D**, the delivery system is withdrawn from the insertion sheath to hook the anchor to its tip. **E**, Correct hook-up is confirmed by the indicator tabs overlapping the insertion sheath hub. **F**, If the anchor passes back into the insertion sheath, the indicator tabs will pass the rear edge of the sheath with no resistance. If this occurs, repeat steps **C** and **D**. (**continued**)

ment) the mechanical hemostasis is probably the only mechanism that stops bleeding. The collagen hemostatic factor becomes much less significant.

Extensive animal research was utilized in the development of the Angio-Seal. More than 350 devices and more than 25 variations were implanted into animals both acutely and chronically [5]. In porcine models, the anchor was found to be coated with fibrin within a matter of hours and totally encapsulated in 7 to 14 days. By 30 days, most of the anchor and collagen

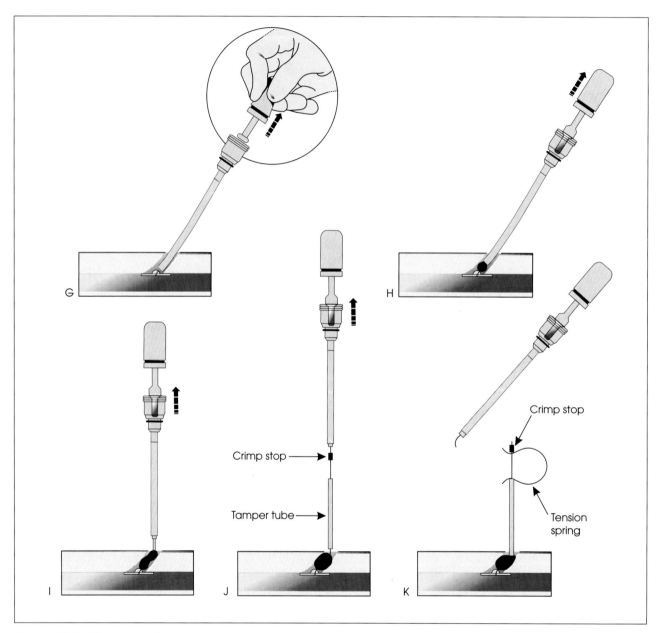

FIGURE 7-3. (CONTINUED)

G, The extensions legs are squeezed together to catch the introducer. **H**, The Angio-Seal and introducer are withdrawn simultaneously and the anchor catches at the artery wall. **I**, The collagen plug is then deployed as the anchor-pulley is activated. **J**, The tamper tube and crimp stop are exposed and the collagen plug compacted.

Gentle tamping of collagen down to the artery wall stops bleeding immediately. **K**, A tension spring is then applied to hold the tamper tube and crimp stop in place. If oozing occurs, further collagen tamping may be helpful. The tension spring should be left in place for no longer than 20 minutes, and then scissors can be used to cut the suture.

were absorbed; by 60 to 90 days, the anchor was completely resorbed. Thirty-day histologic sections showed almost complete resorption of the anchor and collagen with total encapsulation of the anchor by the endothelium (Fig. 7-4).

Another critically important part of this development process was proof that the anchor would not thrombose the artery. The polyglycolic or polylactic acid copolymer was chosen for the anchor material because it has been demonstrated in animals to be a very nonthrombogenic material [6]. In our animal studies, no arterial thrombosis was noted when the anchor was correctly seated on the arterial wall—polyglycolic acid is a very nonthrombogenic agent.

The device has proved safe in animal models, but the degree of efficacy could not be definitely determined in the *in vivo* models. In general, animals are poor models for human vascular anatomy and physiology because the artery walls are thinner and the luminal diameter much smaller. Thus, the success rate of the Angio-Seal in dog models, as measured by immediate hemostasis, was artificially lower than expected (approximately 50%). We believed this was a result of the very thin walls of the dog's artery. In 1991, we passed a major milestone when the decision was made to proceed with human clinical trials.

The first device used in humans was inserted in the femoral artery of the author. Fortunately, the device caused immediate hemostasis and no complications occurred. Ambulation was possible within 1 to 1.5 hours after placement. Ultrasound results, as shown in Figure 7-5, clearly show that the anchor was in the correct position; at 48 hours, we could see that early encapsulation of the anchor had occurred. An ultrasound taken at 2 weeks indicated continued resorption of the anchor, as evidenced by the anchor's reduced opacity.

Results

Clinical investigation of the Angio-Seal indicates that it is effective in substantially reducing the time required to produce hemostasis of the arterial puncture and may also reduce the puncture-site complication rate as compared with manual pressure. Kussmaul and colleagues [7••] studied the device in 310 patients, 157 of whom were randomized to the device and 153 to the control group with manual pressure hemostasis. Despite a significantly higher presheath-removal activated clotting time in the device group, the time up to hemostasis was substantially shorter in the device group (approximately 2.5 min vs 16 min in the control group; $p < 0.001$). In addition, Kussmaul and colleagues demonstrate a lower incidence of hematoma formation in the device group ($p=0.03$) as well as a lower overall complication rate for the patients receiving the Angio-Seal (17 patients vs 32 patients in the control group; $p = 0.02$). The only serious complication was infection of the puncture site and device in one patient that resulted in surgical removal and repair. This incident was traced to a break in sterile technique. Thrombosis of the artery did not occur in any patients. European trials have demonstrated similar results [8••].

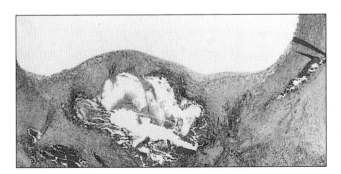

FIGURE 7-4

A cross-section of a porcine aorta stained with hematoxylin and eosin. There was noted cellular inflammatory response with a strong presence of lymphocytes. Polymorphonuclear leukocytes are scarce. Note the wall at the implant site, and the nearly complete resorption of the implant.

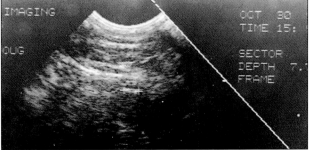

FIGURE 7-5.

An ultrasound study of the efficacy of the Angio-Seal, 2 hours postimplantation. Position and placement of the anchor in the author's femoral artery is noted (*arrows*). Note the small size of the anchor in relation to the diameter of the artery.

Conclusion

Early clinical results suggest that the Angio-Seal HPCD is safe, efficacious, and easy to use. We expect it to be a significant advancement for hemostasis of all arterial puncture sites. It may allow uninterrupted, postprocedure anticoagulation, more aggressive use of thrombolytic agents, and safer use of large-bore catheters. It may also reduce discomfort and complication rates for patients, may allow many inpatient procedures to be performed safely on an outpatient basis, and may decrease the time and cost of interventional procedures. We also expect that the Angio-Seal will significantly reduce hospital personnel's exposure to patient blood. Other companies are also presently developing hemostatic devices to solve the same problem [9].

As initially envisioned, the Angio-Seal HPCD should provide diagnostic as well as post-complex peripheral angioplasty hemostasis without compromising blood flow to the distal extremity by allowing immediate removal of the introducer sheath; and providing puncture hemostasis without the need for manual pressure. This should improve distal blood flow to the leg and is also likely to improve patency rates. Although we initially developed the 8-French size, we are currently developing sizes to meet the demand of other procedures including 10-French, 12-French, 14-French, and 6-French.

The Angio-Seal is currently in clinical trials and has not been approved by the Food and Drug Administration. We are hopeful that this or some yet undiscovered technology will be available in the near future to solve this common, difficult, and costly problem.

References and Recommended Reading

1.• Cragg AH, Nakagawa N, Smith TP, Berbaum KS: Hematoma Formation After Diagnostic Angiography: Effect of Catheter Size. *JVIR* 1991, 2:231–233.
This article explains complications common to manual pressure methods of hemostasis.

2. Bredlau CE, Roubin GS, Leimgruber PP, *et al.*: In-Hospital Morbidity and Morality in Patients Undergoing Elective Coronary Angioplasty. Circulation 1985, 72:1044–1052.

3. Gardiner GA, Meyerovitz MF, Stokes KR, *et al.*: Complications of Transluminal Angioplasty. *Radiology* 1986, 159:201–208.

4. Abbott WM, Austen WG: Microcrystalline Collagen as Topical Hemostatic Agent for Vascular Surgery. *Surgery* 1974, 75: 925–933.

5. Kensey KR, Evans DG, McGill LD, Nash JC: *In Vivo* Feasibility Testing of a Bioresorbable Hemostatic Puncture Closure Device (abstract). *J Am Coll Cardiol* 1991, 17(supplA):263A.

6. Gresiler HP, Kim DU: Vascular Grafting in the Management of Thrombotic Disorders. *Semin Thromb Hemost* 1989, 15:206–213.

7.•• Kussmaul WG, Buchbinder M, Whitlow PL, *et al.*: Randomized Trial of a New Hemostatic Puncture Closure Device (poster presentation). *American Heart Association 66th Scientific Sessions*, Atlanta: November 1993.
A controlled study of phase I clinical trials in the US.

8.•• deSwart H, Dijkman L, van Ommen V, Bar F, Wellens HJJ: Abstract: The Hemostatic Puncture Closure Device Versus a Conventional Pressure Bandage. Preliminary Results of a Randomized Study (poster presentation). *American Heart Association 66th Scientific Sessions*, Atlanta: November 1993.
A phase I study of controlled clinical trials in Europe.

9. Rees MR, Sivananthan UM, Davy-Quinn A, Verma SP: Use of Collagen Vascular Plug in Achieving Hemostasis After Angioplasty. *Radiology* 1993, 146:189.

Select Bibliography

Greenfield AJ: Femoral, Popliteal, and Tibial Arteries: Percutaneous Transluminal Angioplasty. *AJR* 1980, 135:927–935.

Johnston KW, Rae M, Hogg-Johnston SA, *et al.*: 5-Year Results of a Prospective Study of Percutaneous Transluminal Angioplasty. *Ann Surg* 1987, 206:403–413.

Neiman HL, Bergan JJ, Yao JST, *et al.*: Hemodynamic Assessment of Transluminal Angioplasty for Lower Extremity Ischemia. *Radiology* 1982, 143:639–643.

Redman HC: Commentary: Has the Time Come for Outpatient Peripheral Angioplasty. *AJR* 1987, 148:1241–1242.

Interventional Management of Ostial Lesions in the Renal Artery

David Trost
Thomas A. Sos

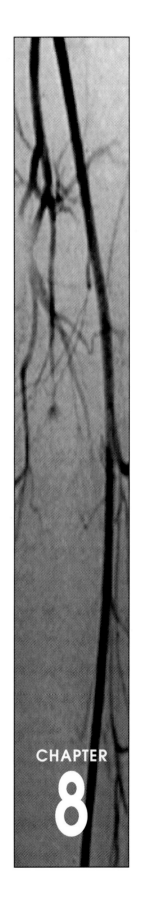

Ostial renal artery stenosis consists of two entities: aortic plaque encroaching on the renal artery orifice and disease of the renal artery origin (Fig. 8-1). These two elements can be difficult or impossible to discriminate on arteriography. Frequently, the disease is a combination of the two types [1].

The Mechanism of Angioplasty

Angioplasty works by controlled trauma. The atheroma is fractured longitudinally and circumferentially and the cracks extend into the intima and media. The muscle fibers of the media are injured and paralyzed, the adventitia is overdilated, and the atheromatous material is redistributed radially and laterally into the overdilated adventitia, thus leaving a large central lumen that is kept open by the increased flow. In true ostial stenoses, the sheet of atheroma surrounding the renal artery ostium is acted upon in a longitudinal rather than a radial fashion by the dilating balloon. Soon after deflation of the balloon, the atheroma recoils and the stenosis recurs. Stenoses truly within the origin of the renal artery respond well to percutaneous transluminal angioplasty (PTA). Unfortunately, origin

stenoses account for relatively few of the total number of angiographic ostial stenoses.

Patient Selection for Renal Angioplasty

The evaluation of patients with suspected renovascular hypertension has been previously described in detail [2,3•]. Because of our patient referral pattern, we usually perform intra-arterial digital subtraction angiography (IADSA) immediately following vein renin (RVR) sampling. If an angiographically significant stenosis is demonstrated, it is treated simultaneously with angioplasty or angioplasty and stent placement. Patients with restenosis of an initially successful ostial lesion angioplasty are stented. Lesions that are not clearly significant by angiographic appearance are either selectively catheterized for pressure gradient measurement or the procedure is terminated. Other factors including a positive peripheral plasma renin activity (PRA), or PRA captopril challenge test, a captopril renal scan suggestive of delayed flow on the affected side and results of the RVR sampling are used to determine if the lesion must be dilated.

CATHETERIZATION OF THE STENOSIS

If a lesion is considered significant or pressure gradient measurement is desired, the artery must be selectively catheterized. Selective catheterization and crossing stenotic renal arteries can be risky, and should not be attempted unless an angioplasty is planned. The vast majority of renal interventions can be performed easily and safely from a femoral approach; however, a minority of patients require an axillary approach.

Catheter choice is difficult to advise because most operators already have preferred catheters. Renal artery interventions are usually performed with a recurve-type catheter such as a Simmons. Cobra catheters are rarely used. They will usually engage the renal orifice and a floppy guidewire can then be advanced across the stenosis. However, it can be difficult to push the cobra catheter across the lesion, especially if it is ostial. In these cases, the catheter and floppy guidewire will tend to buckle up into the aorta.

Because the renal vessels usually have a caudally directed origin, recurve catheters are the desirable choice. Recurve catheters also have another benefit:

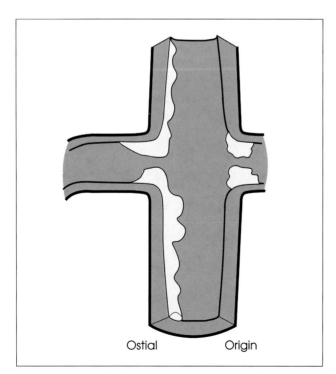

FIGURE 8-1.

True versus ostial disease.

Ostial   Origin

because the catheter is pulled down into the artery rather than pushed across it, the operator can exert more axial force to cross lesions. This leads to increased success in crossing a tight stenosis. One of the most popular recurve designs for cerebral and visceral angiography has been the Simmons series of catheters and their Chuang visceral modification. However, Simmons or other recurve catheters must be reformed in the aortic arch, its branches, or after selective catheterization of the contralateral iliac artery or branches of the abdominal aorta, necessitating a catheter exchange. These maneuvers are often time-consuming and entail the risks of cerebrovascular or distal embolization. There is also a risk of injuring the vessel used to reform the catheter.

We generally use Omni catheters (Angiodynamic, Glen Falls, NY) as our primary choice. These catheters are recurve-style catheters that reform in the descending thoracic aorta just distal to the left subclavian artery, thus eliminating the risks of reforming the catheter in the aortic arch or visceral vessels. However, there is also a risk of injuring the vessel use to reform the catheter. Cope [4] has described a technique to reform Simmons catheters in the aorta by pulling the tip with a suture.

An extremely floppy soft-tip guidewire such as a Bentson (Cook, Bloomington, IN) or a TAD II (Peripheral Systems Group, Mountain View, CA) with the guidewire extending several centimeters out of the end of the catheter tip is the least traumatic way to cross stenoses. Most lesions can be crossed if care is taken to line up the catheter tip with the axis of the stenosis when gently advancing the guidewire. Once the guidewire is across the stenosis, the catheter can be pulled down through or pushed across the lesion. Different techniques for crossing stenoses are illustrated by Figures 8-2, 8-3, 8-4, and 8-5. The soft wire is removed and arterial pressure distal to the stenosis obtained. If there is any question that the catheter is subintimal, then a careful test injection can be performed. Most stenoses and some short occlusions, especially proximal lesions, can be traversed using this method. If initial attempts at crossing the lesion are unsuccessful, the angle of the axis of the stenotic vessel, eccentricity, and irregularity of the plaque are re-evaluated and a different catheter is introduced or positioned. The catheter position can be adjusted to alter the course of the guidewire and respiratory motion can also be used. Sometimes a TAD I guidewire (Medi-Tech, Watertown, MA) with a 0.035-inch shaft

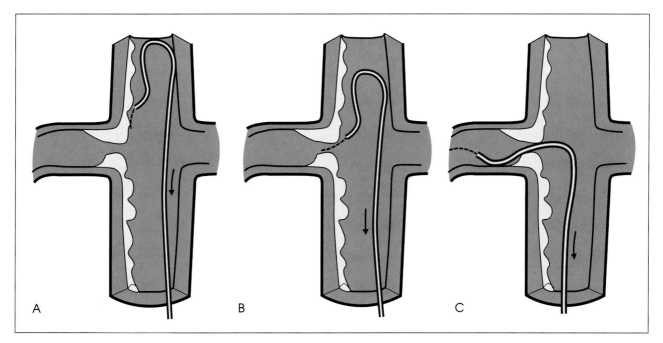

FIGURE 8-2.

The pull-down method. **A**, Starting above the renal ostium, the catheter and the leading guidewire are pulled caudally through **B** and **C**, the stenosis.

and 0.018-inch tip can cross a very tight stenosis, but this wire can be hard to follow with a catheter because of the long floppy portion extending into the aorta. If the angle is appropriate but a soft wire will not cross the lesion, careful use of a hydrophilic or torqueable wire such as a Glidewire (Medi-Tech, Watertown, MA) may be successful. Occasionally, the wire will cross the lesion but the catheter will not follow. In these situations, a Glidecath (Medi-Tech, Watertown, MA) will sometimes work.

If the abdominal aorta is very diseased, a long sheath that extends to the level of the renal arteries can be used to protect the aorta and decrease the risk of thrombo-, athero-, and cholesterol embolization. The use of a sheath will also facilitate the transmission of torque and push to the catheter tip, allowing better catheter control and safety.

Occluded renal arteries can be recanalized using the same basic technique as stenoses. There is little utility in trying to recanalize arteries if the kidney size is less than 7 cm. If the kidney can be successfully revascularized, it will re-expand somewhat. The key to successfully recanalizing an occlusion is to demonstrate the nubbin of the occluded artery. Seeing a reconstituted artery is a desirable feature, but not seeing it does not necessarily mean the artery is completely thrombosed.

The status of the contralateral kidney, the presence or absence of a reconstituted distal artery, and the renal size will help to determine the procedure for recanalization of the artery. Care must be taken to line up the catheter with the nubbin and to carefully probe all areas of the nubbin from various angles with the wire before giving up. If the wire crosses the lesion, its intraluminal position must be assessed. If there is any question about position, advance the catheter slightly into the occlusion and perform a gentle test injection, preferably with the wire left in place through a side-arm adapter or use the over-the-wire injection technique described later. If the position is satisfactory, the lesion is dilated similar to a stenosis. Following successful recanalization and dilation of an ostial occlusion, it is reasonable to primarily place a stent. If the wire has dissected the artery, further attempts can be made at entering the true lumen. However, if a surgical bypass procedure is possible, it is better to stop early rather than to severely dissect the artery and prevent a successful surgical revascularization. Most perforations are self-limiting.

For exchange of the diagnostic for the balloon catheter, a guidewire that has a very soft, atraumatic tip and a rapid transition to a stiff shaft is useful. This type of wire can be safely advanced into the segmental

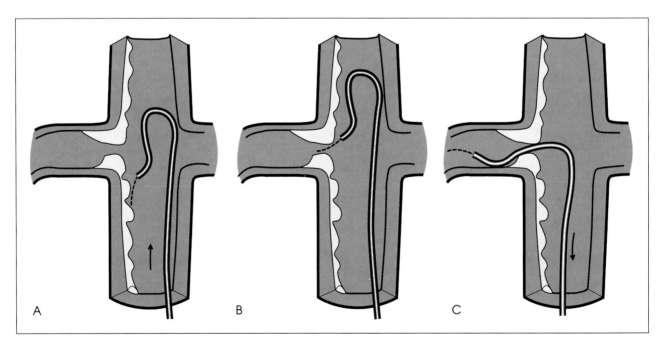

FIGURE 8-3.

The push-up method. **A**, Starting below the renal ostium, the catheter and leading guidewire are advanced cranially until **B**, the wire pops into the ostium. **C**, The catheter shaft is withdrawn, pulling the tip out into the renal artery.

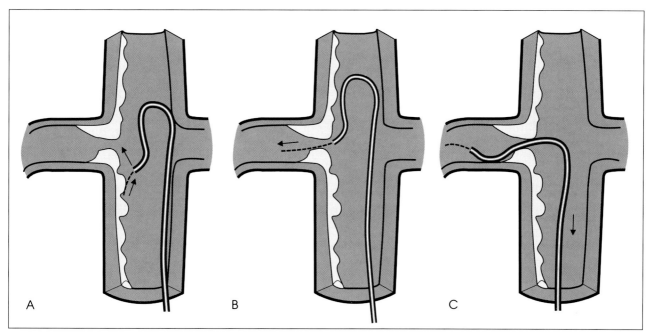

FIGURE 8-4.

The aligned-catheter method. **A**, The catheter and leading guidewire are positioned. **B**, When the catheter is withdrawn, the catheter tip pops up into the renal ositum. **C**, The guidewire is then advanced across the stenosis and the catheter pulled through the stenosis.

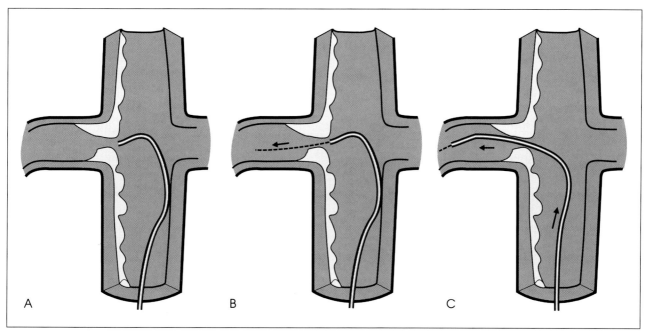

FIGURE 8-5.

The aligned-catheter method. **A**, The cobra catheter is positioned with the axis of the stenosis. **B**, The wire is advanced across the stenosis. **C**, The catheter is advanced into the renal artery.

branches and provide the needed shaft stiffness to facilitate advancing a balloon across the stenosis. The TAD II wire (Peripheral Systems Group, Mountain View, CA) has a stiff 0.035-inch shaft tapering to a floppy 0.018-inch tip. The rigid shaft of the TAD II wire can be shaped to closely match the natural curve of the renal artery and its origin from the aorta, facilitating passage of the balloon catheter (Fig. 8-6). Prior to the placement of the wire, 100 to 200 µg of nitroglycerin should be injected directly into the renal artery to prevent spasm of the vessel during guidewire passage and balloon dilatation. The very tip of the balloon catheter (distal to the balloon) can be gently shaped into a beak to allow it to follow over the wire from the aorta into the renal artery, even through severe rigid proximal stenoses. The rigid shaft of the preshaped TAD II wire also helps prevent shearing forces on the aortorenal junction as the balloon is inflated by forcing the balloon to conform to the aortorenal angle. A technique that helps to decrease the torque force applied to the proximal renal artery during balloon inflation is to play out the catheter slightly (Fig. 8-7). When the balloon is partially inflated, the shaft and wire can be gently and slightly advanced until a more horizontal configuration is achieved. The inflation must be carefully monitored by fluoroscopy. The balloon must not advance during this procedure. If it begins to advance,

the catheter should be withdrawn so the balloon position is stable. During balloon deflation, catheter position should be monitored to prevent the catheter from advancing into the renal artery, possibly injuring it. The wire can be removed to obtain a postdilatation pressure measurement. The soft-tipped, stiff-shaft wire should be readvanced to withdraw the balloon. Withdrawing the balloon over the wire prevents the balloon tip from scraping the cranial wall of the artery as it is withdrawn, possibly inducing spasm or dissection. A control pressure in the aorta can then be obtained.

BALLOON SIZING

A great deal has been written about balloon sizing. The balloon must be large enough to sufficiently dilate the lesion. Many experienced operators gestalt the balloon size by knowing their equipment and its inherent magnification. In the proximal main renal artery, we use 2-cm long, 8-mm balloons for large men, 7-mm balloons for small men and large women, and 6-mm balloons for small women. We have never used a balloon smaller than 6 mm in the proximal main renal artery of an adult. The lesion should be overdilated by 15% to 20% compared with the size of the normal artery [5,6]. The standard method of choosing the correct balloon is to directly measure the normal vessel on a standard cut film arteriogram that has an inherent 20% magnification factor. For this technique to be accurate and reproducible, the film changer distance must be constant and the patient as close to the film changer as possible. Even with careful technique, the exact magnification factor is quite variable. With the advent of good digital subtraction angiographic equipment, many of the interventional procedures and diagnostic angiography are being performed without cut film. The newer digital equipment can provide accurate measurement of the vessel lumen by basing the measurements on the catheter shaft size or other reference sources, eliminating magnification error. A balloon 15% to 20% larger than the measured vessel should be selected. If in doubt, use the smaller size balloon initially and redilate with a larger balloon if necessary.

Patients normally experience mild-to-moderate back or flank pain during the inflation which should resolve quickly following deflation, usually within 1 minute. If the patient experiences severe pain, inflation should not be continued and the balloon immediately deflated. If

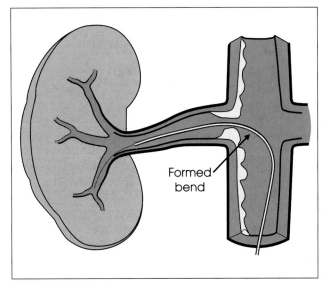

FIGURE 8-6.

A stiff shaft, tapered-tip guidewire can be preshaped to conform to the aortorenal angle to stabilize the wire and help guide the balloon catheter into the artery.

the pain rapidly resolves, it is most likely safe to reinflate with a smaller balloon. If the pain continues or increases, it may be a sign of severe injury to the renal artery, such as rupture or occlusion. If a severe injury is suspected, an angiogram should be performed without losing guidewire position across the lesion.

POSTINTERVENTION IMAGING

A flush aortogram is the best and safest way to image the renal artery after intervention. Selective renal arterial injections for completion angiograms following renal artery angioplasty (PTRA) may produce subintimal contrast injection.

Unfortunately, the flush aortogram requires the removal of the guidewire from across the dilated segment or placement of another aortic catheter by a second arterial puncture. If further intervention is required, the lesion must be recrossed with all the associated additional risks of crossing a recently dilated lesion. Several alternative approaches have been proposed. Tegtmeyer and Sos [7••] describe placing a 0.025-inch guidewire through the balloon catheter with a Y-adapter allowing injection of contrast to monitor the progress of the dilatation. Tegtmeyer and Sos [7••] have previously suggested leaving a guidewire in the

renal artery and placing an aortic pigtail along side of it via the same sheath. It is frequently difficult to simultaneously pass a catheter and a wire through a 5-French sheath; occasionally, the wire in the renal artery advances or pulls out during exchanges.

We recently described a new method of imaging the dilated segment by using a soft-tipped, straight, 5-French, multisidehole catheter over the 0.035-inch guidewire and injecting through a Y-adapter [8]. The technique produces reliable opacification of the renal artery and the aorta when two thirds of the catheter sideholes are placed in the aorta and the tip in the renal artery. This method reduces the number of catheter and guidewire manipulations across the dilated segment, decreasing the associated risk of cholesterol embolization, dissection, and thrombosis.

In a few patients, the guidewire distorts the normal aortorenal angle and as a result the over-the-wire angiogram can be misleading, but we have generally found it to be a reliable technique. If the follow-up angiogram demonstrates a significant residual stenosis and the balloon size was adequate, the artery can be redilated or stented. The decision to redilate or place a stent is mostly an angiographic decision, even in the face of no measured pressure gradient. If the

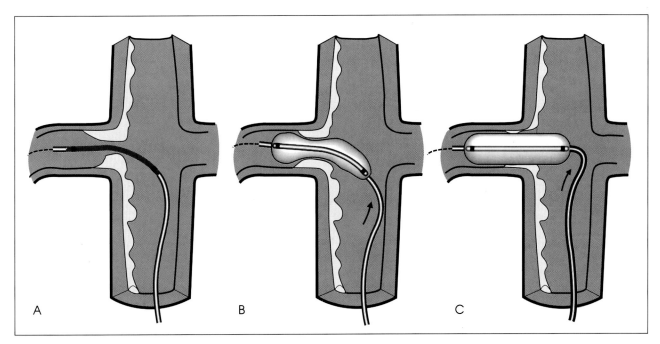

FIGURE 8-7.

Playing out the balloon. **A**, The balloon is advanced across the lesion. **B**, As the balloon is inflated, the catheter is gently pushed cranially. **C**, This results in a more horizontal course for the balloon.

result of the angioplasty with the over-the-wire angiogram technique is satisfactory, we usually still perform a confirmatory standard flush aortogram after removing the wire.

Stenting

Renal stents are currently under evaluation. They are best used for ostial stenoses that have restenosed following PTRA and for ostial lesions which respond poorly to initial angioplasty. Placing renal stents is associated with a new set of considerations. Although angioplasty does not usually affect subsequent surgical renal artery revascularization, stenting can. Stents prevent the performance of an aortorenal endarterectomy, a procedure not widely used. A proximally placed stent will not usually have an effect on most bypass procedures unless the stent extends too far toward the branching of

the artery. Positioning the stent in the stenosis is of utmost importance. It is essential that the artery origin is imaged in the proper oblique so that the origin is exactly in profile. Only in that position can the stent be accurately positioned at the renal origin (Fig. 8-8). The goal is to place the stent so that it extends slightly into the aortic lumen approximately 1 to 2 mm to ensure that it covers the ostium adequately. It is much better to err having too much stent in the aorta rather than risk not adequately covering the renal ostium. Most ostial disease can be treated with a 10- to 15-mm long stent. We routinely use the Palmaz 15-mm nonarticulated stent (Johnson & Johnson, Warren, NJ). This stent can be dilated from 4 to 9 mm. Other stent designs such as the Wallstent (Schneider, Minneapolis, MN) and the Strecker stent (Medi-Tech and Boston Scientific, Watertown, MA) have been used in the renal arteries, particularly in European clinics.

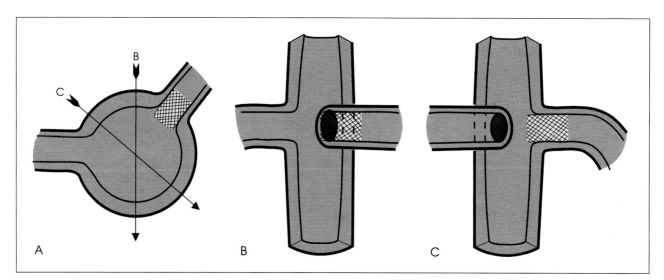

FIGURE 8-8.

A, The importance of imaging the renal artery in the proper oblique. **B,** Note the projected overlap of the stent on the anterior view. **C,** The true overlap is seen on the right anterior oblique view.

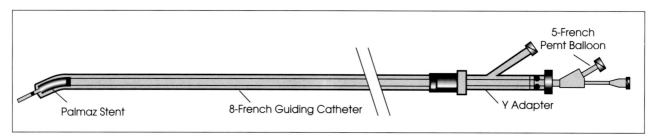

FIGURE 8-9.

The catheter-guide system for renal stent placement.

Performing the completion angiogram following PTRA (or stenting) with a technique that preserves wire position across the stenosis facilitates repeated interventions including stent placement and decreases complications by obviating the need to recross the lesion. For proper placement, the exact position of the stent relative to the balloon markers must be known because occasionally the stent cannot be seen on fluoroscopy. We

prefer to place the proximal (aortic) end of the stent over the proximal balloon marker. The stent or balloon is placed into an angled, 8- or 9-French guiding catheter (the guide must have an inner lumen diameter of 0.081 inches or greater) through a Y-adapter, and positioned so that the tapered tip of the balloon catheter is protruding out of the guide but the stent is kept covered (Fig. 8-9). Stent placement is illustrated in Figure 8-10.

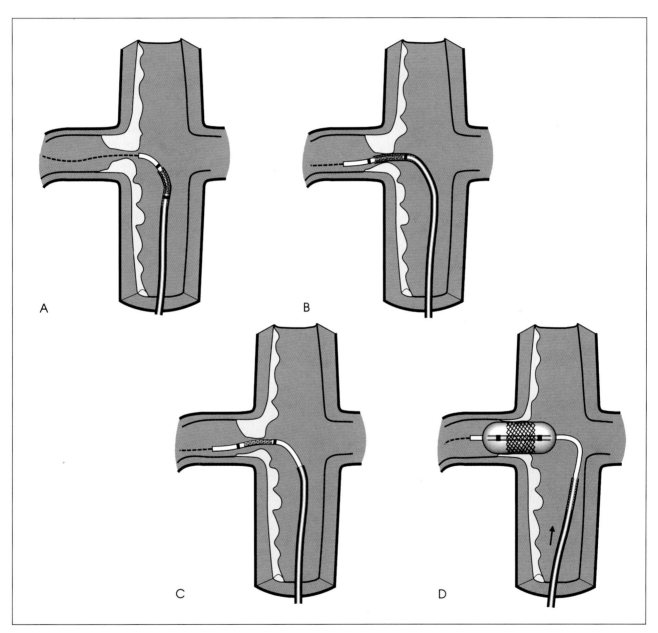

FIGURE 8-10.

A, The stent system in position for placement angiogram through the guiding catheter. **B**, The stent system positioned in the renal artery. **C**, The guiding catheter pulled back for final positioning angiogram. **D**, The stent expanded when balloon is played out (*arrow*).

The balloon and guide combination is advanced to the renal artery ostium and an angiogram in the previously determined optimal oblique is performed through the guide. The balloon and guide are advanced into the renal artery using the arteriogram as a reference. The shortening of the stent as it is expanded must be taken into account when positioning it. When satisfied with the position, the guide catheter is withdrawn to just out of the renal artery. An angiogram through the guiding catheter is performed to confirm positioning. If the positioning is not correct it can usually be easily adjusted. Occasionally, the stent will slide on the balloon as it is moved. Inflating the balloon slightly will usually allow the balloon to grip the stent sufficiently so it can be repositioned. The stent is then expanded, the guidewire left in position, the balloon catheter carefully withdrawn to avoid moving the stent, and a completion angiogram performed through the guiding catheter. If the stent begins to move during balloon withdrawal, the guiding catheter can be used to hold the stent in place as the balloon is withdrawn. If the stent moved but the position is still acceptable, reinflation of the balloon may help to fix the stent in place. An inadequately opened stent or one across an area of motion in the vessel is more prone to migrate. If the stent does not cover the entire lesion, a second stent can be placed to overlap the first.

Potential problems with stent placement include malpositioning, migration, embolization of the stent, and difficult removal of the balloon from the stent. Malpositioning can be minimized by performing the procedure in the proper oblique and taking the time to carefully position the stent as described above.

If the stent slips off the balloon and remains over the wire, it can be retrieved by removing the guiding catheter and placing a 4-French Amplatz Gooseneck snare (Microvena, Vadnais Heights, MN) alongside the guidewire in the sheath. The snare can be placed over the distal (cephalad) end of the wire in the aorta and brought down to grab the proximal (caudal) end of the stent and be pulled out through or funneled into the sheath. The distal (cephalad) end of the stent should not be snared because the proximal (caudal) end will be crushed against the edge of the sheath and form a jagged ball that cannot be pulled through the sheath. The sheath and stent can still be pulled out of the artery, but the risk of injury to the femoral artery is significant.

Atherectomy

Rotational atherectomy of the renal ostium has been performed in very few patients (Dake, personal communication). The technique has a significant risk of cutting through the aortorenal angle unless the catheter is parallel to the proximal renal artery. Tegtmeyer [9] has used the transluminal extraction catheter (TEC) (IVT, La Jolla, CA) to bore a pilot hole through the ostial atheroma, allowing more successful PTRA of the ostium. The benefit of this procedure is not yet clear, and there are theoretic risks of distal embolization.

Complications and Their Prevention

Complications are reported to occur in 5% to 10% of patients. The most frequent major complications in PTRA are initiated by thrombosis and spasm of the renal artery. The manipulation of guidewires in arteries with spasm or thrombosis increases the risks of dissection, occlusion, or perforation. Adjunctive medications can prevent or diminish the incidence and severity of complications.

SPASM

The normal response of the vessel wall to trauma (even to the controlled trauma of angioplasty) is to release serotonin and thromboxane, especially if clot and atheromatous material are present. The renal artery responds to these substances by spasm and thrombosis.

Calcium-channel blockers, such as oral nifedipine, given as little as 20 minutes preprocedure are useful in preventing spasm as is liberal use of intra-arterial nitroglycerine (NTG). The NTG is administered as 100 to 300 μg intra-arterial boluses. Intra-arterial papaverine 15 to 30 mg intra-arterially and verapamil hydrochloride 2.5 mg intra-arterially have also been used [7••].

ACUTE OCCLUSION

Acute occlusion is usually caused by dissection or thrombosis, although rarely severe spasm can simulate total occlusion. For nonocclusive dissection, the balloon can be gently inflated for 2 minutes in an attempt to tack it down. Stents can also be used to treat dissections of the main renal artery but should be used only when surgery is not an option or if their position will not interfere with subsequent surgical repair.

Thrombosis can occur during PTRA from thrombus formation on the catheter and guidewire, low-flow states resulting from spasm, balloon inflation, catheter occlusion of the stenosis, and dissection. The risk of thrombus formation can be reduced by preprocedural administration of antiplatelet agents (ASA 300 mg), intraprocedural heparin, and spasmolytics. Should the procedure last more than 1 hour, heparin should be continued as boluses or a continuous infusion. Inexpensive, activated clotting time (ACT) measuring units are helpful in determining if an adequate level of anticoagulation is present. An ACT value between 250 and 300 seconds is adequate. If thrombus forms, the thrombosed vessels can be frequently opened with urokinase [10]. The pulsed-spray method may be preferred if the occlusion is total, because it will theoretically restore at least partial flow faster than a continuous infusion [11]. For nonocclusive thrombus, a continuous infusion is usually adequate.

PERFORATION AND RUPTURE

The difference between arterial perforation and rupture is important. Frank rupture with retroperitoneal extravasation of contrast requires surgical repair. Perforation by only a guidewire is almost always self-sealing. Perforations that do not stop bleeding can be embolized.

Following rupture, a latex occlusion balloon or an angioplasty balloon can be gently inflated across the tear to tamponade the bleeding. Iced saline can be infused through the catheter to help preserve the kidney when the operating room is being readied. If this does not control the hemorrhage, a large occlusion balloon can be inflated across the renal origin effectively cross-clamping the aorta at that level.

Every patient should be closely monitored following renal intervention. If the patient has persistent or increasing back or flank pain, arterial rupture or impending rupture as well as total occlusion must be considered. Even if the completed angiogram shows no extravasation, a computed tomography (CT) scan is a more sensitive test to look for extravasation around the renal artery and kidney.

MACROEMBOLIZATION

When performing any intravascular procedure, there is always the chance of causing embolization of plaque, thrombus, or cholesterol usually to the lower extremities. The risk of embolization can be minimized by limiting the number of catheter exchanges and using soft-tipped catheters and guidewires. Macroembolization of atherosclerotic plaque or thrombus can usually be treated with surgical embolectomy or bypass. If the emboli are thought to be fresh thrombus, thrombolysis may be attempted.

MICROCHOLESTEROL CRYSTAL EMBOLIZATION

Symptomatic distal embolization of dislodged large plaque is rare. However, as more and more patients with uncomplicated focal atheromatous disease have renal angioplasty in smaller institutions, the ones referred to larger tertiary care centers are more complex. In this patient group, all complications are more frequent. Microcholesterol crystal embolization (CCE), a complication that occurs in approximately 1% of patients, is almost limited to this group [12]. CCE can be the result of simple diagnostic angiography alone; however, it is more frequently seen if multiple catheter manipulations are performed in a diseased aorta. Microemboli can lodge in the kidneys, in the bowel, or in the extremities and can produce permanent renal failure, severe ischemia, or organ necrosis. Unfortunately, these events can be severe and even fatal.

There is no specific treatment for CCE. Some authors believe it is safe to anticoagulate these patients although others feel that because anticoagulation is speculated to be a causative agent, it may make the patient worse [13,14]. Partial function can be regained with time.

Percutaneous transluminal renal angioplasty in patients with diffusely atheromatous abdominal aortas should be performed with the least amount of manipulation. The use of a long sheath introduced just below the renal arteries facilitates transmission of torque and may help prevent microembolization.

CONTRAST-INDUCED RENAL FAILURE

The risk factors for renal failure following administration of iodinated contrast material are well known. They include pre-existing renal insufficiency, dehydration, diabetes mellitus, hyperuricemia, and multiple myeloma. Patients with diabetes and renal disease are at a high risk, particularly if the serum creatinine is greater than 3.5 mg/dL [15,16]. Renal dysfunction is usually temporary; permanent renal dysfunction is a small but real risk. The risks of contrast-induced renal failure can be reduced by liberal patient hydration, if tolerated. Reducing the total contrast load reduces the incidence of contrast-induced renal failure in patients with pre-existing renal disease. Administration of furosemide and mannitol has been widely used to prevent contrast-induced renal failure, but the benefit of these infusions has not been clinically proven [17]. The use of low-osmolality contrast media has not proven to prevent contrast-induced renal failure. CO_2 with IADSA may be the optimal contrast agent in these patients.

Postprocedure Care

Postprocedure patients are immediately hydrated as much as they can tolerate. The heparin given during the procedure is not reversed. Additional doses of heparin are not used directly following PTRA or stent placement. Blood pressure, intake, and output as well as the serum creatinine are monitored closely. Deterioration of the patient's renal status may warrant reangiography, further intervention, or surgical bypass. We recommend that our angioplasty and stent patients receive an antiplatelet agent (usually ASA 80 to 300 mg orally every other day) postprocedure indefinitely. We do not routinely provide systemic anticoagulation except for patients with known hypercoagulable states.

Results

The historic and current literature on renal angioplasty reports a high technical success rate in the treatment of atheromatous renal artery stenosis. It is difficult to separate the results for ostial disease in many of the papers [18–21].

In 1992, Martin and colleagues [22•] reported a series of 110 patients who underwent angioplasty alone for ostial renal artery stenosis at a mean follow-up of 38 months. At the end of follow-up, primary, secondary, and tertiary clinical benefits were 48%, 57%, and 58%, respectively. These data are in conflict with most other operators who feel that almost all true ostial lesions respond poorly to PTA and most will result in restenosis within 1 year. Martin may have classified some proximal renal artery stenoses as ostial, hence the better results.

Early reports of stenting of the renal arteries are now being published. Rees will present the results of a multicenter trial of the Palmaz-Schatz stent (Johnson & Johnson, Warren, NJ) at the 1994 meeting of the Cardiovascular and Interventional Radiological Society of Europe. Three hundred four stents were placed in 296 arteries of 263 patients. Technical success was 95%. Eighty percent of the lesions were ostial. At 6-month follow-up, 64% had improvement or cure of hypertension. In 123 patients with renal insufficiency (creatinine > 1.5 mg/dL), there was improvement in 34%, stability in 39%, and deterioration in 27%. Angiographic follow-up at 6 months was performed in 150 patients. Angiographic restenosis (diameter < 50%) occurred in 32.7%. Restenosis was lower in males (23%, $p < 0.05$), for all stents dilated to greater than 6 mm (26%, $p < 0.05$), and lowest for males dilated greater than 6 mm (10.5%).

Rousseau and Joffre [23•] report experience using the Wallstent for treatment of renal artery stenoses in 21 patients following inadequate PTRA or for recurrent stenosis following PTRA. Fifteen patients had atheromatous lesions, involving the ostium in seven cases. Early benign complications occurred in four patients. Follow-up angiography (12 to 60 months) showed restenosis in four patients. Cumulative primary patency rate (Kaplan-Meier) was 95% at 7 months, 85% at 9 months, and 77% at 15 months. At clinical follow-up (32 ± 15 months), hypertension was cured in three patients and improved in 18. Renal function remained normal in patients without renal failure before stenting. In six patients with renal failure, renal function improved in one patient, stabilized in three, and slightly decreased in two [22•].

We have attempted to place 25 Palmaz stents in 23 arteries of 21 patients. Twenty-two stents were placed for atheromatous ostial stenoses, one for a nonostial atheromatous stenosis, and one for a transplant anastomotic stenosis. In the 21 patients, clinical indications were: hypertension, 100% (21 of 21 patients), creatinine greater than or equal to 1.5 mg/dL, 52% (11 of 21 patients), creatinine greater than or equal to 2.0 mg/dL, 38% (8 of 21 patients), and recurrent flash pulmonary edema, 24% (5 of 21 patients) (some patients had multiple indications). Sixty-seven percent (16 of 24 patients) were placed following one or several failed renal angioplasties. Thirty-three percent (8 of 24 patients) were placed primarily following failed angioplasty. All procedures except one (95%) in a small accessory artery were technically successful. There were two procedural complications (8%, 2 of 25 patients): thrombosis of a renal artery branch (*n* = 1), and embolization of a stent during unsuccessful placement in the accessory artery that was successfully retrieved percutaneously (*n* = 1). Angiographic follow-up has been performed on 48% (11 of 23 patients) of these arteries at a mean of 7.6 months (range 3 to 12

months). Thirty-six percent (4 of 11 patients) had restenosis of greater than or equal to 50%. Clinical follow-up (renal function and blood pressure) reveals improvement in 71% (15 of 21 patients). Mean clinical follow-up was 11.2 months (range 1 to 21 months). Two representative cases are provided in Figures 11 and 12. Accessory renal arteries should be treated

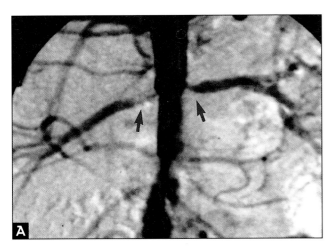

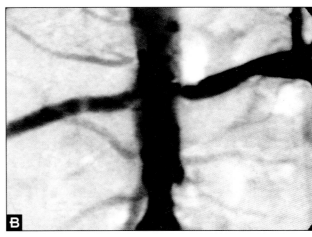

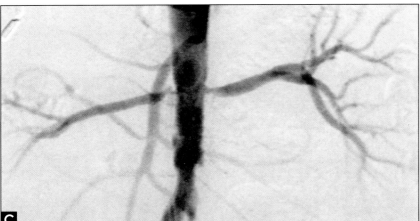

FIGURE 8-11.

A 53-year-old white woman with hypertension, insulin-dependent diabetes mellitus, and an abdominal bruit. **A**, The initial aortogram demonstrating proximal stenoses (*arrows*). **B**, Good results without gradients, postangioplasty. **C**, Recurrent stenoses 5 months postangioplasty. **D**, Excellent results, postbilateral stents. **E**, Partial restenosis 9 months poststenting. The patient continues to do well clinically.

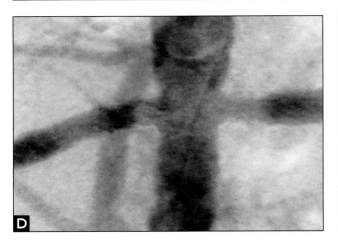

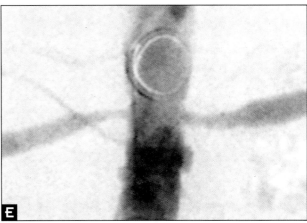

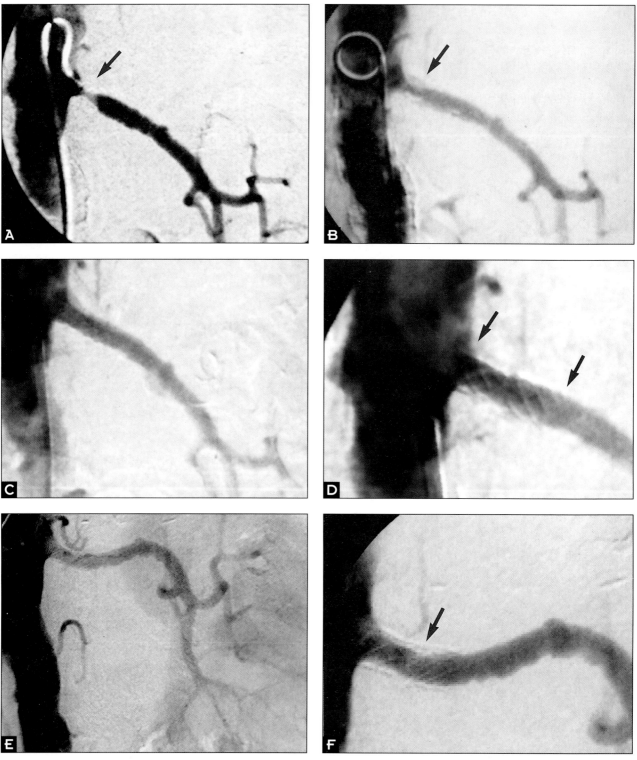

FIGURE 8-12.

A 73-year-old woman, with a 30-year history of hypertension, status post-right nephrectomy. **A**, The initial angiogram shows high-grade proximal stenosis (*arrow*). **B**, Significant residual stenosis is noted postpercutaneous transluminal renal angio-plasty (*arrow*). **C**, The post-stent arteriogram. **D**, A close-up view of the stented site (*arrows*). **E**, A 7-month angiographic follow-up of the patient. **F**, A close-up view of the stent; note minimal intimal growth (*arrow*).

similar to main renal arteries. The smallest balloon we have used in an accessory renal artery is 3 mm in diameter. Arteries 4 mm or smaller in diameter usually supply a relatively small portion of the kidney and can be treated with angiotensin-converting enzyme (ACE) inhibitors if they do not respond to angioplasty. We have had no experience in stenting arteries smaller than 5 mm. Perhaps coronary stents would be useful for this application. If intervention is unsuccessful and hypertension is still a problem, selective embolization of the artery with absolute ethanol can be considered.

We feel that ostial renal artery disease can be effectively treated by percutaneous methods. The patients should initially undergo angioplasty and if the dilation is adequate, the patient should be closely followed clinically. If the angioplasty angiographically appears less than optimal but there is no significant pressure gradient, the patient can be followed-up or undergo stenting. However, only a few of these patients will have a satisfactory long-term result with PTRA alone. If the angioplasty is poor, stenting or surgical revascularization should be performed. Successful long-term results and patient benefit are best served by cooperation and communication between the radiologist, nephrologist, and surgeon.

References and Recommended Reading

Recently published papers of particular interest have been highlighted as:
• Of special interest
•• Of outstanding interest

1. Cicuto KP, McLean GK, Oleaga JA, *et al.*: Renal Artery Stenosis: Anatomic Classification for Percutaneous Transluminal Angioplasty. *AJR* 1981, 137:599–601.

2. Pickering TG, Sos TA, Vaughan ED Jr, *et al.*: Predictive Value and Changes of Renin Secretion in Hypertensive Patients with Unilateral Renovascular Disease Undergoing Successful Renal Angioplasty. *Am J Med* 1984, 76:398.

3.• Vaughan ED Jr, Buhler FR, Laragh JH, *et al.*: Renovascular Hypertension: Renin Measurements to Indicate Hypersecretion and Contralateral Suppression, Estimate Renal Plasma Flow, and Score for Surgical Curability. *Am J Med* 1973, 55:402.
Good description of the value of selective renal vein renin analysis.

4. Cope C: Suture Technique to Reshape the Sidewinder Catheter Curve. *J Interv Radiol* 1986, 63–64.

5. Katzen BT, Chang J, Knox WG: Percutaneous Transluminal Angioplasty with the Gruntzig Balloon Catheter: A Review of 70 Cases. *Arch Surg* 1979, 114:1389–1399.

6. Hessel SJ, Adams DF, Abrams HL: Complications of Angiography. *Radiology* 1981, 138:273–281.

7.•• Tegtmeyer CJ, Sos TA: Techniques of Renal Angioplasty. *Radiology* 1986, 161:577–586.
Excellent discussion of the basic techniques of renal angioplasty.

8. Khilnani NM, Trost D, *et al.*: Multisidehole Catheter Technique for Selective Over-The-Wire Completion Angiography Following Renal Angioplasty. *JVIR* 1994, 5:387–389.

9. Tegtmeyer CJ: Atherectomy and Renal Artery Stenosis (abstract). Presented at IV Course on Vascular and Interventional Radiology as a Therapeutic Alternative. Las Palmas, Spain, 1994.

10. Sos TA: Renal Artery Occlusions and Stenosis: Thrombolysis in Conjunction with Angioplasty. Presented at Sixth Biennial Oakwood Hospital Winter Imaging Conference. Steamboat Springs, CO, 1991.

11. Kandarpa K, Drinker PA, Singer SJ, Cararamore D: Forceful Pulsatile Local Infusion of Enzyme Accelerates Thrombolysis: *In Vivo* Evaluation of a New Delivery System. *Radiology* 1988, 168:739–744.

12. Flory CM: Arterial Occlusions Produced by Emboli From Eroded Aortic Atheromatous Plaques. *Am J Pathol* 1945, 21:549–565.

13. Fuks DF, Griguoli RE, Borracci RA, Sala C: Cholesterol Embolization Following Coronary Angioplasty. *Rev Port Cardiol* 1992, 11:1089–1091.

14. Hollier LH, Kazimer FJ, Ochsner J, *et al.*: "Shaggy" Aorta Syndrome with Atheromatous Embolization to Visceral Vessels. *Ann Vasc Surg* 1991, 5:439–444.

15. Cohan RH, Dunnick NR: Intravascular Contrast Media: Adverse Reactions. *AJR* 1987, 149:665–670.

16. Parfrey PS, Griffiths SM, Barrett BJ, *et al.*: Contrast Material Induced Renal Failure in Patients with Diabetes Mellitus, Renal Insufficiency, Or Both: A Prospective Controlled Study. *N Engl J Med* 1989, 320:143–149.

17. Cruz C, Hricak H, Samhouri F, *et al.*: Contrast Media for Angiography: Effect on Renal Function. *Radiology* 1986, 158:109–112.

18. Sos TA, Pickering TG, Sniderman KW, *et al.*: Percutaneous Transluminal Renal Angioplasty in Renovascular Hypertension Due to Atheroma or Fibromuscular Dysplasia. *N Engl J Med* 1983, 309:274–279.

19. Schwarten DE: Transluminal Angioplasty of Renal Artery Stenosis: 70 Experiences. *AJR* 1980, 135:969–974.

20. Tegtmeyer CJ, Kellum CD, Ayers C: Percutaneous Transluminal Angioplasty of the Renal Artery. *Radiology* 1984, 153:77–84.

21. Martin LG, Price RB, Casarella WJ, *et al.*: Percutaneous Angioplasty in the Clinical Management of Renovascular Hypertension: Initial and Long Term Results. *Radiology* 1985, 155:629–633.

22.• Martin LG, Cork RD, Kaufman SL: Long-Term Results of Angioplasty in 110 Patients with Renal Artery Stenosis. *JVIR* 1992, 3:619–626.

The only published study that specifically discusses ostial renal stenoses.

23.• Rousseau H, Joffre F: Stents in Renal Arteries: Long Term Follow-Up with the Wallstent (abstract). Presented at IV Course on Vascular and Interventional Radiology as a Therapeutic Alternative. Las Palmas, Spain, 1994.

Preliminary data involving the long-term follow-up of the Wallstent in renal arteries.

Select Bibliography

Martin LG, Cork RD, Kaufman SL: Long-Term Results of Angioplasty in 110 Patients with Renal Artery Stenosis. *JVIR* 1992, 13:619–626.

Sos TA, Pickering TG, Phil D, *et al.*: Percutaneous Transluminal Angioplasty in Renovascular Hypertension Due to Atheroma or Fibromuscular Dysplasia. *N Engl J Med* 1983, 309:274–279.

Tegtmeyer CJ, Kellum CD, Ayers C: Percutaneous Transluminal Angioplasty of the Renal Artery. Results and Long Term Follow-up. *Radiology* 1984, 153:77–84.

Tegtmeyer CJ, Sos TA: Techniques of Renal Angioplasty. *Radiology* 1986, 161:577–586.

Review of Devices for Percutaneous Thrombectomy

Jim A. Reekers

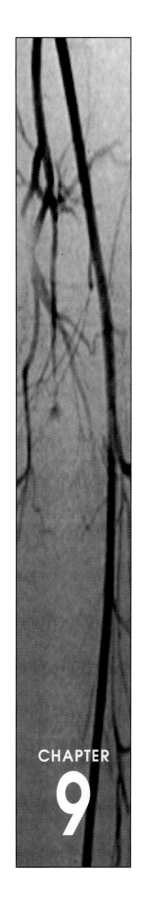

Surgical removal of thrombus from occluded vessels or grafts below the inguinal ligament has a history of more than 30 years. Fogarty and colleagues [1] described this technique for the first time in 1963. Although the technique has been practiced worldwide, the basics for the use of the Fogarty balloon (Baxter Healthcare, Santa Ana, CA) have not changed during these past three decades. In early years, approximately 80% of the acute occlusions below the ligament could be attributed to emboli from a cardiac source. More recently, successful treatment of rheumatic valve disease has changed the etiology of acute vascular occlusion from embolic to arterial thrombosis.

Acute thrombosis in a native vessel is mainly caused by atherosclerosis or stenosis, whereas acute occlusion of a bypass graft is often attributed to a local stenotic lesion. In both native vessels and grafts, the primary therapy before treatment of the underlying pathology is removal of the thrombus. To remove the thrombus, the use of a Fogarty balloon should not be the first treatment of choice because it provides incomplete restoration of flow and can cause significant damage to the intima. Local pharmacologic lysis is the current state-of-the-art technique to treat acute and fresh thrombus below the inguinal ligament. The thrombolytic agent is infused slowly into the clot through a small percutaneous catheter. The main problem with this technique is the prolonged infusion time (sometimes lasting more than 36 hours), which may not be tolerated in patients with a limb at risk. Prolonged infusion time can lead to a systemic lytic effect and an increased risk of bleeding complications. The use of these expensive thrombolytic drugs and the need for patients to be observed in an intensive care unit makes this therapy very costly.

The pulsed-spray lysis technique, first described by Bookstein and colleagues [2] in 1989, can reduce the infusion time considerably (to approximately 1.5 to 2 hours), although not all investigators can produce these results. With this technique, serious bleeding complications were seen in 4% of patients and distal embolization of clot was seen in 10% of patients [3]. For this reason, some authors prefer the conventional local low-flow technique over the more aggressive pulsed-spray technique [4].

A technique that reduces the time to remove or debulk thrombus to only a few minutes and alleviates the necessity of thrombolytic drugs could solve many of the current problems related to lysis.

Theoretically, mechanical removal of thrombus by suction or aspiration is the technique to achieve this goal. Aspiration catheters have been used for treatment of thromboembolic disease for almost 10 years [5]. During the past 7 years, new mechanical devices have been described, many of which have not yet surfaced into clinical practice. They must be simple, safe, and effective to be accepted for clinical use. The percutaneous devices for thrombectomy that are discussed here are relatively new and have shown promising first clinical results.

Experimental Devices

A number of experimental devices for mechanical removal of thrombus have been reported. The Trac-Wright catheter, (Dow Corning Wright, Miami Lakes, FL) formerly known as the Kensey catheter, and the transluminal extraction catheter (TEC) (Interventional Technologies, San Diego, CA) have been used with some success for the removal of thrombus in both animals and humans. These devices were not originally designed for this purpose and have only casuistic importance in mechanical percutaneous thrombectomy.

Two other devices specifically designed for percutaneous thrombectomy have been described by Schmitz-Rode and colleagues [6]. They are the ultrasound-driven, oscillating-probe aspiration thrombectomy device and the electric motor–driven version. The ultrasound-driven device consists of a ball-tipped metal probe of 55-cm length and 1-mm diameter, connected to a piezo-ceramic transducer that provides longitudinal oscillations of the probe with an amplitude of 30 um at a frequency of 27 KHz. The probe is inserted into an 8-French straight catheter so that the ball protrudes 4 mm from the catheter tip. Intermittent suction is applied at the proximal end of the catheter by a roller pump with a maximum suction pressure of -600 mm Hg.

The electric motor–driven device consists of a metal probe with a 0.5-mm diameter that oscillates at a frequency of 40 Hz. All other components are similar to the ultrasound-driven device except that this device has a straight- and an angulated-tip version. Both devices were tested in a hemodialysis graft model. They were able to restore the lumen continuity in 1 to 5 minutes with 10% to 30% wall-adherent residual thrombus. Until now, no *in vivo* evaluation of these devices has been reported.

Clinical Devices

Currently, there are three devices that have been used clinically and that may be of future importance in the treatment of fresh arterial thrombotic occlusion below the inguinal ligament in both grafts and native vessels. These are the rheolytic thrombectomy catheter (Possis Medical, Minneapolis, MN), the Amplatz mechanical thrombectomy device (Microvena, Vadnais Heights, MN), and the Hydrolyser catheter (Cordis, Roden, The Netherlands).

THE RHEOLYTIC THROMBECTOMY CATHETER

A prototype of the system was first described in 1991 by Drasler and colleagues [7•]. The improved version of the rheolytic thrombectomy catheter consists of a 5-French dual lumen tubing (Fig 9-1). The smaller lumen contains a high-pressure stainless-steel tubing used to supply high-pressure water jets. The jets are oriented such that direct close-range impingement onto the vessel wall is avoided and thrombus is removed from the vessel wall primarily by fluid mixing and recirculation. One jet is directed toward the catheter's large lumen to promote the evacuation of debris.

The remnant thrombus particles then pass into a second larger lumen provided for the evacuation of debris.

To operate the catheter, a special pump is required to achieve the pressure of 10,000 psi required to remove the thrombus. The exhaust lumen is operated by a roller pump. This device can be applied in vessels between 6 and 9 mm in diameter. The catheter is flexible and can follow a 0.0018-inch guidewire. *In vitro* testing of the device demonstrated a prompt removal of fresh thrombus with little to no vessel wall damage. Concurrent removal of thrombotic debris, achieved during fragmentation of the thrombus, is a definite advantage of this device which is provided without a thrombectomy catheter. However, there are no reported *in vitro* studies on distal embolization with the use of this device.

Clinical Experience

To date, there has been limited reported clinical experience with only three patients having been treated with

this device—two in native vessels and one in a femoropopliteal graft [8]. In all three patients, a partial thrombolysis was seen, but two of these patients eventually required a secondary surgical intervention. No distal embolization was observed in any of these patients. Residual thrombus with this device currently remains a clinical problem.

THE AMPLATZ MECHANICAL THROMBECTOMY DEVICE

The catheter is 100-cm long and 8-French in size [9]. At the distal tip is a 1-cm, open-ended metal capsule with two sideholes. The capsule contains a rapidly spinning helical screw propeller. Torque to the helix is transmitted by a cable-driven air motor at approximately 100,000 rpm. The mode of action of this device is identical to that of a blender; the sideholes allow the material to recycle (Fig. 9-2). There is a direct relation

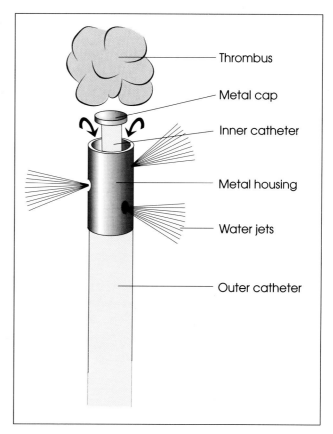

FIGURE 9-1.

The 5-French rheolytic thrombectomy catheter. The catheter tip is shown with three shooting jets of water. These jets create a stagnation pressure that forces the thrombotic debris out through the effluent lumen.

between the speed of rotation and the time needed to achieve dissolution of the thrombotic material. In essence, this device resembles a Kensey catheter (Dow Corning Wright, Miami Lakes, FL), but has a distal housing. It cannot be inserted over a guidewire. The outflow distal to the diseased vessel must be interrupted by a blood-pressure cuff downstream. After the procedure and prior to releasing the compressing cuff, the fragmented residue must be aspirated. It is assumed that small resdiual particles will not produce any clinical sequelae, although there is no real evidence to verify this assumption.

Clinical Experience

In a recent publication by Coleman and colleagues [10], five patients were included in a study of this device. Two patients had occluded lower-extremity synthetic grafts and three patients had occluded native superficial femoral arteries. The duration of clinical occlusion was 2 days to 2 weeks. An 8- or 9- French introducer sheath was used. A blood-pressure cuff was placed on the proximal calf and inflated to 20 mm Hg above systolic pressure to prevent distal embolization of particulate matter. After the thrombus was homogenized, an 8- or 9-French large-bore guiding catheter was advanced to aspirate the macerated clot. The blood-pressure cuff was then deflated. Thrombus could be completely removed in the two bypass grafts and in one native vessel. In the two other native vessels, thrombus was only partially removed. It is important that the thrombus be fresh for adequate mechanical maceration. This device is less efficacious when the clot becomes partially adherent to the vessel wall. The main limitation of this device is that binding of the impeller can cause breakage of the unit cable (in this small series, the cable broke in two cases). Another limitation is that it is impossible to perform the procedure from the contralateral side, as it is not an over-the-wire instrument. Although not encountered in this series, the potential risk of distal embolization of particles is worrisome. More clinical investigations must be performed before the true clinical value of this device can be established.

THE HYDROLYSER CATHETER

The Hydrolyser catheter is a 65-cm long, straight, 7-French double lumen catheter, with a 6-mm, oval-shaped sidehole located 4 mm from the closed distal tip (suction nozzle) [11•]. The catheter is made of nylon, has a stiff body, and the closed distal tip of the catheter is round. The Hydrolyser accepts a 0.0025-inch guidewire and is introduced through a 7-French sheath. Using a conventional contrast injector, 150 mL of physiologic saline is injected through the 0.6-mm diameter supply (injection) channel at 4 mL/s and 750 psi (Fig. 9-3). Due to the resultant pressure reduction (Venturi effect) at the catheter tip, thrombus is sucked toward the sidehole, fragmented, and removed as a mixture of thrombotic material and physiologic saline through the second larger (1-mm radius) exhaust lumen into a collection bag (Fig 9-4 and Fig. 9-5). *In vitro* experiments demonstrate that the volume of fluid removed is approximately equal to the volume injected; this means there is no overload danger.

Clinical Experience

In the past 12 months we have treated 28 patients with arterial thrombus below the infraguinal ligament with the Hydrolyser catheter [12•]. There were 11 native vessels and 17 bypass grafts. The estimated mean age of the thrombus 12 days (range of 1 to 68 days). Mean length of the thrombus was 33 cm (range of 8 to 65 cm); in seven patients, the thrombus also occluded the outflow arteries.

The Hydrolyser Technique

Infrainguinal arterial thrombosis is usually approached through an ipsilateral antegrade common femoral puncture; in two of our patients, a contralateral puncture was used. Thereafter, a 0.035-inch guidewire was

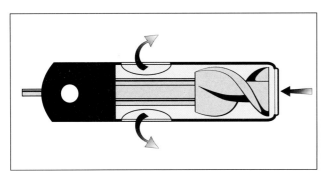

FIGURE 9-2.

The Amplatz thrombectomy catheter tip. Note the tip has no exposed cutting edges (*arrow*). Its recirculation systems reduces significant blood loss and the infusion sideholes allow the injection of contrast or thrombolytic agents (*curved arrows*).

passed through the thrombus. If there was no passage of the wire through the occlusion, thrombosuction was not attempted. When the guidewire traversed the thrombotic occlusion, a 7-French vascular sheath was placed in the common femoral artery and 5000 units of heparin administered intra-arterially. The Hydrolyser catheter was then advanced through the sheath and positioned 2 cm proximal to the thrombus; clot fragmentation was activated by the injection of saline through the smaller catheter lumen with the aid of a standard mechanical contrast injector. After a 6-second delay (the time between the initiation of the injection and the moment of effective funtioning), the catheter was slowly and steadily advanced through the thrombus at a rate of approximately 1 cm/s. After each run of 150 mL of saline, the catheter was withdrawn from within the clot and a control angiogram performed through the sideport of the sheath (Figs. 9-6 and Figs. 9-7). The fluid balance was controlled by checking the volume in the collection bag. This

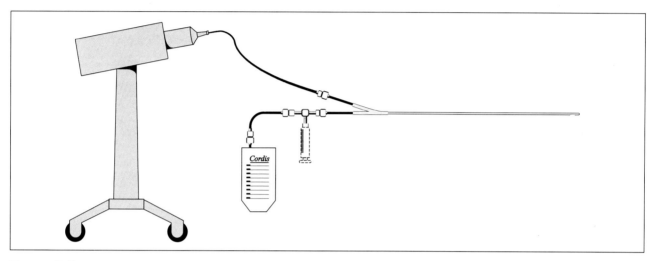

FIGURE 9-3.

Proper connection of the Hydrolyser catheter. The small injection lumen is connected to a standard-power contrast injector. The syringe is filled with saline.

Settings are 750 psi and 4 mL/s at maximum syringe volume. The larger exhaust lumen is connected to a collection bag.

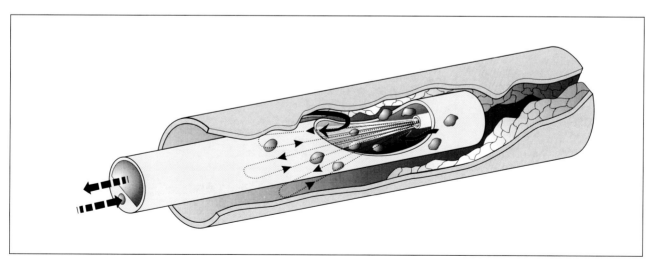

FIGURE 9-4.

The tip of the Hydrolyser catheter. The broken arrows indicate the injection lumen ($\rightarrow$) and the exhaust lumen ($\leftarrow$).

Within the nozzle, suction, fragmentation, and removal of thrombus occurs as a result of the local Venturi effect.

ensured no danger of fluid overload. The procedure was repeated until all thrombus was removed or no further improvement seen.

The overall initial thrombectomy result of the Hydrolyser catheter was 82.2% in the treated segment (72.7% for native vessels and 88.2% for synthetic or composite grafts). In three patients, there was residual thrombus of more than 10%. In two patients, the Hydrolyser was not able to remove any thrombus, although there was easy guidewire passage. In both patients, the clinical history of vascular occlusion was older than 14 days.

To achieve the above results, a mean of 4.2 runs was required. The underlying vascular stenosis was treated by percutaneous transluminal angioplasty (PTA) (n=17), PTA and stenting (n=5), and local surgical revision (n=1). Three patients did not require any local therapy after thrombosuction. Seven patients were also treated with additional lysis for thrombus below the popliteal trifurcation (local low-dose urokinase, 50,000 units/h with systemic intravenous heparin).

The overall clinical result showed improvement in 67.9%, no change in 28.6%, and worsening of complaints in 3.6% (1 patient). When assessed per vessel type, there was 81.8% improvement for the native vessels and 58.8% for the grafts. In two patients, proximal displacement of thrombotic material was seen at the beginning of the procedure, whereas distal embolization of thrombotic material was seen in five patients (17.9%). All but one of these complications were successfully treated in the same session by standard percutaneous procedures.

The distal embolization of thrombotic material was only seen in graft-related procedures and never in

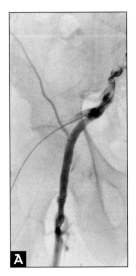 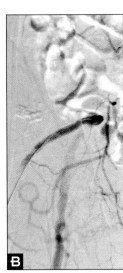 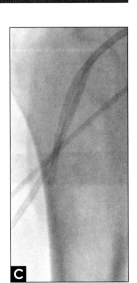 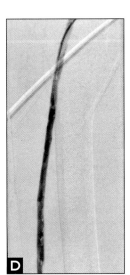 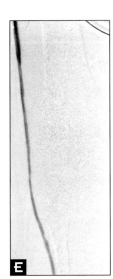

FIGURE 9-5.

The Hydrolyser with water jet action.

FIGURE 9-6.

A 72-year-old man with acute occlusion of an iliac-crural venous composite graft. The graft is tunneled subcutaneous. The patient presented with critical ischemia for 1 day. There are no longer pulsations of the graft. **A**, Direct retrograde puncture in the graft shows the occlusion of the graft and a patent deep femoral artery. **B**, The thrombectomy of the promixal part of the graft, shown after one run with the Hydrolyser catheter. **C**, A second antegrade puncture in the graft performed with a 7-French sheath. **D**, Complete thrombectomy of the graft after two Hydrolyser runs. **E**, A satisfactory distal result after PTA of a local stenosis.

thrombosed native vessels. Thrombectomy was achieved in 17 of 28 patients (60.8%) using only the Hydrolyser; in the remaining 11 of 28 patients (39.2%), local lysis was used in addition. The initial problems of distal and proximal migration of clot fragments encountered with the Hydrolyser were related to the way the procedure was first performed, at which time we neglected to position the device 2 cm proximal to the thrombus and did not ensure a good inflow to the treated vessel. The current limitation of this device is that it can only be used in vessels between 5 mm and 9 mm in diameter. Although the initial peripheral embolization can most likely be attributed to initial incorrect technique, some concern still remains.

Recent clinical experience with this device in thrombosed hemodialysis grafts by Vorwerk and colleagues (unpublished data) also shows very promising results.

Special Devices

There are two devices for local thrombectomy that are limited to the iliofemoral vein and the inferior vena cava because of their large 12-French diameter.

The Ponomar transjugular clot-trapper device consists of a 12-French double lumen catheter that necessitates a venous cutdown in the right internal jugular vein for introduction of a 18-French sheath [13]. The smaller channel extends 15 cm beyond the distal catheter end and contains a stainless-steel wire whose distal end emerges at a 90° angle to the shaft. The loop is attached to the distal end of a 15-cm long funnel-shaped polyvinyl bag. The proximal end of the bag can be opened or closed by advancing or retracting the wire. The thrombus is fed into the opening of the bag with an occlusion balloon. Once the thrombus is trapped in the bag, the balloon is deflated, withdrawn, and the bag is closed. The first preliminary *in vitro* and *in vivo* results are encouraging.

The saline-jet aspiration thrombectomy catheter (Clinical Supply, Hajima, Japan) has also been developed for the treatment of large thrombi in the central veins [14]. The catheter consists of two tubes. A 75-cm long outer tube with a 4-mm diameter is distally tapered to 3.3 mm, and a 1.3-mm inner tube is bent 180° at the distal end to created a proximally directed nozzle. The distal 10 cm of the inner tube are tapered to 1.0 mm, and

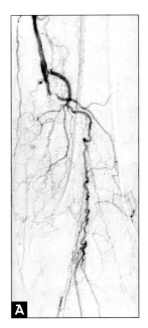 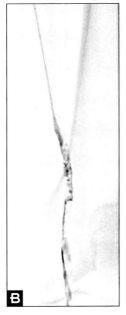 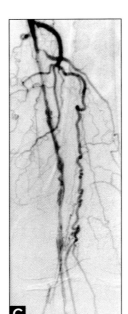 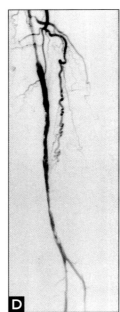 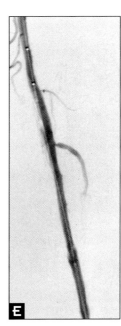

FIGURE 9-7.

A 68-year-old man presented with acute restpain lasting 4 days. The patient had a previous history of mild claudication with a walking distance of 300 m. **A**, Occlusion of the popliteal artery with collaterals. **B**, Fresh thrombus in the popliteal artery. **C**, Popliteal artery thrombus after one run with the Hydrolyser catheter. **D**, The end result after three runs with the Hydrolyser. There was no change in condition after one additional run. This was considered to be the endpoint for thrombectomy. **E**, Successful angiographic result and good flow after PTA and a proximal Palmatz stent. The patient became clinically asymptomatic.

the diameter of the nozzle is 0.6 mm. The nozzle is 2 mm proximal to the tip of the catheter. Saline is injected under pressure to the inner tube with the use of a power injector. The maximum flow rate of saline at the inner tube is 9 mL/s. The negative pressure generated at the distal end of the outer tube causes the clot to be aspirated and flushed out with the aid of the saline jet. One patient with inferior vena cava thrombosis has been reportedly treated with this device. Restoration of flow was re-established after two sessions; however, significant blood loss of 1090 mL occurred. The tip of the catheter must be in direct contact with the thrombus to avoid significant blood loss.

Conclusion

Although both continuous-drip infusion and pulsed-spray pharmacomechanic thrombolysis work well,

a safe and effective method of rapid thrombolysis can shorten costs, angiographic room-time, and inpatient hospital days. For this reason, mechanical methods of thrombolysis offer a promising area. The three clinical devices that have been described all have this potential but also show the need for modification to increase their safety. The optimal device must be safe, effective, and easily incorporated into a standard interventional procedure without too much cost and time increase. Based on current experience, the Hydrolyser catheter, which consists of a standard 7-French catheter and operates only with a standard-power contrast injector without any extra hardware, is the device that has the potential to match these goals.

Although clinical testing will continue to determine the future role of these devices, it is anticipated that new concepts will emerge to meet this challenge.

References and Recommended Reading

Recently published papers of particular interest have been highlighted as:

• Of interest

•• Of outstanding interest

1. Fogarty TJ, Cranley JJ, Krause RJ, *et al.*: A Method for Extraction of Arterial Emboli and Thrombi. *Surg Gynecol Obstet* 1963, 116:241.

2. Bookstein JJ, Fellmeth B, Roberts A, *et al.*: Pulsed-Spray Pharmacomechanical Thrombolysis: Preliminary Clinical Results. *AJR* 1989, 152:1097–1100.

3. Valji K, Roberts A, Davis GB, Bookstein JJ: Pulsed-Spray Thrombolysis of Arterial and Bypass Graft Occlusions. *AJR* 1991, 156:617–621.

4. LeBlang SD, Becker GJ, Benenati JF, *et al.*: Low-Dose Urokinase Regimen for the Treatment of Lower Extremity Arterial and Graft Occlusions: Experience in 132 Cases. *JVIR* 1992, 3:475–483.

5. Starck EE, McDermott JC, Crummy AB, *et al.*: Percutaneous Aspiration Thromboembolectomy. *Radiology* 1985, 156:61–66.

6. Schmitz-Rode T, Pfeffer JG, Bohnderf K, Gunther RW: Percutaneous Thrombectomy of Acute Thrombosed Dialysis Grafts: *In Vitro* Evaluation of Four Devices. *Cardiovasc Intervent Radiol* 1993, 16:72–75.

7.• Drasler WJ, Jenson ML, Wilson GJ, *et al.*: Rheolytic Catheter for Percutaneous Removal of Thrombus. *Radiology* 1992, 182:263–267.
This article describes the initial model and the proposed indications for the rheolytic catheter.

8. Becker GJ: Initial Results with a Rheolytic Thrombectomy Catheter for Rapid Thrombolysis (abstract). Presented at the Sixth Annual International Symposium of Vascular Diagnosis and Intervention 1994, 187–188.

9. Bildsoe MC, Moradian GP, Hunter DW, *et al.*: Mechanical Clot Dissolution: New Concept. *Radiology* 1989, 171:233–321.

10. Coleman CC, Krenzel C, Dietz CA, *et al.*: Mechanical Thrombectomy: Results of Early Experience. *Radiology* 1993, 189:803–805.

11.• Reekers JA, Kromhout JG, Van der Waal K: Catheter for Percutaneous Thrombectomy: First Clinical Experience. *Radiology* 1993, 188:871–874.
This study contains the first reported clinical trials and results of the Hydrolyser catheter.

12.• Reekers JA, Spithoven HG, Kromhout JG, *et al.*: Percutaneous Thrombectomy Below the Inguinal Ligament with the Use of the Hydrolyser Catheter (abstract). Presented at the RSNA 1993, 1321C:333.
A most recent trial with the Hydrolyser catheter in patients with arterial thrombosis.

13. Ponomar E, Carlson JE, Kindlund A, *et al.*: Clot-Trapper Device for Transjugular Thrombectomy from the Inferior Vena Cava. *Radiology* 1991, 179:279–282.

14. Yamauchi T, Furui S, Irie T, *et al.*: Acute Thrombosis of the Inferior Vena Cava: Treatment with Saline-Jet Aspiration Thrombectomy Catheter. *AJR* 1993, 161:405–407.

Percutaneous Drainage of Postoperative Intra-abdominal Abscesses and Collections

Dean A. Nakamoto
John R. Haaga

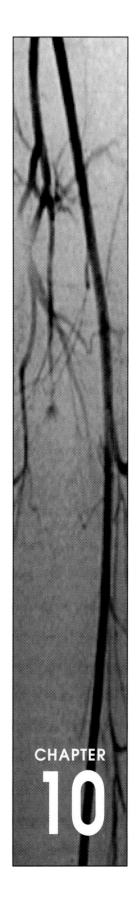

Postoperative, intra-abdominal abscess is a serious surgical complication. Despite modern techniques and the use of antibiotics, mortality rates for intra-abdominal abscess are still as high as 30% [1–5]. Fortunately, the frequency of postoperative, intra-abdominal abscess is low, approximately 3.4% in one series of 499 laparotomies [3]. The management of this complication is controversial because there are many advocates of both percutaneous and surgical drainage. Most authors will agree that simple, unilocular, peripheral abscesses are best managed percutaneously. However, the treatment of the multilocular or complicated abscess is more problematic, particularly in critically ill patients. We advocate a cautious approach and consider each case individually with the referring surgeon. We will aggressively perform diagnostic aspiration of a suspicious fluid collection as there is little risk involved and a sample can almost always be obtained [6]. The decision to proceed to percutaneous drainage is then made in conjunction with the referring surgeon. The goals such as cure, temporization, or palliation are determined. Interdisciplinary cooperation and close follow-up are essential for successful treatment.

The comparative benefits of percutaneous drainage versus operative drainage continue to be debated. Assessment is difficult because the early results of percutaneous drainage have been compared with older surgical techniques not having the benefits of new antibiotics. Most older series do not separate patients based on severity of illness and only few series have long-term follow-up data. Earlier series of percutaneous drainage also used very strict criteria and were often limited to unilocular abscess. The success rates ranged from 82% to 92% [6]. As inclusion criteria expanded to include complex abscesses and critically ill patients, the success rates for percutaneous drainage decreased.

Critics of percutaneous drainage correctly suggest that some cases are not suitable for a nonoperative approach. McLean and colleagues [3] studied 17 consecutive postoperative patients with intra-abdominal abscesses. Three patients were excluded, ie, two with obvious anastomotic dehiscence and one with a retroperitoneal abscess believed inappropriate for percutaneous drainage. The remaining 14 patients were divided between percutaneous drainage and percutaneous drainage with surgery. Only 33% were successfully managed by percutaneous drainage alone. McLean and colleagues' literature review on operative versus percutaneous drainage suggests that the efficacy of percutaneous drainage is only about 30%.

However, several errors have been noted in the McLean review. For example, in their review of Johnson and colleagues [7] who studied 43 operative drainage and 27 percutaneous drainage patients, they indicate that there had been no mention of the number of postoperative abscesses. However, the article reports that 52% of the patients in the percutaneous drainage group were postoperative patients; 60% (26 of 43 patients) were postoperative patients in the surgically drained group.

It is clear that location of abscesses and patient selection influence the success of percutaneous drainage, which may account for different reported outcomes and opinions. In McLean and collegues' review of Deveney and colleagues [8], they state that the location of the abscesses influenced the success of percutaneous drainage. They state that 78% of patients who underwent percutaneous drainage had good risk subphrenic abscesses. In reality, the percentage of subphrenic abscesses was only 48% (14 of 29 patients). Of these 14 patients, 78% were cured by percutaneous drainage. The McLean group also states that 85% of the surgical drainage group had difficult pelvic abscesses. Actually, only 32% (12 of 37 patients) of the surgical group had pelvic abscesses and 85% of those 12 patients were cured by surgical drainage. Therefore, although the two groups are somewhat different, they are much more similar than described by McLean and colleagues. Thus the McLean group properly asserts that abscesses with anastomotic dehiscence are difficult to cure using percutaneous drainage, but probably underestimates the utility of percutaneous drainage when they state that only 30% of the patients with postoperative, intra-abdominal abscess benefited from the percutaneous drainage alone.

Current data suggest that outcomes of percutaneous drainage and operative drainage of postoperative, intra-abdominal abscesses are similar with regard to cure, complications, and mortality rates [4,8,9]. Critical factors include the status of the patient and early accurate localization and drainage; the method of drainage seems less important [10]. Both Hemming and colleagues [9] and Levison and Zeigler [4] used the Acute Physiology and Chronic Health Evaluation (APACHE) II scoring method to assess the severity of illness. This method combines physical examination, complete blood count, arterial blood gas, and electrolyte determination. Also included are patient age and immunodeficiency or chronic organ insufficiency.

When selecting patients or considering results, the physician must also take into account the patient's clinical and immune status. Hemming and colleagues [9] examined 83 patients; 41 had operative drainage and 42 had percutaneous drainage. The groups were matched for age and abscess location. Although percentages of postoperative abscesses are not known, the abscesses were similar in etiology. The APACHE II scores did not differ significantly between the two groups. Morbidity was similar—26% complications for operative drainage and 29% for percutaneous drainage. The mortality rates were also similar at 14% for operative drainage and 12% for percutaneous drainage. However, those patients who died had significantly higher APACHE II scores, regardless of the drainage method. Levison and Zeigler [4] studied 91 patients with postoperative, intra-abdominal abscesses. Forty-five patients had percutaneous drainage and 46 patients had operative drainage. Again, these groups were similar with respect to age, abscess location, severity of illness, percent mortality, and percent success. There was no difference for multiloculated abscess, multiple abscesses, or abscesses with enteric communication. In Levison and Zeigler's study [4], patients grouped according to their APACHE II scores had significant differences in mortality rates. Using a cut-off score of 15, there was only one death in the group of patients with a score below 15 (1.7% mortality rate). In those patients with scores of 15 or greater, the mortality rate was 78%. Lambiase and colleagues [11••] reviewed 335 consecutive abscesses and found an overall cure rate of 62.4%. However, when they studied the immune status of their patients, there was a significant difference in cure rates. The immuno-compromised patient population that represented 53.1% of the total patients studied had a cure rate of 53.4% (95 of 178 abscesses), compared with the immunocompetent patients who had a cure rate of 72.6% (114 of 157 abscesses). Included in the immunocompromised population were patients with absolute neutropenia (< 500 granulocytes per µL), cancer with distant metastases, local disease with complications requiring surgery, chemotherapy or radiation therapy, diabetes, splenectomy, HIV, and others. These data suggest that the status of the patient determines the probability of cure, regardless of whether an operative or percutaneous drainage procedure is performed.

In reality, to compare percutaneous drainage with surgical drainage one must remember that percutaneous drainage is a nonsurgical procedure requiring only local anesthesia. This suggests that if percutaneous drainage can be performed, it is worthwhile to

attempt in order to avoid a second operation with the inherent risk of anesthesia on a postoperative patient. As more and more complicated abscesses are drained percutaneously in critically ill patients, one would expect the success rate to decline. A final point related to economics is also relevant. Although no cost analysis has been made, it is more likely that percutaneous procedures would be more cost effective because of the absence of surgical intervention.

Diagnostic Aspiration

Infected fluid collections in postoperative patients may or may not produce the typical signs and symptoms of infection. Because such collections can usually be aspirated without significant risk, we aggressively obtain samples if there is any clinical concern for infection. We have aspirated more than 500 collections with no secondary infection and only one with hematoma as a complication [6]. To sample these collections, it is important to avoid traversing bowel loops and normal organs. If the liver is involved, then the cuff of the normal tissue should be included before entering the collection.

If the aspirated fluid appears clear, we usually send a small sample for culture and leave most of the fluid in the collection. If the sample turns out to be culture-positive, the collection is then re-entered and drained. If the aspirated fluid is slightly turbid or only questionably infected, a drainage catheter may be left after consultation with the referring surgeon. If the cultures are negative after 48 hours, the catheter can be withdrawn.

Patient Selection
As previously noted, the indications for percutaneous drainage are expanding. Patients with loculated abscesses, abscesses with enteric communication, or multiple abscesses are now candidates for percutaneous drainage [12]. Not only are patients referred for cure, but also for temporization or palliation to reduce toxic load [13].

However, some abscesses may require operative drainage. These include fungal abscesses, infected hematomas, abscesses with anastomotic dehiscence or larger enteric communication, most pancreatic abscesses, and failed percutaneous drainages [6,14,15]. A drainage is a failure if there is an incomplete response, such as persistent sepsis, in the 2 to 4 days following percutaneous drainage. In such cases surgical intervention or a second percutaneous drainage must be considered [14,15].

Abscess Drainage

The following are the steps for percutaneous abscess drainage:

1) Abscess detection
2) Trajectory planning
3) Selection of guidance modality
4) Diagnostic aspiration
5) Catheter selection and insertion
6) Sinogram and catheter adjustment
7) Catheter management and irrigation
8) Follow-up diagnostic evaluation
9) Catheter removal

Although any modality may be used to detect an abscess and guide the aspiration, most physicians agree that computed tomography (CT) is the modality of choice [1,2,6,11••,16,17], particularly in complicated cases. The trajectory should be carefully planned to avoid bowel loops, uninvolved organs, and uninvolved body cavities not crossing the diaphragm. The catheter should traverse the entire length of the abscess. Patient positioning is also important. For example, some fluid collections are better approached with the patient in a decubitus position, which may allow the colon to shift out of the planned needle pathway. Changing patient position also helps to determine if fluid collections are loculated or actually free (Fig. 10-1). In addition, unlike surgical drainage where an extraperitoneal approach is preferred for an intraperitoneal process, a peritoneal

approach can be used with proper technique. The potential for contamination is minimal because only the puncture site and tube tract are exposed to potential pathogens, unlike a wide area of peritoneum in an open surgical procedure [6].

As stated before, we are very aggressive with diagnostic aspiration of suspicious fluid collections. Typically, a 19-gauge needle with an 18-gauge teflon sheath (Longdwel catheter; Becton, Dickenson & Co, Rutherford, NJ) is used. The 18-gauge sheath permits easier aspiration of thick fluid. Again, collections that appear clear and not obviously purulent should only have a small amount of fluid aspirated; aspiration of the entire collection is not recommended as there will be no later target should the fluid have a positive culture result.

If the fluid appears purulent, a standard, 0.035-inch angiographic guidewire can be advanced into the abscess cavity through the 18-gauge teflon sheath. A modified Seldinger technique can then be performed to introduce a 5-French, angiographic pigtail catheter (Cook, Bloomington, IN) into the cavity over the guidewire.

When draining abscesses, we use either angiographic catheters or single-step catheters on trocars. The 8.3-French, single-step trocar catheters (Medi-Tech, Watertown, MA) are ideal for large, peripheral abscesses. However, for small abscesses or those located in critical areas, a two-step procedure may be preferable using the modified Seldinger technique with introduction of a guidewire into the abscess, followed

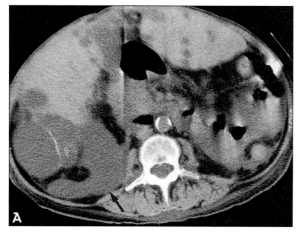 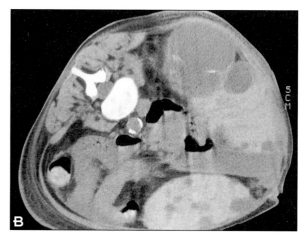

Figure 10-1.

A, This patient, who is status post-bilateral nephrectomy for autosomal, dominant polycystic kidney disease, had a suspicious fluid collection in the right renal fossa (*arrow*) seen on the supine examination. Multiple liver cysts are also identified. **B**, When the patient was placed in the left-lateral decubitus position, the fluid flowed freely out of the right renal fossa and toward the dependent left side. Thus the fluid represented ascites, not a loculated collection. This fluid was subsequently aspirated; however, no drainage catheter was placed.

by catheter insertion over the guidewire. The small catheter can subsequently be up-sized to an 8- to 14-French self-retaining catheter in 2 to 3 days following a sinogram. Larger catheters (8- to 14-French in size) are preferred, as these drain abscesses more quickly. Because the entire length of an abscess should be covered, multiple catheters may be necessary. If the abscess cavity contains loculations, we do not advocate the mechanical disruption of the septae because of concern regarding spreading infection or sepsis. We prefer to use injected fibrinolytics in such situations.

To check drainage progress, sinograms are performed initially from 48 to 72 hours, then every 4 to 5 days thereafter. If catheter output suddenly stops, a sinogram should be performed to determine catheter location (as it may have become dislodged from the abscess cavity) and to check for patency and possible catheter kinking.

For most abscesses, gravity drainage is sufficient as the fluid flows out the path of least resistance. Active suction is usually not required unless there is communication to the bowel or biliary system. In such situations, several catheters (as large as possible) may be needed. To keep the catheter patent, approximately 10 mL of saline are injected every 6 to 8 hours. For thick, purulent material or for an abscess with septations, urokinase can be instilled for 3 to 4 days.

The catheter can be removed when the cavity heals. As the abscess heals, the amount of drainage decreases and gradually becomes sterile and serous in character. On sinograms, the cavity appears smooth and small. A second CT scan should be obtained prior to catheter removal to verify that no other undrained abscess collections exist.

COMPLICATIONS AND FAILURES

The complication rates usually vary from 5.9% to 13% [11••,15,17]. One of the most common complications reported by Lambiase and collegues [11••] is sepsis (4.2%) that can be treated with antibiotics. Other complications include hemorrhage, traversing normal bowel or pleura, and catheter-placement errors.

Abscess Drainage by Location

Abscess drainage can be classified by specific location. Because postoperative abscesses, especially intra-abdominal abscess, are relatively rare, data on specific locations are not abundant. However, based on experience and trends in the literature, certain principles are apparent.

INTRAPERITONEAL ABSCESSES

We include subphrenic, subhepatic, omental bursa, and pericolonic abscesses in this category. Percutaneous drainage of subphrenic abscesses has a very high success rate of nearly 80% [6,11••]. It is important to avoid the diaphragmatic pleura and to insert a catheter (as large as possible) at the most inferior aspect of the collection. The approach should be anterior or midaxillary; a posterior approach is less desirable because of the location of the diaphragmatic slips. A patient can also be placed with the abscess in the nondependent position which will accentuate the intrathoracic space (Fig. 10-2).

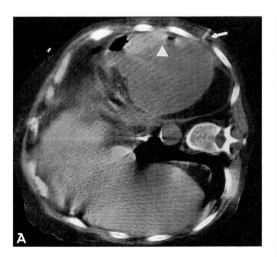
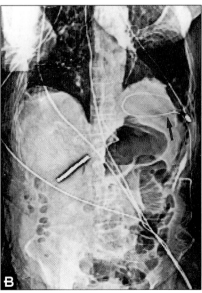

FIGURE 10-2.

A, This patient is status post-splenectomy and distal pancreatectomy with development of a left subphrenic or splenic-bed abscess. The abscess was aspirated (*arrow*) and drained with the patient in the right-lateral decubitus position, which exaggerates the left thoracic space. This position helps to ensure that the placement of the catheter is below the diaphragmatic insertion. Because the patient's splenic flexure of the colon (*arrowhead*) was located adjacent to the splenic bed, the approach was more posterior than is usually necessary. **B,** Note the drainage tube on the topogram (*arrow*) in the left upper quadrant.

It is also important to check contiguous areas, (subhepatic and pericolonic spaces) which may also be involved and may require additional drainage catheters.

The right subhepatic space can be approached laterally or posterolaterally, avoiding the colon, gallbladder, and duodenum. The left subhepatic space is best approached anteriorly between the stomach and the liver.

Fluid collections in the omental bursa or lesser sac can be drained using several approaches, depending on the fluid location. Fluid in the inferior recesses can be drained via an anterior approach inferior to the greater curve of the stomach. Fluid in the splenic portion of the lesser sac can be drained via an antero-lateral approach through the gastrosplenic ligament. Any varices must be identified and avoided. Other approaches include the transgastric route, preferably through a percutaneous endoscopic gastrostomy (PEG), or less desirably, the transhepatic approach. Traversing a normal liver to drain an abscess is not an optimal approach because of possible tracking of purulent material. However, other physicians have recommended this method [17].

The pericolonic areas are usually best approached laterally. It is important for the catheter to traverse the entire length of the abscess, using two catheters if necessary (Fig. 10-3).

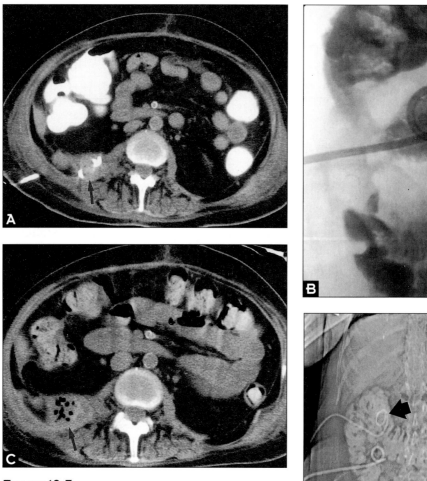

FIGURE 10-3.

A, This patient is status postrenal and pancreas transplant, and subsequently developed a right paracolic abscess. This was drained from a lateral approach (*arrow*). B, On sinogram, this abscess had a communication to the small bowel. Note filling of the large cavity in the superior aspect of the abscess (*arrow*). C and D, The superior cavity of the collection (*arrow*) did not decrease in size, and a second catheter was placed (*arrowhead*).

LIVER ABSCESSES

Liver abscesses are best drained using the shortest possible trajectory, yet including a cuff of normal liver to prevent spillage of purulent material into the peritoneum. Such abscesses should be approached anteriorly or laterally to avoid traversing the diaphragm. Any visible vessels or bile ducts should be avoided (Fig. 10-4).

Liver abscesses with communication to the intrahepatic biliary system appear to respond well to percutaneous drainage and require no special techniques [11••]. However, those abscesses with communication to the extrahepatic biliary system may require biliary diversion in addition to percutaneous abscess drainage [11••].

RETROPERITONEAL ABSCESSES

Intrarenal abscesses and abscesses in the para- and perirenal spaces can be drained using a posterolateral approach, avoiding the erector spinal muscles. The retroperitoneal spaces extend from the diaphragm to the pelvis; the catheter should extend the entire length of the cavity. CT should be used to monitor for any undrained areas.

PELVIC ABSCESSES

Pelvic abscesses are best approached anteriorly or laterally [6]. However, deep pelvic abscesses may not be accessible from these routes. Some physicians have used the sciatic notch for deep abscesses. Although this may be satisfactory for biopsies or diagnostic aspiration, this approach has drawbacks because of possible complications including sciatic neuritis and the tracking of purulent fluid into the gluteal muscles (Fig. 10-5) [6,18]. For deep pelvic abscesses close to the rectum, a transrectal approach is preferred [19]. This can be performed using CT guidance. The patient is placed in either the right- or left-lateral decubitus position. The 19-gauge needle with an 18-gauge teflon sheath is partially covered with a short plastic tube and inserted into the rectum. Axial images are performed to align the tip of the needle with the inferiormost aspect of the abscess. The needle is then advanced into the abscess and a catheter is placed into the abscess using the modified Seldinger technique. This is facilitated using the short plastic tube (Fig. 10-6).

Miscellaneous Procedures

The inferior mediastinum is continuous with the retroperitoneum of the abdomen and can have postoperative fluid collections whether from local procedures or from fluid tracking along soft-tissue planes, *ie*, pseudocysts or abscesses. Aspirations and drainage can be performed from a posterior paraspinal approach, even between the aorta and spine (Fig. 10-7). It is important to remain extrapleural and not cross the pleural space.

Infection of prosthetic vascular grafts is a serious complication with high mortality rates of up to 75% for aortic grafts [20,21]. Treatment may require surgical removal of the graft. Because a sample of suspicious perigraft fluid collection can usually be obtained without significant risk, diagnostic aspiration should be performed for any suspected vascular graft infection. For aortic grafts, the approach should be posterolateral, avoiding the erector spinal muscles and the kidneys. Intravenous bolus enhancement may be necessary to demonstrate the lumen.

Surgical treatment of graft infection is a very complex procedure, often entailing the removal of the

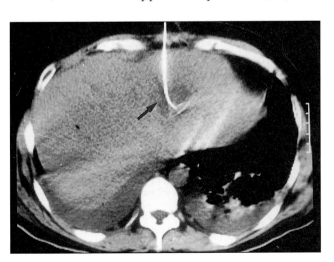

FIGURE 10-4.

This patient is status post-previous biliary diversion and subsequently developed a liver abscess. The approach is anterior and subxyphoid (*arrow*) through the left lobe of the liver. On sinogram, this abscess was multiloculated. However, this abscess was resolved with a single catheter.

graft, wide debridement, and extra-anatomic reanastomosis [20]. Therefore, percutaneous drainage is an attractive alternative, particularly for midgraft infections where the anastomoses are intact. Lambiase and colleagues [22] and Cherry and colleagues [23] have had some success with percutaneous treatment. Cherry and colleagues [23] found that reinfection and mortality rates were similar in both the surgical and nonexcisional percutaneous methods. However, limb salvage rate was significantly greater with the nonexcisional approach. A patient with a midgraft infection of an aortobifemoral bypass graft was recently treated by our group using percutaneous drainage. To enhance drainage, we instilled urokinase into the abscess cavity for 4 days. This resulted in resolution of the abscess with no evidence of recurrence for more than 1 year (Sabatinos, unpublished data).

ASPIRATION AND DRAINAGE OF POST-TRANSPLANT FLUID COLLECTIONS

Abnormal abdominal fluid collections are relatively common following renal, hepatic, or pancreas transplantation [24•]. To determine their etiology and the possibility of infection, diagnostic aspiration should usually be performed.

The most common fluid collections following renal transplantation are lymphocele, hematoma, urinoma, and abscess [24•]. Although there is little data regarding abscess drainage, an initial percutaneous attempt with close follow-up may be helpful to avoid a major surgical procedure [25]. Urinomas can usually be resolved with percutaneous urinary diversion [24•,26]; however, lymphoceles can be very difficult [24•].

Fluid collections involving liver transplants include abscess, hematoma, and bilomas. Hepatic abscess can be managed in the usual fashion, and hematomas usually need not be drained unless infected. Bilomas may be intra- or extrahepatic and may also be infected. Although biloma formation may not appear serious, it is often indicative of hepatic-artery thrombosis [24•,27,28]. The treatment may often require retransplantation; some success may be obtained from external drainage, internal biliary diversion to bowel, antibiotics, and hyperoxygenation [24•].

Fluid collections following pancreas transplantation include abscess, pseudocysts, urinary or pancreatic anastomotic leaks, duct leaks, and hematomas. Successful drainage depends on the location of the allograft (ie, intra- or extraperitoneal). Those patients with

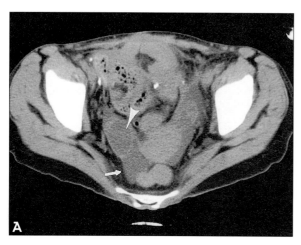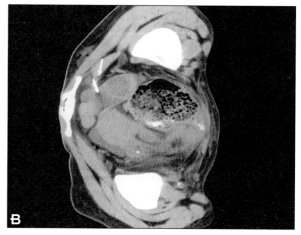

FIGURE 10-5.

A, This patient has a history of multiple previous abdominal procedures with a new pelvic fluid collection in the cul-de-sac and a rising leukocyte count (*arrow*). This small amount of fluid did not flow freely when the patient was placed in either the prone or the left-lateral decubitus position. Note that the uterus is anteromedial to the fluid, and the right ovary with a follicular cyst is anterolateral to the fluid (*arrowhead*). B, This fluid collection was then aspirated through

the right sciatic notch (*arrow*). Because the aspirate was clear, only a small amount was sent for culture and the needle was removed. If the aspirated fluid appeared purulent or if cultures became positive, a drainage procedure would have been performed, possibly through a transrectal approach. Although the transsciatic approach is appropriate for aspirations or biopsies, this is the least-preferred approach for percutaneous catheter drainage of pelvic abscesses.

intraperitoneal allografts have been shown to experience a relatively low success rate for percutaneous drainage. However, for approximately 25% to 33% of these patients surgery may be avoided; this suggests than an attempt is probably indicated if clinically feasible [24•].

One small series of six patients showed a success rate of 50% for those patients with extraperitoneal allografts [29]. Although this represents a small number, the extraperitoneal allografts are theoretically better suited to percutaneous drainage because the infectious process may be more confined.

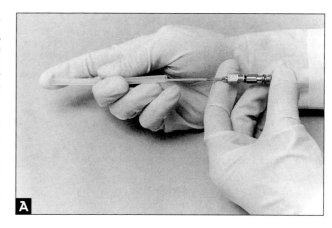

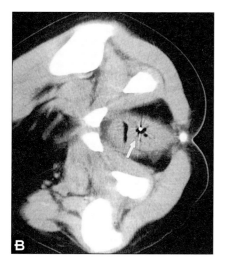
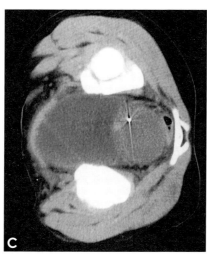
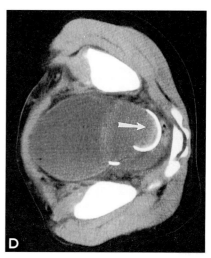

FIGURE 10-6.

A young woman, status post-appendectomy for perforated appendicitis, who subsequently developed a pelvic abscess. **A**, The Longdwel needle (19-gauge needle with an 18-gauge teflon sheath) partially covered by a short plastic tube, which can be found covering many biopsy needles. This plastic tube protects the Longdwel needle and the operator's fingertip during insertion of the needle into the rectum. The tube is left in place to facilitate guidewire insertion and subsequent catheter exchange. **B** and **C**, The tip of the needle is inserted inferior to the abscess and then advanced into the collection (*arrow*). **D**, A guidewire followed by a catheter is then advanced into the cavity using the modified Seldinger technique and the short plastic tube (*arrow*).

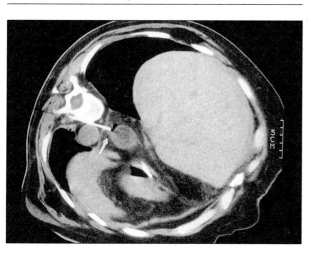

FIGURE 10-7.

This patient is status post-esophagectomy and gastric pull through and subsequently developed a small postoperative fluid collection in the inferior mediastinum (*arrow*). This was aspirated from a posterior approach between the aorta and the spine. The aspirate was clear; only a small amount was sent for culture and was subsequently negative.

Pancreatic Fluid Collections

Pancreatic abscess and the complications of pancreatitis are potentially life-threatening situations that may require both surgical and radiologic intervention. Percutaneous versus operative management of these disorders is a very controversial issue. Although some well-defined, infected pseudocysts are amenable to percutaneous drainage, the ill-defined pancreatic abscess and pancreatic necrosis are probably better managed surgically.

The success rates for infected pseudocysts vary and range between 69% and 94% [30–33]. These collections should be approached directly without traversing the normal bowel or other organs. Either a retroperitoneal approach anterior to the kidney or an anterior approach is best (Fig. 10-8). If necessary, a transgastric route through a previously placed PEG can be used.

In contrast, a noninfected pseudocyst should preferably be drained via a transgastric route, ideally through a PEG. Drainage of a noninfected pseudocyst may be necessary if the pseudocyst is symptomatic, increasing in size, or persistently large. Complications occur in approximately 13% of cases [30,31] and include bacterial superinfection, bleeding, and empyema. The placement of a PEG prior to pseudocyst drainage provides several advantages compared with a direct transgastric approach through both walls of the stomach. With the PEG, the

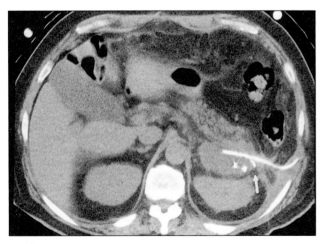

Figure 10-8.

This patient had a large leiomyosarcoma resected from the left upper quadrant and subsequently developed an infected pseudocyst. This was drained from a lateral approach (*arrow*). No connection to the pancreatic duct was noted.

anterior wall of the stomach is in direct contact with the anterior wall of the abdomen, thereby reducing the possibility of leaking gastric contents into the peritoneal cavity. An 18-gauge Longdwel needle (Becton, Dickenson & Co, Rutherford, NJ) can easily be placed through the 22-French PEG. The PEG acts as a fulcrum for the Longdwel needle that facilitates puncture of the pseudocyst through the posterior wall of the stomach. Without the PEG, puncture of both walls of the stomach can be difficult. The transgastric approach allows pancreatic secretions to enter the stomach, decreasing the possibility of fistula formation. However, if there is recurrence, surgery may be required.

Most authors agree that ill-defined pancreatic abscess and necrosis are probably best managed surgically, although percutaneous aspiration and subsequent drainage may temporize a critically ill patient [6,11••,30,31,33]. A diagnostic aspiration may also be very helpful in determining the bacterial etiology of a pancreatic abscess. Lang and colleagues [33] found that diagnostic aspiration in septic patients revealed a microorganism that was different from the organisms grown in concomitant blood cultures in 29 of 85 patients.

The percutaneous approach may be most useful in a patient who has had a surgical drainage and later develops a postoperative collection. Because the second surgical procedure may be difficult in such a patient, percutaneous drainage should be attempted as indicated [6,34,35]. Again, either a direct anterior approach or a retroperitoneal approach anterior to the kidney should be used. The transgastric method through a PEG can also be used, if necessary.

Spleen Abscesses

Macroabscesses of the spleen are fairly uncommon; this is fortunate because the spleen is a vascular organ and any percutaneous manipulation may lead to a potential complication. Although some authors have had success with percutaneous drainage and are advocates of this method, the majority of splenic macroabscesses are probably best managed surgically [16,36]. This is in contradistinction to microabscesses of the spleen that are usually small, disseminated fungal abscesses (often in immunocompromised patients) and are usually treated medically with antifungal agents [37].

Percutaneous drainage of the spleen may be indicated only in certain high surgical-risk patients, such as the elderly or patients of recent postoperative status. In such cases, conservative criteria should be used, such as a superficial location and a unilocular appearance [37,38]. As little splenic parenchyma as possible should be traversed.

Fibrinolytic Agents

Although success rates for percutaneous drainage of unilocular abscesses are high, the multilocular abscess and infected hematoma have lower rates of successful percutaneous drainage [13,17]. Our group has been investigating the use of intracavitary urokinase as an adjunct to percutaneous drainage (Fig. 10-9).

Fibrin is one of the important factors of the host-defense mechanism for intra-abdominal infection. Fibrinogen and proteins leak from surrounding vessels in response to histamine release from neutrophil aggregation. The fibrinogen is then converted to fibrin, which helps prevent dissemination of the infection. However, fibrin also increases the viscosity of the abscess fluid, may form septations, and helps to trap bacteria, all of which may make percutaneous drainage difficult. Fibrin is degraded by plasmin and plasminogen activators such as urokinase convert plasminogen to the active plasmin form. In an *in vitro* study, Park and colleagues [39] show that urokinase decreases both the viscosity of purulent fluid and the flow times of purulent fluid through catheters.

Urokinase has been used clinically to treat infected hematomas and loculated empyema [40,41]. Recently, Lahorra and colleagues [42•] evaluated the safety of intracavitary urokinase during routine percutaneous abscess drainage. They studied 26 patients with 31 abscesses and found no significant alteration in hematocrit or any of the measurable coagulation factors, including prothrombin time, partial thromboplastin time, fibrinogen level, platelets, or levels of fibrin-degradation products. No bleeding complications were observed. In addition, urokinase (and plasmin) appears to remain active within the purulent fluid of the abscess cavity, based on measurements of increased levels of fibrin-degradation products and decreased levels of fibrinogen in the purulent fluid. The plasmin levels could not be easily measured because of lack of a commercial assay. Further data from an animal model show that urokinase has a synergistic effect with systemic antibiotics in treating infected vascular graft material implants. The combination of intra-abscess urokinase and systemic antibiotic was significantly better than either intra-abscess urokinase alone or systemic antibiotic alone [43]. Thus, it would appear that intra-abscess urokinase is safe and may be a valuable adjunct to routine percutaneous abscess drainage.

We are currently compiling a prospective, multi-center trial that randomizes patients to percutaneous drainage with or without intracavitary urokinase

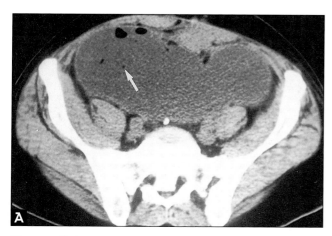
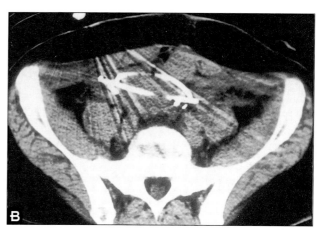

FIGURE 10-9.

A, This patient, status post-laparotomy, developed a large pelvic abscess with thick, purulent fluid. Note the air bubbles suspended with the abscess (*arrow*). **B**, This abscess was successfully treated with two catheters and installation of intra-abscess urokinase for 4 days. The catheters were placed on each side of the abscess and crossed in the midline.

(Haaga, unpublished data). The dosage of intracavitary urokinase depends on the size of the abscess, assuming a spherical shape. The dosages are:

- 12,500 units for 0 to 3 cm
- 25,000 units for 3 to 5 cm
- 50,000 units for 5 to 10 cm
- 100,000 units for greater than 10 cm

These amounts are given every 8 hours for 4 days. The urokinase is injected into the catheter and flushed with 3 to 5 mL of saline, and the catheter is clamped. After 15 minutes, the catheter is unclamped and allowed to drain. There are few contraindications to intracavitary urokinase. These include: 1) a known coagulopathy with a prothrombin time of 4 seconds or more above normal; 2) platelet count of less than 50,000; 3) any pancreatic abscess in which no bacterial etiologies are established; 4) a known central nervous system tumor or bleed; 5) hepatic failure; 6) a pregnant female or nursing mother; and 7) known hypersensitivity to urokinase.

References and Recommended Reading

Recently published papers of particular interest have been highlighted as:
- Of interest
- • Of outstanding interest

1. Levison MA: Percutaneous vs. Open Operative Drainage of Intra-abdominal abscesses. *Infect Dis Clin North Am* 1992, 6:525–544.

2. Adam EJ, Page JE: Intra-abdominal Sepsis: The Role of Radiology. *Baillieres Clin Gastroenterol* 1991, 5:587–609.

3. McLean TR, Simmons K, Svensson LG: Management of Postoperative Intra-abdominal Abscesses by Routine Percutaneous Drainage. *Surg Gynecol Obstet* 1993, 176:167–171.

4. Levison MA, Zeigler D: Correlation of APACHE II Score, Drainage Technique and Outcome in Postoperative Intra-abdominal Abscess. *Surg Gynecol Obstet* 1991, 172:89–94.

5. Butler JA, Huang J, Wilson SE: Repeated Laparotomy for Postoperative Intra-abdominal Sepsis. *Arch Surg* 1987, 122:702–706.

6. Haaga JR, Lanzieri CF: CT-guided Procedures. In *Computed Tomography of the Whole Body*, edn 3. Edited by Haaga JR, Lanzieri CF. St. Louis: CV Mosby; 1994: in press.

7. Johnson WC, Gerzof SG, Robbins AH, *et al.*: Treatment of Abdominal Abscesses: Comparative Evaluation of Operative Drainage vs. Percutaneous Catheter Drainage Guided by Computed Tomography or Ultrasound. *Ann Surg* 1984, 194:510–520.

8. Deveney CW, Lurie K, Deveney KE: Improved Treatment of Intra-abdominal Abscess: A Result of Improved Localization, Drainage, and Patient Care, not Technique. *Arch Surg* 1988, 123:1126–1130.

9. Hemming A, Davis NL, Robins RE: Surgical vs. Percutaneous Drainage of Intra-abdominal Abscesses. *Am J Surg* 1991, 161:593–595.

10. Malangoni MA, Shumate CR, Thomas HA, Richardson JD: Factors Influencing the Treatment of Intra-abdominal Abscesses. *Am J Surg* 1990, 159:167–171.

11. •• Lambiase RE, Deyoe L, Cronan JJ, Dorfman GS: Percutaneous Drainage of 335 Consecutive Abscesses: Results of Primary Drainage with 1-year Follow-up. *Radiology* 1992, 184:167–179.
The authors provide an excellent review of their experience from 1985 to 1990, with follow-up of 1 year or more on all of their patients. The rates for cure, complication, and recurrence are determined and the importance of the patient's immune status is emphasized.

12. Lambiase RE, Cronan JJ, Dorfman GS, *et al.*: Postoperative Abscesses with Enteric Communication: Percutaneous Treatment. *Radiology* 1989, 171:479–500.

13. Haaga JR: Imaging Intra-abdominal Abscesses and Nonoperative Drainage Procedures. *World J Surg* 1990, 14:204–209.

14. Brolin RE, Flancbaum L, Ercoli FR, *et al.*: Limitations of Percutaneous Catheter Drainage of Abdominal Abscesses. *Surg Gynecol Obstet* 1991, 173:203–210.

15. Lent WM, Goldman MJ, Bizer LS: An Objective Appraisal of the Role of Computed Tomographic Guided Drainage of Intra-abdominal Abscess. *Am Surg* 1990, 56:688–690.

16. van Sonnenberg E, D'Agostino HB, Casola G, *et al.*: Percutaneous Abscess Drainage: Current Concepts. *Radiology* 1991, 181:617–626.

17. Gerzof SG, Johnson WC, Robbins AH, Nabseth DC: Expanded Criteria for Percutaneous Abscess Drainage. *Arch Surg* 1985, 120:227–232.

18. Casola G, van Sonnenberg E, D'Agostino HB, *et al.*: Percutaneous Drainage of Tubo-ovarian Abscesses. *Radiology* 1992, 182:399–402.

19. Gazelle GS, Haaga JR, Stellato TA, *et al.*: Pelvic Abscesses: CT Guided Transrectal Drainage. *Radiology* 1991, 181:49–51.

20. Edwards MJ, Richardson JD, Klamer TW: Management of Aortic Prosthetic Infections. *Am J Surg* 1988, 155:327–330.

21. Calligaro KD, Veith FJ: Diagnoses and Management of Infected Prosthetic Aortic Grafts. *Surgery* 1991, 110:805–813.

22. Lambiase RE, Dorfman GS, Cronan JJ: Percutaneous Management of Abscesses that Involve Native Arteries or Synthetic Grafts. *Radiology* 1989, 173:815–818.

23. Cherry KJ, Roland CF, Pavolero PC, *et al.*: Infected Femorodistal Bypass: Is Graft Removal Mandatory? *J Vasc Surg* 1992, 15:295–305.

24. • Letourneau JG, Ferral RCB, Finlay DE, *et al.*: Percutaneous Aspiration and Drainage of Fluid Collections Complicating Solid Organ Transplants. *Semin Intervent Radiol* 1992, 9:305–314.
The authors compile data on the diagnosis and management of intra-abdominal fluid collection following organ transplantation.

25. Letourneau JG, Day DL, Ascher NL, Castaneda-Zuniga WR: Imaging of Renal Transplants. *AJR* 1988, 150:833–838.

26. Matalon TAS, Thompson MJ, Patel SK, *et al.*: Percutaneous Treatment of Urine Leaks in Renal Transplantation Patients. *Radiology* 1990, 174:1049–1051.

27. Hoffer FA, Teele RL, Lillehei CW, Vacanti JP: Infected Bilomas and Hepatic Artery Thrombosis in Infant Recipients of Liver Transplants. *Radiology* 1988, 169:435–438.

28. Kaplan SB, Zajko AB, Koneru B: Hepatic Bilomas Due to Hepatic Artery Thrombosis in Liver Transplant Recipients: Percutaneous Drainage and Clinical Outcome. *Radiology* 1990, 174:1031–1035.

29. Patel BK, Garvin PJ, Aridge DL, *et al.*: Fluid Collections Developing After Pancreas Transplantation, Radiologic Evaluation and Intervention. *Radiology* 1991, 181:215–220.

30. Freeney PC, Lewis GP, Traverso LW, Ryan JA: Infected Pancreatic Fluid Collections: Percutaneous Catheter Drainage. *Radiology* 1988, 167:435–441.

31. van Sonnenberg E, Wittich GR, Casola G, *et al.*: Percutaneous Drainage of Infected and Noninfected Pancreatic Pseudocysts: Experience in 101 Cases. *Radiology* 1989, 170:757–761.

32. van Sonnenberg E, Casola G, Varney RR, Wittich GR: Imaging and Interventional Radiology for Pancreatitis and Its Complications. *Radiol Clin North Am* 1989, 27:65–72.

33. Lang EK, Paolini RM, Pottmeyer A: The Efficacy of Palliative and Definitive Percutaneous vs. Surgical Drainage of Pancreatic Abscesses and Pseudocysts: A Prospective Study of 85 Patients. *South Med J* 1991, 84:55–64.

34. Steiner E, Mueller PR, Hahn PF, *et al.*: Complicated Pancreatic Abscesses: Problems in Interventional Management. *Radiology* 1988, 167:443–446.

35. Rotman N, Mathieu D, Aglade MC, Fagniez PL: Failure of Percutaneous Drainage of Pancreatic Abscesses Complicating Severe Acute Pancreatitis. *Surg Gynecol Obstet* 1992, 174:141–144.

36. Hadas-Halpren I, Hiller N, Dolberg M: Percutaneous Drainage of Splenic Abscesses: An Effective and Safe Procedure. *Br J Radiol* 1992, 65:968–970.

37. Faught WE, Gilbertson JJ, Nelson EW: Splenic Abscess: Presentation, Treatment Options and Results. *Am J Surg* 1989, 158:612–614.

38. Gleich S, Wolin DA, Herbsman H: A Review of Percutaneous Drainage in Splenic Abscesses. *Surg Gynecol Obstet* 1988, 167:211–216.

39. Park JK, Kraus FC, Haaga JR: Fluid Flow During Percutaneous Drainage Procedures: An *In Vitro* Study of Effects of Fluid Viscosity, Catheter Size, and Adjunctive Urokinase. *AJR* 1993, 160:165–169.

40. Vogelzang RL, Tobin RS, Burstein S, *et al.*: Transcatheter Intracavitary Fibrinolysis of Infected Extravascular Hematoma. *AJR* 1987, 148:378–380.

41. Lee KS, Im JG, Kim YH, *et al.*: Treatment of Thoracic Multiloculated Empyemas with Intracavitary Urokinase: A Prospective Study. *Radiology* 1991, 179:771–775.

42. • Lahorra JM, Haaga JR, Stellato TM, *et al.*: Safety of Intracavitary Urokinase with Percutaneous Abscess Drainage. *AJR* 1993, 160:171–174.
In this phase I study, the authors demonstrate the safety of instilling urokinase into an abscess cavity. No changes in any measured coagulation factors are noted. All of the abscesses, including multiloculated abscesses, were successfully drained.

43. Nakamoto DA, Rosenfield ML, Haaga JR, *et al.*: *In Vivo* Treatment of Infected Prosthetic Graft Material with Urokinase: An Animal Model. *JVIR* 1994, in press.

Select Bibliography

Dougherty SH, Simmons RL: The Biology and Practice of Surgical Drains Parts I and II. *Curr Probl Surg* 1992, 29:559–730.

Gallinaro RN, Polk HC: Intra-abdominal Sepsis: The Role of Surgery. *Baillieres Clin Gastroenterol* 1991, 5:611–637.

Strategies for Maintaining Dialysis Access Patency

Kevin L. Sullivan
Anatole Besarab

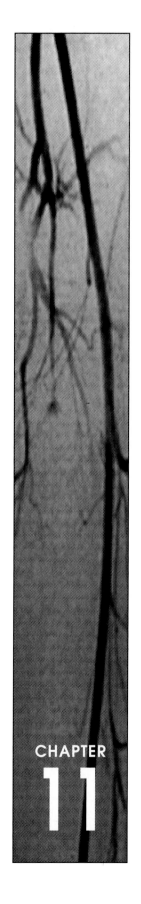

CHAPTER

11

Maintaining access for hemodialysis is a major challenge. As the hemodialysis population ages, the proportion of patients with Brescia-Cimino (B-C) shunts relative to synthetic bridge grafts decreases, because of diseased peripheral arteries and veins. The shorter primary patency of synthetic bridge grafts has fostered the search for methods to maximize graft longevity and preserve veins as sites for future grafts [1]. Angioplasty has become the treatment of choice in the management of grafts that have failed as a result of stenosis.

One successful strategy for maintaining graft patency requires detection and treatment of stenoses prior to graft thrombosis. Techniques used to identify stenoses prior to occlusion include venous dialysis pressures, true intra-access pressures, Doppler ultrasound, and recirculation. This review presents a protocol that has successfully decreased the incidence of graft thrombosis, the number of inpatient hospital days required for patients with vascular access problems, and prolonged-access life in a chronic hemodialysis population. The approach involves screening for stenoses with true intra-access pressures and managing significant stenoses with angioplasty prior to graft thrombosis.

Methods of Measuring Pressures During Dialysis

Venous dialysis pressures measured in line with the dialyzed blood return have been used to screen dialysis accesses for stenoses [2••]. However, these pressures are determined by a number of factors, including blood flow rate through the needle, diameter of the needle, the patient's hematocrit, and true intra-access pressure [3]. The latter can be more accurately determined by the measurement of static pressures, ie, no flow through the needle. To accomplish this with current technology, a pressure transducer is intro-

duced into the tubing used to return dialyzed blood to the patient. To record access pressure, the dialysis pump is stopped for less than 1 minute. This method of measuring pressure generally requires less than 3 minutes, and does not significantly reduce dialysis time or efficiency. We routinely measure such pressures three times per year in each chronic hemodialysis patient.

Graft pressure depends in part on systemic pressure. Normalizing graft pressures with systemic pressures eliminates variation caused by differences in patient systemic blood pressures. For this reason, we express graft pressures as a ratio: systolic graft pressure to systolic systemic pressure.

Sensitivity and Specificity of Screening Criteria

A normalized pressure ratio of greater than 0.4 has a sensitivity and specificity of 91% in detecting stenoses greater than or equal to 50% in synthetic grafts (Table 11-1). Recirculation is not as sensitive nor as specific in detecting stenoses in synthetic grafts. However, in B-C shunts, recirculation is a better method for detecting stenoses than are normalized pressure ratios [4•]. A lower pressure threshold in B-C shunts might improve the sensitivity, but could also lower the specificity. Collateral formation around native vein stenoses probably accounts for the low sensitivity of normalized pressures in detecting stenoses in B-C shunts.

The Role of Dialysis Graft Hemodynamics in Guiding Interventions

There is a normal drop in pressure between the artery and vein draining a synthetic dialysis graft. Knowledge of the pattern of pressure decrements is necessary to interpret gradients pre- and postintervention.

Table 11-1. Comparison of Normalized Pressure Ratios (>0.4%) Versus Recirculation (>15%) in Detecting Stenoses (>50%)				
	Synthetic		Native	
	Normalized pressures	Recirculation	Normalized pressures	Recirculation
Sensitivity, %	91	29	46	71
Specificity, %	91	75	100	100

Grafts with low-grade stenosis (< 40%) or with no stenosis lose 50% or more the systolic arterial pressure between the artery and the arterial limb of the graft. By the venous limb of the graft, the pressure drops to less than one third of systolic pressure. Central venous pressure in these patients is 13% of systolic pressure,

on the average. A similar pattern was seen in normal canine synthetic dialysis grafts [5]. Thus, in a patient with a systolic pressure of 150 mm Hg, a normal graft or one with a low-grade stenosis will have a pressure gradient of 75 mm Hg across the arterial anastomosis, a further 26 mm Hg over the length of the graft, and a final pressure drop of 30 mm Hg across the venous anastomosis. If hemodynamic parameters are used to select patients for intervention or to evaluate the results of an intervention, these gradients must be taken into account [6•].

Graft pressure rises in proportion to the severity of outflow stenosis [7]. The relationship is best described by a sigmoid-shaped curve, with the steepest part of the curve between 30% and 70% diameter stenosis. The pressure gradient normally present between the artery and graft is gradually eliminated with increasing stenosis severity (Fig. 11-1). However, stenosis location influences the rise in pressure. A high-grade stenosis at the venous anastomosis or within a synthetic graft will almost invariably lead to a rise in graft pressure proximal to the stenosis (Fig. 11-2). This is not always the case in central-vein stenoses with well-developed collaterals. Such stenoses probably pose little risk of graft thrombosis, although they may lead to arm edema or central-vein thrombosis (Fig. 11-3).

Hemodynamic evaluation of grafts can be used to guide interventions. Stenosis severity can be underestimated with angiography, particularly at the venous

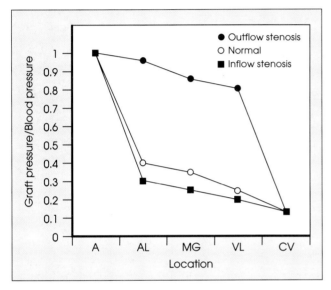

FIGURE 11-1

Outflow stenoses at the venous anastomosis or within the graft progressively eliminate the drop in pressure that normally occurs between the artery and synthetic graft. Inflow stenoses reduce graft pressures. A—artery; AL—arterial limb of graft; MG— midportion of graft; VL—venous limb of graft; CV—central vein.

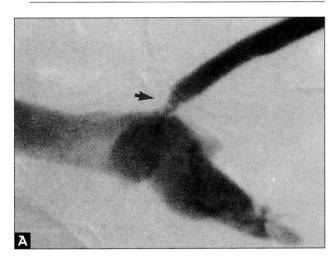

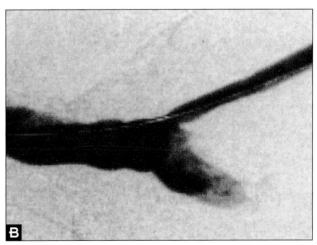

FIGURE 11-2.

A, Angiography of this synthetic graft, performed for elevated screening pressures, revealed a 70% stenosis at the venous anastomosis (*arrow*). The arterial-limb pressure was 109/56 (77), and the blood pressure was 115/68 (93).

The systolic ratio was therefore 0.95 (109/115). **B,** Following a good result with angioplasty, the pressure dropped to 29/19 (22), and the blood pressure was 122/78 (95), yielding a systolic ratio of 0.24.

anastomosis because of overlap with the vein. Patients with elevated pressures and without apparent high-grade stenoses should be studied in multiple obliques to search for such stenoses. In patients with multiple stenoses, pressures can be used to determine an endpoint for intervention because some stenoses may be hemodynamically insignificant (Fig. 11-4). Normal or low pressures in a patient presenting with graft thrombosis should prompt careful examination of the arterial anastomosis.

Based on patients with low-grade or no stenoses, as well as previously published animal studies, the goal of intervention should be to achieve a pressure less than 50% of systemic pressure in the arterial limb of the graft, and less than 33% of systemic pressure in the venous limb of the graft.

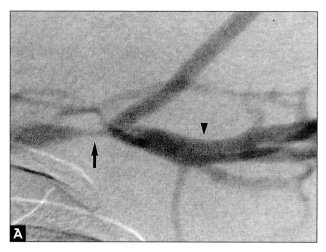
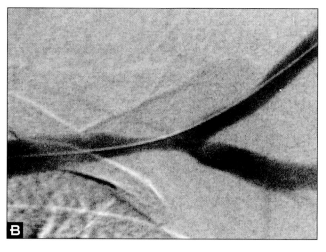

FIGURE 11-3.

A, This patient was evaluated for arm edema. Access angiography revealed an 80% stenosis of the axillary vein, just central to the venous anastomosis (*arrow*). The pressure in the arterial limb was 66/43(54), and the blood pressure was 187/88(116), producing a ratio of 0.35. Note that there is no significant stenosis extending into the graft. Thus, there is unimpeded flow from the graft retro-grade into venous collaterals (*arrowhead*). This pattern of flow is responsible for the normal graft pressures and for the arm edema. **B**, Angioplasty leads to moderate reduction of the stenosis and resolution of the edema. The pressure ratio remained essentially unchanged at 0.32.

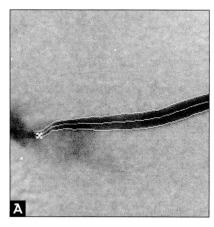
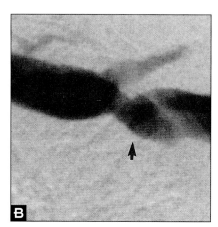
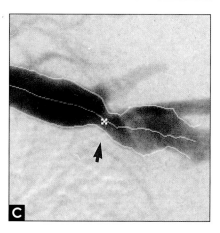

FIGURE 11-4.

A, Access angiography performed for elevated pressures revealed a 62% venous anastomotic stenosis (X). Graft pressure in the arterial limb was 95/51(67), and blood pressure was 116/69(86), yielding a systolic pressure ratio of 0.82. **B**, Following angioplasty, the region of the venous anastomosis is difficult to evaluate because of overlap with the vein (*arrow*). However, the arterial-limb pressure dropped to 57/40(49), and blood pressure was 132/70(103), giving a systolic ratio of 0.43. **C**, A 58% central-vein stenosis remained at the level of the venous anastomosis (*arrow*). However, because of the favorable pressure response, no further intervention was performed.

Pressure Monitoring and Early Dialysis Access Angioplasty: Influence on Thrombosis, Hospitalization Rates, and Graft Longevity

The influence of angioplasty rates on access thrombosis, inpatient hospital days required for vascular access problems, and graft age were assessed over a 69-month period. The first 51 months were retrospective. During a 24-month historic control period (beginning in 1986), little angioplasty was done. A 15-month transitional period followed, when the amount of angioplasty began to rise based on positive published reports. A 12-month high-utilization period followed. Because of the high restenosis rate, a prospective study was designed. During a 9-month period, angioplasty was performed only where it was required to continue dialysis, such as in postgraft thrombosis or arm edema. This was followed by a 9-month period, when regularly monitored patients with systolic graft pressures greater than 40% of systemic pressure were evaluated with dialysis angiograms; angioplasty was performed

if stenosis greater than or equal to 50% was detected. These patients did not necessarily have symptoms of access dysfunction. Angioplasty was performed in many cases based on stenosis greater than or equal to 50%, causing an elevated graft pressure. Patients with access problems were also managed with angioplasty during this period (Fig. 11-5).

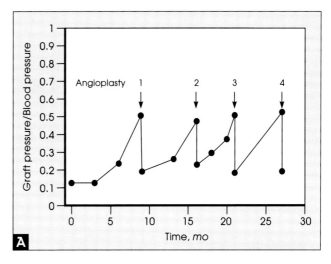

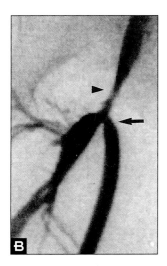 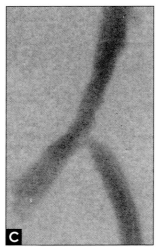 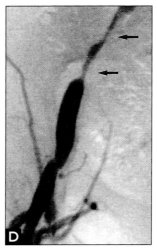 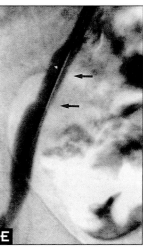

FIGURE 11-5.

This patient with polyarteritis nodosa presented with elevated pressures in the sixth synthetic graft. The first three grafts, in both arms and the left thigh, failed during a 2-month period. No hypercoaguable state could be identified. The fourth access, placed in the left arm, clotted five times over 5 months, despite an increase in prothrombin time of 2.5 to 3.0 seconds with warfarin sodium. The fifth access, placed in the right thigh, clotted three times over 13.6 months, and the sixth, also placed in the right thigh, was monitored closely with normalized pressures as described. **A**, After 9 months, the pressure rose above the threshold of 0.4. **B**, Angiography indicated a moderate stenosis at the venous anastomosis (*arrow*) and a high-grade stenosis in the femoral vein (*arrowhead*).

C, Angioplasty 1 of both stenoses via the graft led to improved morphology and pressure. **A**, At 16 months, the pressure rose above 0.4 and angiography revealed the same stenosis pattern. Angioplasty 2 produced similar results to angioplasty 1. At 21 months, the patient developed elevated pressure and lower-extremity edema. Common femoral and venous anastomotic stenoses were both approximately 40%. **D**, A new high-grade, external iliac vein stenosis (*arrows*) was **E**, successfully dilated as shown following angioplasty 3 (*arrows*). At 27 months, the patient again experienced elevated pressure and leg edema. **A**, A recurrent high-grade, external iliac vein stenosis was redilated (angioplasty 4). The graft remains patent at 31 months and monitoring continues.

During the prospective part of the study, there was a significant drop in the rate of access thrombosis and in the number of inpatient hospital days required to treat vascular access problems. Linear regression was used to determine the relationship between the rate of angioplasty and access thrombosis and hospitalization for access problems (Fig. 11-6). Based on the prospective and retrospective data, there was a loss of 1.4 episodes of access thrombosis and 4.8 inpatient hospital days associated with each angioplasty.

This program of screening and early intervention has also increased access longevity. During the historic control period, the average access age was 2 years. Currently, with screening and early intervention, the average access age is 2.8 years, despite increased patient age and proportion of the population with synthetic grafts compared with B-C shunts. During the historic control period, only one third of accesses were greater than 2 years in age. Currently, half of the accesses are greater than 2 years in age.

Conclusion

The strategy that we propose for maintaining hemodialysis access patency is both simple and effective. Measurement of true intra-access pressures is less expensive than Doppler ultrasound. It is also less time consuming and can be measured easily during a routine dialysis session. Flow rate through the needle does not influence true intra-access pressure measurements as it can with venous dialysis pressures that are measured when dialyzed blood flows through the venous return needle. Recirculation is neither as sensitive nor as specific as normalized intra-access pressures in detecting significant stenoses in synthetic dialysis grafts.

Although not directly addressed in this report, there is a need to control intimal hyperplasia following angioplasty of dialysis graft–related stenoses. Stents may play a role in salvaging an unsuccessful angioplasty, but they do not prevent intimal hyperplasia. Unfortunately, they do not appear to achieve better long-term patency than a successful angioplasty [8]. Thus, early intervention with angioplasty is the only viable method for prolonging synthetic access longevity at this time.

There are a number of advantages to the approach discussed here aside from prolonged-access patency. A formal cost-benefit analysis has not been performed, but the loss of almost 5 inpatient hospital

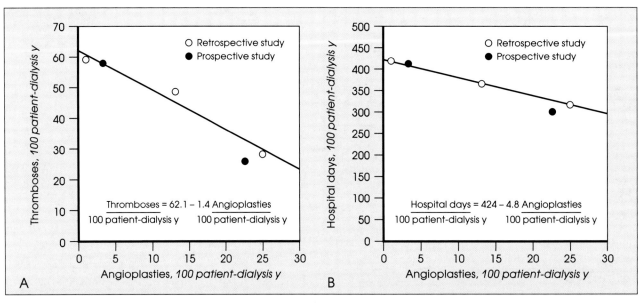

FIGURE 11-6.

The number of angioplasties per 100 patient-dialysis years is indicated on the horizontal axis. **A**, On the vertical axis are the number of access thromboses, or **B**, inpatient hospital days for access problems per 100 patient-dialysis years. The upper left and lower right data points are the periods with low and high angioplasty utilization, respectively. The data point in the middle is the retrospective transitional period. **A**, Using linear regression, a slope of -1.4 indicates that for each angioplasty, there was a loss of 1.4 thrombotic episodes. **B**, Similarly, a slope of -4.8 indicates that each angioplasty was associated with a decrease of 4.8 inpatient hospital days for vascular access problems.

days for each angioplasty would argue strongly in favor of a cost advantage for early intervention with angioplasty. Additional benefits include an improved quality of life, as a result of less inpatient hospital time, and a reduced need for central-venous hemodialysis catheters when awaiting graft declotting or maturation of a new graft with the attendant risk of central-vein stenosis.

References and Recommended Reading

Recently published papers of particular interest have been highlighted as:
• Of interest
•• Of outstanding interest

1.   Zibari GB, Rohr MS, Landreneau MD, *et al.*: Complications from Permanent Hemodialysis Vascular Access. *Surgery* 1988, 104:681–686.

2.•• Schwab SJ, Raymond JR, Saeed M, *et al.*: Prevention of Hemodialysis Fistula Thrombosis. Early Detection of Venous Stenoses. *Kidney Intern* 1989, 36:707–711.
This article demonstrates both the ability of venous-dialysis pressure monitoring to detect significant dialysis-access stenoses, and the efficacy of angioplasty of these stenoses in decreasing the thrombosis rate in a chronic hemodialysis population.

3.   Besarab A, Dorrell S, Moritz M, *et al.*: Determinants of Measured Dialysis Venous Pressure and Its Relationship to True Intra-access Venous Pressure. *ASAIO Transactions* 1991, 37:M270–M271.

4.•   Besarab A, Moritz M, Sullivan K, *et al.*: Venous Access Pressures and the Detection of Intra-access Stenosis. *ASAIO Journal* 1992, 38:M519–M523.
This article discusses the high sensitivity and specificity of normalized pressures in the detection of significant dialysis-access stenoses.

5.   Zamora JI, Gao ZR, Weilbaecher DG, *et al.*: Hemodynamic and Morphologic Features of Arteriovenous Angioaccess Loop Grafts. *Trans Am Soc Artif Intern Organs* 1985, 31:119–122.

6.•   Sullivan KL, Besarab A, Bonn J, *et al.*: Hemodynamics of Failing Dialysis Grafts. *Radiology* 1993, 186:867–872.
This manuscript describes the role of hemodialysis-access pressures in directing percutaneous interventions.

7.   Sullivan KL, Besarab A, Dorrell S, Moritz MJ: The Relationship Between Dialysis Graft Pressure and Stenosis. *Invest Radiol* 1992, 27:352–355.

8.   Beathard GA: Gianturco Self-expanding Stent in the Treatment of Stenosis in Dialysis Access Grafts. *Kidney Intern* 1993, 43:872–877.

Select Bibliography

Fan P, Schwab SJ: Vascular Access: Concepts for the 1990s. *J Am Soc Nephrol* 1992, 3:1–11.

Swedberg SH, Brown BG, Sigley R: Intimal Fibromuscular Hyperplasia at the Venous Anastomosis of PTFE Grafts in Hemodialysis Patients. *Circulation* 1989, 80:1726–1736.

Windus DW: Permanent Vascular Access: A Nephrologist's View. *Am J Kidney Dis* 1993, 21:457–471.

Esophageal Stenting

Wojciech Cwikiel

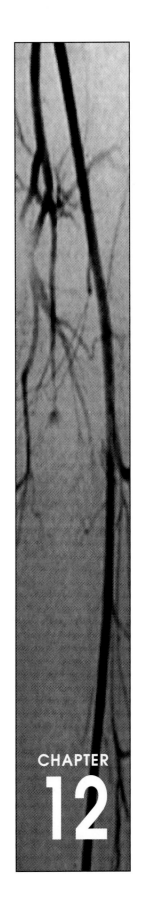

The idea of esophageal endoprosthesis is not new. Intubation of the esophagus using decalcified ivory was suggested by Leroy d'Etiolles of France in 1845, and the first successful insertion of an esophageal tube was reported by Sir Charles Symonds in 1887 [1]. The introduction of plastic materials has been essential for the further development of esophageal endoprosthesis. In 1959, Celestin presented a new plastic tube, which subsequently modified, was widely used in the palliative treatment of malignant esophageal strictures [2–7]. Access tract and diameter of the stricture limits the lumen of the plastic tube. An expandable stent can be inserted easily and can restore the diameter of an obstructed part of the esophagus.

Narrowing of the esophageal lumen is most often caused by disease in the esophageal wall, and less frequently by mediastinal pathology. The common symptom is dysphagia followed by malnutrition and chest pain. Malignant strictures in the proximal and middle part of the esophagus are usually caused by squamous cell carcinoma, and in the distal third by gastric adenocarcinoma. The diagnosis of malignant esophageal disease is often delayed because of lack of early symptoms, making curative therapy impossible. Resection may be performed in approximately 50% of patients, but only about 10% will survive more than 5 years after surgery [8,9]. Mediastinal tumors may compress the esophagus, and may also infiltrate the esophageal wall. Palliation of dysphagia and malnutrition is the primary goal for the treatment of patients with unresectable tumors or recurrence of cancer. Bypass surgery is rather complicated with a high mortality rate [9,10]. Radiotherapy or chemotherapy have relatively limited effects and endoscopic laser treatment must be repeated at short intervals in a majority of patients [11–15]. Endoscopic insertion of plastic tubes requires general anesthesia, has several complications, and is impossible to use in a number of patients [3–7,16].

Benign esophageal strictures are caused by ingestion of concentrated alkali or acids and reflux esophagitis. Destroyed esophageal mucosa is subsequently replaced by fibrotic and connective tissues, resulting in constriction of the wall and narrowing of the lumen. Patients experience dysphagia and several present with a poor nutritional condition. Dilatation is usually tried first, and a bouginage using stiff dilators or balloon dilatation are commonly used techniques [17–20]. No matter which method is used, dilatation must be repeated frequently in a large number of patients because of its relatively short-lasting effect. Also, long-term intubation using plastic tubes has been reported in the treatment of benign strictures, but a relatively high complication rate limits the usefulness of this method [21]. Esophageal resection with interposition of the stomach or bowel is the surgical alternative in patients when other therapeutic methods fail. However, surgical reconstruction has a limited effect on dysphagia in nearly 50% of patients.

Expandable Esophageal Stents

The esophageal tube of German silver wire proposed by Souttar in 1924 is probably the first prototype in the history of expandable esophageal metallic endoprostheses [22]. Endoscopic insertion of an expanding metallic spiral in the human esophagus was reported by Frimberger [23] in 1983. Complications, foremost high migration rate, halted further use of this device. During recent years, different expandable esophageal stents have been tested predominantly by radiologists. The following stents are presently available for treatment of esophageal strictures:

Self-expanding nitinol Strecker stents, (Boston Scientific, Watertown, MA) also called Elastoy stents, are knitted of a 0.15-mm nitinol wire (Fig. 12-1) [24,25•]. Flexible in the long axis, the fully expanded stent measures 18 mm in diameter, with its proximal end flared into a 5-mm long collar with a 20-mm diameter. The delivery system includes a 95-cm long (2-mm outer diameter) teflon catheter with a distal, olive-shaped widening and a soft, 4-cm long tip to simplify insertion, and a covering sheath. To minimize the diameter of the stent at insertion, it is stretched, compressed, and encased in gelatin. Thus, in the delivery device, 10- and 15-cm long stents are stretched to 14 and 19 cm, respectively. The 60-cm long (8-mm outer diameter), proximally tapered, covering teflon sheath prevents contact of the stent with fluid inside the esophagus during insertion. The delivery system with the stent is introduced over a 0.038-inch guidewire. When in position, the sheath covering the stent is quickly removed and the stent expands within 2 to 4 minutes immediately after dissolution of the gelatin. A new, simplified delivery system that allows direct controllable deployment of the stent is presently being tested.

Gianturco stents (William Cook Europe, Bjaeverskov, Denmark) are made of a 0.5-mm, stainless-steel wire that is bent in a zigzag configuration with ends soldered to form a cylinder [26•,27–30]. Several stents covered with polyethylene film form an expandable tube with 16-mm inner diameter (Fig. 12-2). The stents at the edges of this tube have flanged proximal (22.5 mm), respectively distal (18 mm) ends to prevent migration. Barbs soldered to the stent wires may also increase the stability of the stent. Such an expandable tube is compressed within an 8-mm outer diameter introducer catheter. The tube is preloaded into the introducer catheter and inserted to the intended position through the previously placed introducer sheath. By use of a pusher, the stents are kept in place and thereafter released by simultaneous retraction of the introducer catheter with the sheath. The tube has relatively poor longitudinal flexibility and its shortening after delivery is negligible.

The Wallstent (Schneider AG, Böulach, Switzerland) is woven in a multifilament net cylinder, comprised of a high-performance, medical-grade, 0.12-mm stainless-steel alloy (Fig. 12-3) [31–35,36•]. The stents for esophageal strictures are 40-, 70-, or 100-mm long and 20 to 22 mm in diameter when fully open. When stretched and constrained, the stent is mounted in a 4-mm outer diameter delivery device and simultaneously elongated respectively to 66-, 115-, and 165-mm. For delivery, the stent is advanced in position over a 0.038-inch guidewire, and deployment is accomplished by withdrawal of a membrane covering the stent. Controllable progressive deployment of the stent from the delivery instrument permits the prosthesis to expand spontaneously and to affix itself to a wall as the stent simultaneously shortens. Longitudinal flexibility depends on the degree of expansion of the esophageal Wallstent. A new type of Wallstent, covered by a nylon membrane, is also presently being tested.

Choice of the Stent

In patients with malignant strictures, the stent may be approximately 4 cm longer than the stricture to prevent subsequent tumor overgrowth at the stent edges. Thus, the stent should be positioned with the edges at least 2 cm proximal and distal to the stricture.

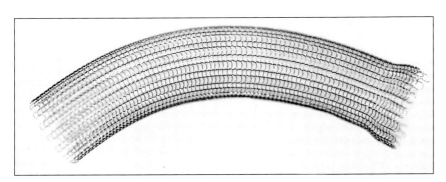

FIGURE 12-1.

The expanded nitinol Strecker stent, 18 mm in diameter. The stent is knitted of one nitinol wire.

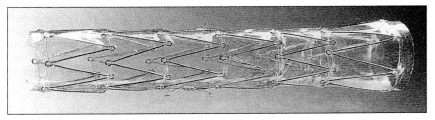

FIGURE 12-2.

The Gianturco stent tube, 16 mm in diameter. The coating prevents tumor ingrowth and is also able to close an esophagorespiratory fistula.

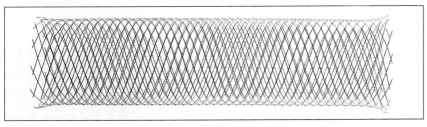

FIGURE 12-3.

The esophageal Wallstent, 20 mm in diameter. The stent is woven of stainless-steel wires.

Because insertion of multiple stents increases discomfort in the patient and cost of the treatment, use of a single stent with adequate length is advisable. Good longitudinal flexibility of the stent is important in patients with tortuous strictures, particularly in the distal esophagus. Substantial shortening of the stent is a serious disadvantage in patients with high strictures where an exact placement of the proximal end of the stent is very important, so as not to disturb the act of swallowing. In patients with esophagorespiratory fistula or tumor abscess connecting esophageal lumen to the mediastinum, placement of coated stents may be advisable. However, uncoated stents may be inserted in patients with a small fistula or tumor abscess without connection to the mediastinum.

Insertion Technique

Before stent insertion, extension of the tumor is evaluated at radiography and the position of the stricture may be indicated with metal markers on the patient's chest. Topical anesthesia in form of spray or gel lidocaine is given, and a mild sedative (*eg*, diazepam) may be given intravenously when necessary. Under fluoroscopic guidance, a 5- to 8-French feeding tube and a 0.035- to 0.038-inch guidewire are jointly manipulated through the stricture (Fig. 12-4). In patients with tortuous or fibrotic strictures, a super-stiff Amplatz guidewire (Medi-Tech and Boston Scientific, Watertown, MA) may be left in place. Dilatation of the stricture, using a 10- to 12-mm angioplasty balloon introduced over the guidewire, is performed to facilitate placement of the stent. The delivery system containing the stent is advanced over a guidewire into the stricture. When the stent has been released in an adequate position, it may be further expanded with a balloon catheter, to fix the stent to the esophageal wall. If necessary, additional stents may be positioned adjacent to or overlapping with the first stent to include the whole stricture. The patency of the stents is checked with injection of contrast medium through the dilatation catheter, positioned with the distal end above the stent. Ingestion of fluids is permitted after the effects of the anesthesia wear off.

Patient Follow-up

All patients are examined by esophagography after 24 hours. If the stent is not fully expanded, further fluoro-scopic or endoscopic follow-up examinations may be performed at intervals of 5 to 7 days, until the stent is adequately expanded. During this time, only ingestion of liquids and a mashed-food diet is advisable. As soon as the stent is fully expanded, a regular diet is permitted, and carbonated drinks recommended after meals. Endoscopic or fluoroscopic follow-up examinations should be performed every 4 months for evaluation of stent function and early diagnosis of possible tumor ingrowth or overgrowth.

Clinical Reports

Clinical reports describing treatment of esophageal strictures with expandable stents are summarized in Table 12-1. Although the number of treated patients is

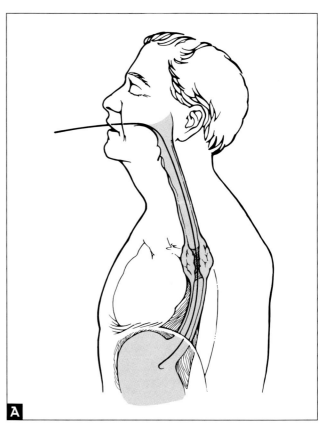

FIGURE 12-4.

The guidewire insertion technique. **A**, A guidewire is placed through the stricture. **B**, Balloon dilatation of the stricture prior to the stent insertion. **C**, The delivery system containing the stent is placed in position. **D**, The released stent is partially compressed and left for self-expansion. **E**, The stent is completely expanded the day following insertion.

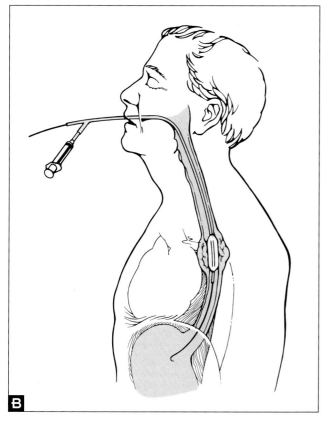

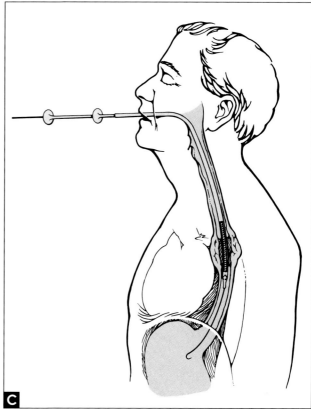

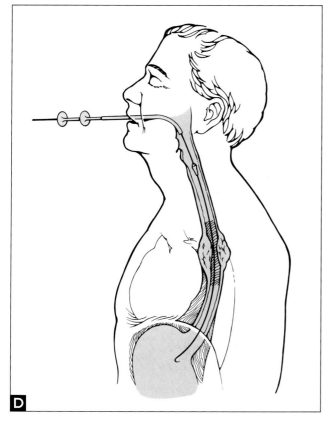

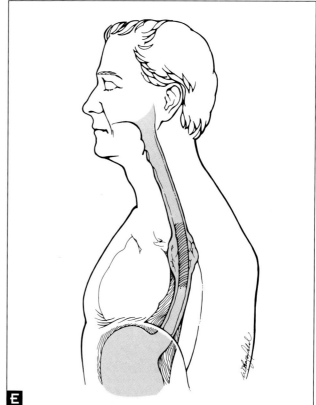

rather small, the results are quite similar. Except for the group of patients treated with the expanding spiral stent, the number of patients treated with other stents is comparable. Insertion of a different self-expandable stent was possible in all patients, and procedures could be performed using only topical anesthesia in most patients. There were no serious procedure-related complications and the improvement of dysphagia in the patient was described as good or very good by the majority of authors. Maximum observation time was less than 10 months, with a mean of 6.6 months, in 10 of 14 reports. However, a majority of patients died without recurrent dysphagia. The number of late complications was similar for the different stents with exception of the expanding spiral stents, which had a relatively high migration rate. Penetration of the stent through the esophageal wall occurred in two patients [27,28]. In addition to stent migration, food impaction and tumor ingrowth were other dominating complications.

Personal Experience

TREATMENT OF PATIENTS WITH MALIGNANT STRICTURES BY INSERTION OF WALLSTENTS

Twelve patients, one woman and 11 men with carcinoma of the esophagus and significant dysphagia, were treated. Because of the use of relatively short (60 mm) prototype stents, one to six stents were initially inserted, depending on the length of the stricture. In

Table 12-1. Results of Treatment of Esophageal Strictures with Self-expandable Stents

Study	Patients, n	Type of stent	Stent diameter, mm	Follow-up, mo	Effect on dysphagia	Complications					
						Migra-tion	Food impact	Chest pain	Tumor ingrowth	Tumor over-growth	Perfora-tion
Frimberger (23)	10	Spiral	13–15	9	Good	3	–	–	–	–	–
Domschke et al. (32)	1	Wallstent	10	4	Very good	–	–	–	–	–	–
Lindberg et al. (33)	12	Wallstent	16–20	11	Good	1	1	–	2	1	–
Song et al. (29)	9	Gianturco	18	8	Very good	–	–	2	–	–	–
Bethge et al. (31)	8	Wallstent	14	3	Good (75%)	–	–	–	1	1	–
Schaer et al. (28)	6	Gianturco	15	8	Good	1	1	1	–	–	1
Neuhaus (35)	8	Wallstent	16–20	7	Good	–	1	–	–	–	–
Neuhaus et al. (34)	10	Wallstent	Not known	9	Good	–	3	–	2	–	–
Kozarek et al. (27)	5	Gianturco	15	6	Not known	1	–	–	–	–	1
Song et al. (30)	21	Gianturco	18–20	9	Very good	1	2	–	–	–	–
Do et al. (26)*	8	Gianturco	20	6	Good	–	–	–	–	1	–
Cwikiel et al. (24)	40	Nitinol-Strecker	18	15	Good	1	1	–	8	–	–
Cwikiel et al. (25)†	5	Nitinol-Strecker	18	16	Good	–	–	1	–	–	–
Knyrim et al. (36)†	21	Wallstent	16	7	Good	–	3	–	3	2	–
Total	164					8(5%)	12(7%)	4(2.5%)	16(10%)	5(3%)	2(1.3%)

*All patients were treated for benign strictures.
†All patients were treated for esophagorespiratory fistulae.
†A prospective comparison of expandable stents versus plastic tubes.

two patients, additional stents had to be inserted on separate occasions because of tumor overgrowth. In another patient, separation and angulation between the initial stents necessitated supplementary stent insertion after 5 days. In another procedure-related complication, one distal coaxial stent separated from the proximal stent during balloon dilatation immediately after insertion, migrated into the stomach, and had to be removed by laparotomy. The functional effect of these stents on dysphagia was estimated as successful in seven patients and improved in the other four patients. All patients were able to receive oral nutrition during the remaining observation time.

TREATMENT OF PATIENTS WITH MALIGNANT STRICTURES BY INSERTION OF GIANTURCO STENTS

Eight patients, seven men and one woman, received one stent tube and one of these patients received two coaxial tubes. Reduction of dysphagia was achieved in all patients. Migration of the inserted stent tubes occurred in three patients. In the first patient, the coaxial stent tube migrated to the stomach after delivery and had to be replaced during laparotomy. In the second patient, the stent tube inserted close to the proximal esophagorespiratory fistula migrated after 4 weeks to the distal part of the esophagus. In the third patient, migration of the stent tube to the stomach occurred after 8 weeks.

TREATMENT OF PATIENTS WITH MALIGNANT STRICTURES WITH SELF-EXPANDING NITINOL STENTS

Seventy patients, 48 men and 22 women, with significant dysphagia were treated. The strictures were caused by primary squamous cell carcinoma ($n=32$), primary adenocarcinoma ($n=21$), recurrent anastomotic carcinoma ($n=9$), and mediastinal tumors ($n=8$). Successful stent placement was achieved in all patients. Placement of two coaxial stents was necessary in six patients; all other patients received a single stent. During delivery, one coaxial stent was fixed in large-tumor masses involving the stomach and was left misplaced. Twelve stents could be dilated directly to the maximum stent diameter and 21 other stents self-expanded within 24 hours after insertion (Fig. 12-5).

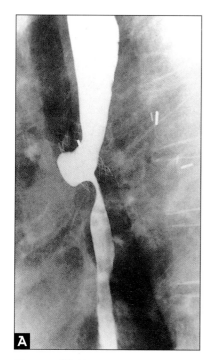
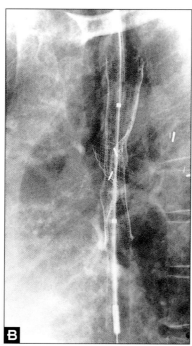
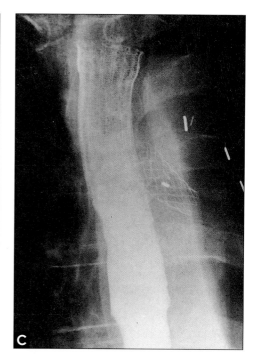

FIGURE 12-5.

Pulmonary carcinoma. **A**, A Palmaz stent positioned in the main left bronchus to combat a stricture of the esophagus. **B**, A delivered esophageal stent after balloon dilatation. **C**, Twenty-four hours following insertion the stent is completely expanded.

The other stents all eventually expanded completely during further observation (Fig. 12-6), except for three stents that did not fully open, as a result of technical failure. Substantial reduction of dysphagia was noted in all patients. Stent migration subsequently occurred in one patient with recurrent cancer in an esophagojejunal anastomosis. The stent passed through the gastrointestinal tract 1.5 months after insertion without causing any serious complications. Tumor ingrowth through the stent mesh was seen at endoscopy in nine patients 4 to 11 months after stent insertion. Tumor ingrowth necessitated secondary intervention in two patients at 6 and 18 months, respectively, after insertion.

TREATMENT OF PATIENTS WITH BENIGN STRICTURES WITH SELF-EXPANDING NITINOL STENTS

Two men and three women 13 to 82 years of age were treated. The strictures were secondary to reflux esophagitis in two patients and to ingestion of alkali in three patients. Repeated dilatation had incomplete and short-lasting effects and none of the strictures could be dilated to the maximum angioplasty balloon diameter of 12 mm before stent insertion. All stents self-expanded to their maximum diameter within 2 to 14 days, with improvement of dysphagia. During the observation time

of up to 20 months after insertion, three patients developed new strictures at the edges of the stents. In two of these patients, additional treatment was required.

Conclusion

The ability to ingest food normally is one of the basic factors determining the patient's quality of life. Metallic expandable stents offer new options in the treatment of esophageal strictures. Insertion of esophageal stents is both easy and safe. All patients treated could receive oral nutrition and a majority followed a normal diet during stent treatment. Contrary to the reported experience with plastic tubes, insertion of the esophageal stents is easy, safe, and cost effective [36•]. The subsequent, complete self-expansion of the majority of nitinol stents demonstrated that their radial expansive force is sufficient to successfully dilatate both benign and malignant esophageal strictures [24,25•]. Such a gradual dilatation most likely reduces traumatic injury to the esophageal wall and diminishes the risk of rupture. Ingrowth of a tumor through the stent wall was observed in several patients. It is likely that a majority of patients with esophageal cancer will die before the stent can be occluded. Coating of the stents may prevent ingrowth of tumors and, more importantly, may lead to closure of

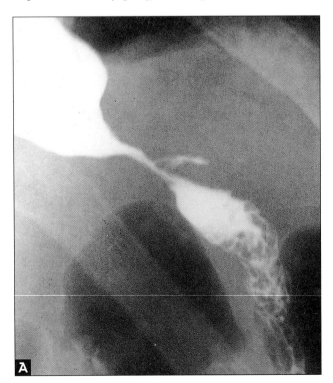

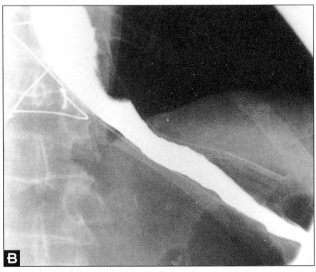

FIGURE 12-6.

Recurrence of the adenocarcinoma. **A**, A pronounced stricture in the esophagojejunal anastomosis, appearing as a small fistula. **B**, The results on the day following stent insertion. The stent, still partially compressed, allows ingestion of fluids and mashed food.

esophagorespiratory fistulae [26•,28–30]. Coated stents may be less adherent to the esophageal wall than plain stents, and may also migrate more frequently.

The number of patients treated for benign strictures is small [25•]. Because of the frequent development of new stenoses at the edges of the stents in these patients, it is advisable to insert stents only in patients requiring preoperative nutritional support or in selected elderly patients. However, we find that self-expanding stents are safe and efficacious and we recommend them for use in the palliative treatment of patients with malignant esophageal strictures.

References and Recommended Reading

Recently published papers of particular interest have been highlighted as:
• Of interest
•• Of outstanding interest

1. Celestin LR: Permanent Intubation in Inoperative Cancer of the Esophagus and Cardia. *Ann R Coll Surg Engl* 1959, 25:165–170.

2. Saunders NR: The Celestin Tube in the Palliation of Carcinoma of the Oesophagus and Cardia. *Br J Surg* 1979, 66:419–421.

3. Atkinson M, Ferguson R: Fibreoptic Endoscopic Palliative Intubation of Inoperable Oesophagogastric Neoplasms. *Br J Med* 1977, 1:266–267.

4. Foutch PG, Talbert G, Sanowski RA: Nonoperative Traction Method for Placement of Esophageal Stents: A New Use for the Percutaneous Endoscopic Gastrotomy. *Gastrointest Endosc* 1988, 34:259–262.

5. Gasparri G, Casalegno P, Camandona M, *et al.*: Endoscopic Insertion of 248 Prostheses in Inoperable Carcinoma of the Esophagus and Cardia: Short-Term and Long-Term Results. *Gastrointest Endosc* 1987, 33:354–356.

6. Lux G, Wilson D, Wilson J, *et al.*: A Cuffed Tube for the Treatment of Oeso-Phago-Bronchial Fistula. *Endoscopy* 1987, 19:28–30.

7. Tytgat GNJ, Bartelsman JFWM, Den Hartog Jager FCA, *et al.*: Upper Intestinal and Biliary Tract Endoprosthesis. *Dig Dis Sci Suppl* 1986, 31:57S–76S.

8. Möuller JM, Erasmi H, Stelzner M, *et al.*: Surgical Therapy for Oesophageal Carcinoma. *Br J Surg* 1990, 77:845–857.

9. Sons HU, Streicher HJ: Palliative and Curative Surgical Therapy of Malignant Stenoses of the Esophagus and Cardia. *J Surg Oncol* 1989, 40:162–169.

10. Earlam R, Cunha-Melo JR: Oesophageal Squamous Cell Carcinoma: I. A Critical Review of Surgery. *Br J Surg* 1980, 67:381–390.

11. Albertsson M, Evers S-B, Widmark H, *et al.*: Evaluation of the Palliative Effect of Radiotherapy for Esophageal Carcinoma. *Acta Oncol* 1989, 28:267–270.

12. Earlam R, Cunha-Melo JR: Oesophageal Squamous Cell Carcinoma: II. A Critical Review of Radiotherapy. *Br J Surg* 1980, 67:457–461.

13. Ell C, Demling L: Laser Therapy of Tumor Stenoses in the Upper Gastrointestinal Tract: An International Inquiry. *Lasers Surg Med* 1987, 7:491–494.

14. Murray FE, Bowers GJ, Birkett DH, *et al.*: Palliative Laser Therapy of Advanced Esophageal Carcinoma. An Alternative Perspective. *Am J Gastroenterol* 1988, 83:816–819.

15. Santhi-Swaroop V, Desai PB: Palliative Management of Esophageal Cancer. *Sem Surg Oncol* 1989, 5:373–375.

16. Tytgat GNJ, Den Hartog Jager FCA, Bartelsman JFWM: Endoscopic Prosthesis for Advanced Esophageal Cancer. *Endoscopy* 1986, 18:32–39.

17. Broor SL, Kumar A, Chari ST, *et al.*: Corrosive Oesophageal Strictures Following Acid Ingestion: Clinical Profile and Results of Endoscopic Dilatation. *J Gastroenterol Hepatol* 1989, 4:55–61.

18. London RL, Trotman BW, DiMarino AJ, *et al.*: Dilatation of Severe Esophageal Strictures by an Inflatable Balloon Catheter. *Gastroenterology* 1981, 80:173–175.

19. Owman T, Lunderquist A: Balloon Catheter Dilatation of Esophageal Strictures–A Preliminary Report. *Gastrointest Radiol* 1982, 7:301–305.

20. Tytgat GNJ: Dilation Therapy of Benign Esophageal Stenoses. *World J Surg* 1989, 13:142–148.

21. Winter J, Jung M, Saeger H-D, *et al.*: Long-Term Results of Palliative Endoscopic and Surgical Intubation of Benign Oesophageal Stenoses. *Surg Endosc* 1990, 4:168–172.

22. Souttar HS: A Method of Intubating the Oesophagus for Malignant Stricture. *Brit J Med* 1924, 1:782–783.

23. Frimberger E: Expanding Spiral–A New Type of Prosthesis for the Palliative Treatment of Malignant Esophageal Stenoses. *Endoscopy* 1983, 15:213–214.

24. Cwikiel W, Stridbeck H, Tranberg H-G, *et al.*: Malignant Esophageal Strictures: Treatment with Self-expanding Nitinol Stent. *Radiology* 1993, 187:661–665.

25. • Cwikiel W, Willén R, Stridbeck H, *et al.*: A New Self-expanding Stent in the Treatment of Benign Esophageal Strictures. An Experimental Study in Pigs and Presentation of Clinical Cases. *Radiology* 1993, 187:667–671.
The only report describing clinical treatment of benign esophageal strictures. Findings from the animal trial are presented.

26. • Do YS, Song H-Y, Lee BH, *et al.*: Esophagorespiratory Fistula by Esophageal Cancer: Palliation With a Modified Gianturco Stent Tube. *Radiology* 1993, 187:673–677.
Treatment of these fistulas is a very serious problem. Reported results open new options for such treatment.

27. Kozarek RA, Ball TJ, Pattersson DJ: Metallic Self-expanding Stent Application in the Upper Gastrointestinal Tract: Caveats and Concerns. *Gastrointest Endosc* 1992, 38:1–6.

28. Schaer J, Katon RM, Ivancev K, *et al.*: Treatment of Malignant Esophageal Obstruction with Silicone-Coated Metallic Self-expanding Stents. *Gastrointest Endosc* 1992, 38:7–11.

29. Song H-Y, Choi K-C, Cho B-H, *et al.*: Esophagogastric Neoplasms: Palliation with a Modified Gianturco Stent. *Radiology* 1991, 180:349–354.

30. Song H-Y, Choi K-C, Kwon H-C, *et al.*: Esophageal Strictures: Treatment with a New Design of Modified Gianturco Stent. *Radiology* 1992, 184:729–734.

31. Bethge N, Knyrim K, Wagner HJ, *et al.*: Self-expanding Metal Stents for Palliation of Malignant Esophageal Obstruction - A Pilot Study of Eight Patients. *Endoscopy* 1992, 24: 411–415.

32. Domschke W, Foerster EC, Matek W, *et al.*: Self-expanding Mesh Stent for Esophageal Cancer Stenosis. *Endoscopy* 1990, 22:134–136.

33. Lindberg G-C, Cwikiel W, Ivancev K, *et al.*: Laser Therapy and Insertion of Wallstents for Palliative Treatment of Esophageal Carcinoma. *Acta Radiol* 1991, 32:345–348.

34. Neuhaus H, Hoffmann W, Dittler HJ, *et al.*: Implantation of Self-expanding Esophageal Metal Stents for Palliation of Malignant Dysphagia. *Endoscopy* 1992, 24:405–410.

35. Neuhaus H: Metal Esophageal Stents. *Sem Intervent Radiol* 1991, 8:305–310.

36. • Knyrim K, Wagner H-J, Bethge R, *et al.*: A Controlled Trial of an Expansile Metal Stent for Palliation of Esophageal Obstruction Due to Inoperable Cancer. *New Engl J Med* 1993, 329:1302–1307.

Advantages of the self-expandable esophageal metallic stents compared with plastic tubes are presented. Cost effectiveness of stent treatment is also discussed.

Select Bibliography

Cwikiel W, Stridbeck H, Tranberg K-G, *et al.*: Malignant Esophageal Strictures: Treatment with a Self-expanding Nitinol Stent. *Radiology* 1993, 187:661–665.

Knyrim K, Wagner H-J, Bethge R, *et al.*: A Controlled Trial of an Expansile Metal Stent for Palliation of Esophageal Obstruction Due to Inoperative Cancer. *N Engl J Med* 1993, 329:1302–1307.

Song H-Y, Choi K-C, Kwon H-C, *et al.*: Esophageal Strictures: Treatment with a New Design of Modified Gianturco Stent. *Radiology* 1992, 184:729–734.

Self-expanding Stents in the Management of Tracheobronchial Stenosis

Herve P. Rousseau
Phillipe Carré
Francis Joffre
Simon Martel
Alain Didier
Ignatio Bilbao

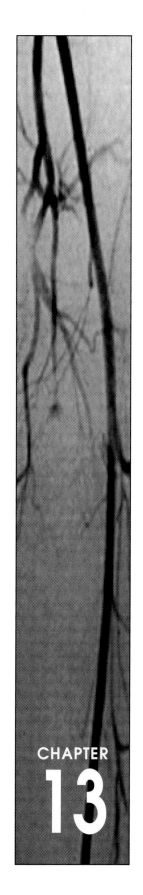

CHAPTER

13

There are numerous causes of benign and malignant tracheobronchial obstructions. Tracheobronchial tumor obstruction can occur as a result of endoluminal invasion or extrinsic compression. Prolonged intubation and tracheobronchial surgery are the leading causes of tracheobronchial obstruction. Treatment of these lesions by surgery, radiation therapy, or endobronchial therapy is frequently unsatisfactory [1,2].

Radiation therapy can lead to reduction in size of malignant obstructions, but its toxic effects on surrounding tissues limits its efficacy and is therefore rarely applicable for tumor recurrence. Endoscopic techniques using resection with diathermy, lasers, cryotherapy, or balloon dilatation have been proposed but they all have short-term beneficial effects [3–7].

Benign lesions, stenosis, or malacia are better treated by surgical resection, but this technique can only be proposed for short lesions. Alternative surgical techniques that use substitution materials of autologous or synthetic origin to replace or support the airway wall are not widely accepted [8–10].

Silicone rubber tubes provide a safe, relatively trouble-free airway in a variety of acquired benign or malignant obstructive lesions of bronchi by maintaining tracheobronchial lumen continuity and providing a barrier for tissue ingrowth and preventing tumor invasion [11•, 12•, 13, 14•].

However, conventional prostheses are poorly tolerated in the short term because of the lack of epithelialization. They are plagued with complications such as obstruction by dried secretions, distal migration leading to occlusion of lobar bronchi, and repeated pulmonary infections [11•, 12•, 14•]. Therefore, regular bronchoscopic checks are necessary with this type of prostheses.

A simple atraumatic approach that could help to reestablish airway caliber would be the implantation of an endoluminal scaffolding device or a self-expandable stent. The theoretic advantage of auto-expandable stents is two-fold: 1) the endoluminal introduction requires no surgery and is a rapid and simple procedure; and 2) the stents are rapidly incorporated into the airway wall and are covered with functional neoepithelium because they are highly porous.

Historic Notes and Experimental Background

The use of metallic endoprostheses in the treatment of tracheal and bronchial stenoses was described 20

years ago by Belsey [15] and Bucher and colleagues [16]. One of the most interesting publications was written by Pagliero and Shepherd [17] in 1974. These authors demonstrate that after the implantation of a stainless-steel coil across a tracheal anastomotic disruption, 80% of metallic filaments were covered after only 21 days. Subsequently, dilation sessions were required for the first 8 months to treat granulomas further developing nonprogressive tissue membranes over the following 16 months. This first observation suggested that even with a rapid inflammatory reaction, metallic endoprostheses could be well tolerated on a longer follow-up. We had to wait until the mid-1980s to see the re-emergence of tracheobronchial metallic endoprostheses.

Experimental studies show, both for the Gianturco and the Wallstent device, that the stents are well tolerated experimentally by the trachea [18–20]. Histologically, there develops a covering of ciliated, pseudostratified epithelium, characteristic of the airway. In addition, we and Wallace and colleagues [18], found that epithelial hyperplasia also occurred with a mild localized inflammatory reaction.

An experimental study performed in our institute on 21 rabbits using the Wallstent showed that this reaction attained a peak at 1 month and subsided gradually thereafter, becoming a simple epithelial hyperplasia covered by normal ciliated epithelium (Fig. 13-1). In their experimental studies with the Gianturco stent, Rauber and colleagues [19] observed significant granulomas at the points of maximum contact pressure of the filaments. This could be explained by overdilation of the trachea by too large a stent diameter or to the type of filament stiffness chosen. One would believe that by using a stent caliber better adapted to the tracheal diameter and with a better load distribution over the stent filaments, this problem could be avoided. In the latter respect, the Wallstent would appear to be the better choice.

Technical Aspects

TYPES OF PROSTHESES: THE WALLSTENT MODEL

This device (Schneider Europe, Zurich, Switzerland), extensively used in vascular, biliary, and urethral applications, is composed of 20 surgical-steel monofilaments each 100 µm in diameter, braided into a cylindrical tube (Fig. 13-2A) [21–23]. The prosthesis can be longitudinally stretched to a small diameter format, spontaneously springing back to its original diameter when removed from its delivery catheter. When mounted on the 7- to 9-French delivery catheter, the prosthesis is constrained by a rolling membrane that protects the device during insertion and progressively deploys it from the instrument. The prosthesis diameter is greater than that of the target airway so that the device molds itself to the passage wall by residual radial pressure. Its inherent flexibility allows it to conform to airway curves and bends. The prostheses used in this indication are 6 to 20 mm in diameter; the size is chosen so that it is at least 2 mm greater than the larger lumen diameter measured at the proximal region of the normal bronchus. Implanted lengths range from 3 to 5 cm, according to the length of the lesion.

Types of Prostheses: The Gianturco Model

This device (DK 4632; Cook, Bjaeverskov, Denmark) is comprised of 0.018-inch, stainless-steel monofilaments made into a double zigzag format introduced via a 12-French teflon sheath (Fig. 13-2B). The double pros-

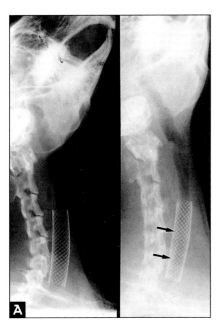
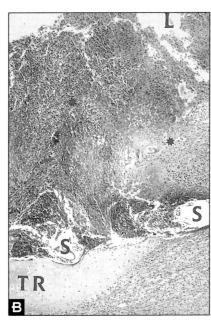
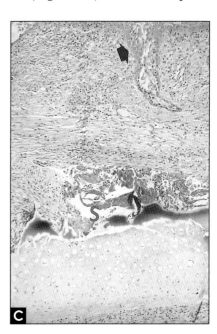

Figure 13-1.

Experimental studies show that the Wallstent is experimentally well tolerated by the rabbit trachea. **A,** Three months after stenting, an endoluminal defect inside the lumen can be seen corresponding to epithelial hyperplasia (*arrows*). **B,** Histologically, we note the disappearance of epithelial covering replaced by a localized inflammatory reaction (❋) 2 weeks after stenting. This reaction attained a peak at 1 month, and subsided gradually thereafter. **C,** Two months later a covering of ciliated pseudostratified epithelium developed characteristic of the airway (*arrow*) (Hemalun Eosin Safran coloration). L—lumen; S—stent filaments; TR—tracheal ring.

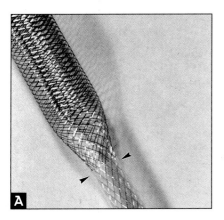
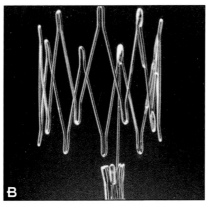

Figure 13-2.

A, The Wallstent endoprosthesis. The controlled withdrawal of the external membrane allows the progressive release of the endoprosthesis (*arrowheads*). **B,** The double-zigzag Gianturco stent. The first stent is totally extruded from the teflon sheath. Further retraction of the sheath releases the second stent.

theses modified by Uchida are equipped with fixation hooks for engaging the airway wall [24]. Stents 30 mm in diameter and 5-cm long are used for tracheal stenoses and those 30 × 25 mm for bronchial stenoses. Other authors have recently described the successful utilization of balloon-mounted prostheses for this indication, the Strecker prosthesis in particular [25]. In our experience, we prefer to use auto-expandable prostheses that seem more stable in view of the wide tracheobronchial diameter variation observed in the respiratory cycle. There is also a higher risk of migration when coughing with the nonauto-expandable prostheses.

Other than these two prostheses (Gianturco and Wallstent), additional auto-expandable prostheses made of nitinol could also be used for this indication, such as the Memotherm (Angiomed, Karlsruhe, Germany) and the Cragg (Mintec, La Ciotat, France) prostheses.

THE IMPLANTATION TECHNIQUE

A flexible bronchoscopy and a computed tomography (CT) scan are performed a few days prior to implantation to document the length of the lesions and the diameter of the airway as well as to confirm its noninflammatory character. These implantations are performed with only mild sedation and topical anesthesia. The patient is given nasal oxygen 2 to 5 L per minute and monitored continuously with pulse oximetry and electrocardiography. Appropriate antibiotic and anti-inflammatory steroid prophylaxis are given for 1 week. The implantation technique depends on the lesion location.

Tracheal Implants

The exact position of the stenosis is established using a combination of endoscopic and fluoroscopic guidance. The bronchoscope is positioned above the stenosis, and metallic markers are placed on the skin, specifying the distal and proximal limits of the lesion. A 0.035-inch, 145-cm long guidewire is then inserted through the channel of the bronchoscope, past the lesion, and the bronchoscope is then removed. Under fluoroscopic control, the stent delivery system is advanced over the guidewire until radiovisible markers on the edges of the prosthesis are aligned with skin markers that indicate the limits of the lesion. The prosthesis is then progressively deployed and removed from its delivery catheter.

Bronchial Lesions

Implantation is performed after opacification of the bronchial tree with Iopidol (Hytrast; Guerbet Laboratories, Villepinte, France) (Fig. 13-3). The bronchi are then selectively catheterized using conventional radiologic vascular techniques and balloon dilatation (performed in patients with stenosis only) is performed under fluoroscopy. The balloon is gradually inflated to its maximum dimensions as visualized by fluoroscopy and held inflated at 6 to 12 atmospheres for 10 to 30 seconds, depending on the clinical tolerance and consequences of cutaneous oxygen saturation. A further one

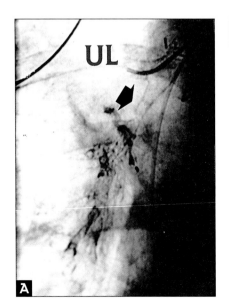
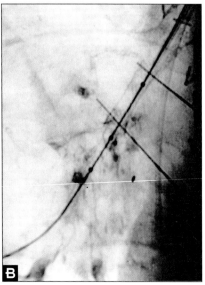

FIGURE 13-3.

A, A Wallstent has been used to treat post–double-lung transplantation stenosis (*arrow*). Implantation was performed after opacification of the tracheobronchial tree with Iopidol. **B**, A 2-cm long prosthesis was implanted on the intermediate bronchus between the two radioopaque skin markers, without covering proximal and distal bronchi. UL—upper lobe.

or two dilatations are performed at 3-minute intervals before removing the balloon catheter and advancing the prosthesis into position.

The implantation can be performed under either endoscopic or radiologic guidance but the technique is more precise and much easier when both guidance methods are used. By using radiologic guidance alone, the characteristics of the lesion cannot be precisely determined, particularly the noninflammatory types. On the other hand, it is often difficult to go through the bronchial obstruction with the bronchoscope to evaluate the full extent of the lesion before the prosthesis implantation. Moreover, it is difficult to place the prosthesis in good position to ensure that it straddles the lesion accurately and does not obstruct the segmental bronchi. Proper placement of the stent is vital to the success of the procedure, because the stent position cannot be subsequently modified.

Indications

Following preliminary trials, many studies have been published in the past 2 years.

MALIGNANT LESIONS

Obstruction of large airways is major cause of morbidity and mortality in patients with lung cancer. In such patients, radiotherapy or endoscopic methods can be effective, but these procedures may themselves be distressing and are usually effective only in the short term.

Metallic endoprostheses can efficaciously treat tracheal or bronchial extrinsic compression by malignant tumors, but they are least effective when there is wall invasion by the tumor because they cannot stop endoluminal tumor proliferation. However, these prostheses can be proposed for patients with life-threatening or severely disabling breathlessness for which conventional treatments have been unsuccessful or were not feasible [25, 26, 27••, 28••, 29]. Furthermore, patency of the airway can be maintained by additional therapeutic options such as intraluminal or percutaneous after-loading irradiation and laser or diathermic resection [25]. Tumor ingrowth through the metal stent continues to be problematic.

Silicone-covered metallic endoprostheses have also been used for this indication, either to prevent endotracheal tumor proliferation or, when placed in the esophagus, to treat esophagotracheal fistula caused by tracheal tumor invasion [30••, 31••, 32]. These prostheses have two main advantages compared with standard silicone prostheses: 1) wider internal lumen; and 2) more reliable parietal fixation that lowers the risk of migration and secondary obstruction.

BENIGN LESIONS

In the majority of patients, benign stenoses are secondary to intubation or tracheotomy and present a significant therapeutic problem, especially when the lesions are extensive. Surgery is often debilitating for lesions in excess of 6 cm in length and the anastomoses can be the source of recurrent stenosis [1]. Conventional prostheses, because of the lack of epithelialization, are poorly tolerated in the short term and are plagued with complications such as obstruction or migration, leading to occlusion of lobar bronchi and recurring pulmonary infections [11•]. Dilatation has been proposed for these types of lesions, but seems limited to benign pediatric stenoses and is of little or no value for dyskinesia or extrinsic compression that recoils immediately [3–5]. Alternatives such as cryotherapy or laser photoresection often have only transient success [6,33].

Different reports demonstrate that self-expandable endoprostheses can be very attractive solutions to the treatment of long, noninflammatory stenoses and tracheobronchial dyskinesias [18, 26, 27••]. This technique offers a good alternative to surgical correction of extrinsic compressions, whether of vascular or extrinsic tumoral origin. For inoperable patients with poor life expectancy, the prostheses offer an atraumatic improvement in the quality of life. Other benign lesions have been treated, associated with extreme mediastinal shift and with rotation after pneumonectomy, as well as anastomotic strictures following sleeve resection, posttracheostomy strictures, idiopathic chondritis, postinfectious lesions, emphysematous processes, and Wegener's syndrome [27••, 34•, 35].

Another potential indication for stent use is in stenosis secondary to lung transplantation. After transplantation, the bronchial anastomotic site is at risk for ischemic complications [36]. Although recent improvements in graft preservation and surgical techniques have reduced their prevalence, airway complications, including necroses and fibrous strictures with malacia or prolific granulation, remain a major problem [7, 12•, 14•, 37–40, 41•].

Different alternative therapies with a rigid broncho-scope have been proposed for the relief of such stenoses [7, 40, 41•]. These procedures can alleviate distressing symptoms but are usually only effective in the short term. Therefore, subsequent bronchial widening has been proposed using silicone stents [7, 12•, 14•]. Potential disadvantages of these stents necessitate regular endoscopic checks, include a tendency for distal migration, a relatively unfavorable wall-to-lumen ratio risking mucus retention, and a possible tendency to stimulate formation of granula-tion tissue distal to the stent.

In lung recipients, these complications may be particularly troublesome and more frequent than in other causes of bronchial obstruction. Indeed, in the patient who has undergone pulmonary transplantation, the presence of secretions distal to the tracheobronchial anastomosis will not elicit a cough reflex. Furthermore, stent obstruction may provoke respiratory distress, particularly in single-lung transplant patients. These limitations have led to a recent interest in expanding metal stents for this indication [42, 43, 44••].

INFLAMMATORY LESIONS
The greatest drawback of metallic stents is the stim-ulation of granulomata in inflammatory lesions. In our experience, Wallstent prostheses were placed on fibroinflammatory lesions in two patients [44••]. During the following months, granulation tissue grew through the interstices of the stents which further necessitated repeated balloon dilatations inside the stent.

In the presence of inflammation, it seems advisable to postpone implantation in favor of a sequential stenting approach—using a silicone stent with anti-inflammatory therapy as the first stage to provide a barrier to tissue ingrowth as the inflammatory tissue matures, and then replacing it with a self-expanding metal stent [45••]. However, because the silicone stent hides the stenotic lesion, it is difficult to determine when the stricture has become completely fibrous and suitable for metal stenting.

As reported by Carré and colleagues [44••] patients with inflammatory stenoses can be prepared for subse-quent metal stenting using balloon dilatation. These early observations led us to adopt the following strategy: balloon dilatation is performed as soon as granulomata are present and the Wallstent prosthesis is inserted when the stenosis relapses and is no longer granulomatous. As indicated above, four post-lung transplantation stenoses were successfully treated in this manner at our institution.

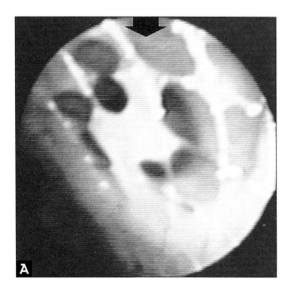
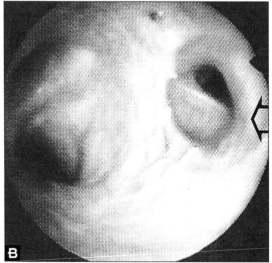

FIGURE 13-4.

A, Endoscopic view of a Wallstent crossing the uper lobe orifice. This prosthesis was implanted to treat a long lesion of the truncus intermedius and the right main bronchus. Sputum retention was observed 4 days after the implantation in the upper lobe bronchus. An endoscopic laser (Nd:YAG) was successfully used to remove the filaments of the stent crossing the orifice (*arrow*). **B**, Endoscopy 3 months later shows a translucent tissue evocative of epithelialization that appears complete on the truncus intermedius and the right main bronchus; the upper lobe bronchus is patent (*open arrow*).

PEDIATRIC LESIONS

After surgical correction of cardiovascular defects in a child, there is a high incidence of tracheomalacia that is sometimes fatal. Using metallic endoprostheses for this indication could be very tempting, but we are perplexed about the future of these nonexpandable prostheses because their caliber would not fit a normal-size adult trachea.

Spatenka and colleagues [46] experimented on growing animal auto-expandable prostheses made of a weak-resistance metal so they could be remodeled with wider prostheses when the animal had grown. With this animal model, the authors demonstrated that in time, the tracheal diameter increased concurrently with the growth of the animal and there was no need for another prosthesis.

Subsequently, three clinical cases on tracheal endoprostheses used in children have been published with promising results [47].

Clinical Results

Self-expandable stenting appears to be a safe procedure and is a good alternative to silicone-stent insertion for the treatment of tracheomalacia or purely fibrous stenosis. With a mean follow-up of 10.35 months, ranging from 3 to 27 months, we observed an improvement in the respiratory status of 49 of 55 patients (89%) with excellent tolerance of the device [27••].

RESULTS WITH THE WALLSTENT

Because of their excellent flexibility and conformability, this prosthesis allows accurate placement and conforms extremely well to the bronchial anatomy, making it very suitable for this indication. Wallstents were initially available in too small a diameter for stenting the trachea, but this problem has now been resolved by the availability of stents in excess of 30 mm in diameter.

In two cases, the stenosis was so located that the lower end of the Wallstent overlapped the upper-lobe bronchial orifice; to prevent subsequent obstruction, 3 to 4 days after stent insertion the filaments of the stent crossing the lobar orifice were vaporized by laser (Fig. 13-4). A Nd:YAG laser (Multilase 2500; Technomed International, Bron, France) was used to administer 40-watt pulses per second at a dose of approximately 500 J.

All patients demonstrated a good tolerance and improvement in respiratory status after Wallstent insertion [27••]. No patients reported any pain, discomfort, or foreign body sensations. An irritation-type cough occurred in a few patients within the first month, but settled under temporary inhaled steroid therapy. Sputum retention and secondary infection did not occur in any patients.

One instance of hemoptysis was observed following prosthesis implantation. This complication was observed in a patient in which the stent diameter was too small and did not approximate the bronchial wall in all areas.

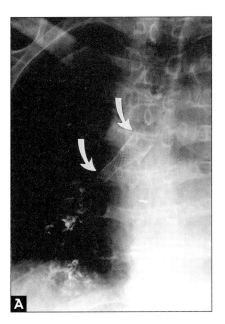

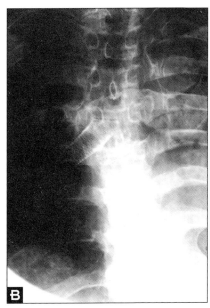

FIGURE 13-5.

Chest radiograph taken just after Wallstent implantation and 1 week later. **A**, Note stent extremities (*arrows*). As can be seen, immediately after stenting the bronchus diameter has improved, although it is not normalized. **B**, One week later, radiologic studies confirmed the progressive prosthesis expansion to the predetermined diameter of the stent, substantially increasing the diameter of the lumen.

Radiologic studies confirmed no device migration and progressive prosthesis expansion during the first week (Fig. 13-5) to the predetermined diameter for each stent, substantially increasing the diameter of the lumen and resulting in maintenance of an adequate airway (Fig. 13-6). Endoscopic inspection showed rapid covering of the epithelium by translucent tissue, beginning from the twentieth day; it appeared complete after 6 months of follow-up.

However, this type of prosthesis has two disadvantages: 1) problems may supervene when placing the prosthesis because of its weak opacity; and 2) the lesion may be inadequately covered because of its significant shortening occurring either during placement of the prosthesis or after its insertion.

Four of five patients who presented with tumoral compressions died from their conditions at a mean of only 3 months. They all had normal respiratory function during their survival. In one patient with tracheal carcinoma, tumoral proliferation inside and above the prosthesis was seen and successfully treated endoscopically with a laser.

Carré and colleagues [44••] show that combined or sequential use of balloon dilatation and self-expanding metal stents can resolve most of the airway obstruction problems following lung transplantation. Wallstent placement after lung transplantation resulted in expansion of stenoses to a diameter large enough to normalize pulmonary function parameters. In 10 patients with a mean ± SE time with the stent in place for 15.3 ± 2.7 months, six were functionally evaluated before, and at 1 and 6 months after Wallstent insertion. The mean forced expiratory volume in 1 second (FEV_1) was 1288 ± 433 mL, 1728 ± 658 mL, and 1874 ± 658 mL, respectively. Of the 10 patients managed for airway complications, three single-lung transplant recipients died 3, 10, and 12 months respectively, after prosthesis positioning. Deaths were not believed to be airway-related complications because no abnormality was endoscopically noted (Fig. 13-7).

In our experience with 39 Wallstents, six complications were observed: one tumoral proliferation within the stent previously described; two early restenoses at a stent extremity, caused by insufficient covering by the prosthesis which were successfully treated by overstenting; and three bronchial late restenoses within the stent, successfully treated by balloon dilatations or a second stent with a persistent clinical benefit (Fig. 13-8) [26].

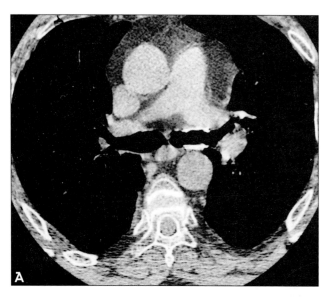

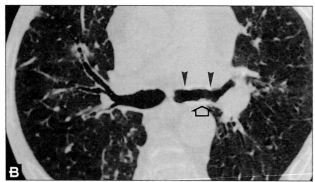

FIGURE 13-6.

A, Computed tomography scan 9 months after Wallstent implantation. **B,** The slightly radiodense stent (*arrowheads*) is seen within the lumen of the left mainstem bronchus where it maintains patency across the mainstem structure. Note hyperplasia reaction inside the lumen (*open arrow*).

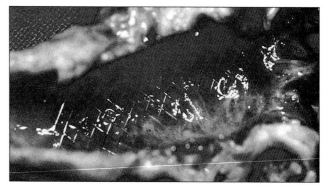

FIGURE 13-7.

Macroscopic view of a Wallstent implanted 12 months before for a left bronchial stenosis following transplantation (specimen was obtained after a second transplantation for a chronic rejection).

RESULTS WITH THE GIANTURCO STENT

This stent seems well suited to tracheal lesions, given its very large diameter. However, because the pressure exerted on the wall is small, this device appears better indicated for tracheomalacias than fibrotic stenoses.

Prosthesis implantation of the Gianturco stent is simple, but positioning problems can occur if there is a sudden opening of the prosthesis when releasing it into the tracheal lumen, thus increasing the risk of distal migration before the fixation hooks can adequately adhere to tracheal walls. Finally, kinking of the prosthesis can be observed when placed in a tortuous trachea.

In our experience, this stent was used exclusively for tracheo- and bronchomalacia. No coughing or syncope episodes were noted in any patients. Endoscopic controls observed no expiratory collapse in 65% of patients. A cellular covering was visible by the third week and stabilized at 6 months without signifi-

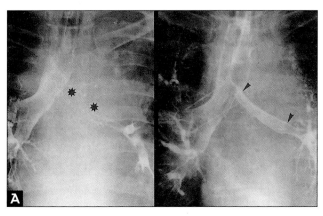

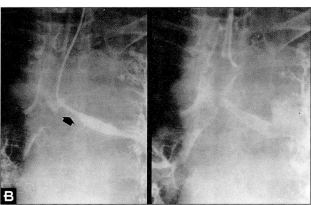

FIGURE 13-8.

A, Postinfectious stenosis (✳) of the left main bronchus. A first stent (*arrowheads*) was implanted following balloon dilatation. **B**, A restenosis (*arrow*) inside the stent 9 months later was successfully treated by balloon dilatation and a second stent.

cant epithelial hyperplasia (Fig. 13-9) [26]. With respect to the advantages of the Gianturco stents in tracheomalacia, the main impact was in the improvement in cough efficiency in 66% of patients.

The functional values observed in a 1-year follow-up in 10 random patients were essentially unchanged. Similar to surgical or previous silicone-stent insertion in tracheomalacia, we observed a slight decrease in FEV_1 after 1 month. This decrease is most likely a result of an endoscopically observed local inflammatory process within the stent, causing a temporary increase in bronchial obstruction. The inflammatory process in these stent placements peaks at approximately 1 month and then gradually subsides.

When using this type of prosthesis, Sawada and colleagues [28••] observed an increase in tracheal and bronchial diameter (89.7% and 63.2%, respectively) in 14 patients with nine extrinsic compressions and 10 tumor invasions. Concurrently, with this increase in endoluminal diameter, a clinical improvement of at least one degree on the Hugh Jones classification scale was observed in 12 of 14 patients [28••]. Tumor ingrowth through the metal stent remained problematic in two patients; however, the incidence of palliative interventions required seemed to be markedly reduced after stenting.

Routine flexible endoscopies further confirmed excellent patency of the stent in most of the patients, but the problem of migration observed in animal and early clinical trials is not totally solved by the tissue-engaging hooks.

Gianturco stents had a high complication rate (*eg*, breaks in the filament branches with or without migration that potentially led to obstruction or wall perforation). In our experiment, this was observed in six of 19

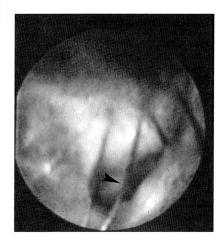

FIGURE 13-9.

Endoscopic study of a Gianturco stent crossing the upper lobe orifice revealed no significant epithelial hyperplasia and a cellular covering was visible at 6 months. Note stent filaments crossing the upper lobe orifice (*arrowhead*).

patients (31%). Two of these patients required extraction of the prosthesis and there was one case of respiratory distress that was fatal (Fig. 13-10).

In lung transplant recipients, spontaneous fractures of stents have recently been described in two patients 2 to 4 months after implantation. In one of these patients, circulatory arrest and death occurred at the time of bronchoscopic removal and an autopsy revealed a tracheal perforation [46]. Additionally, one patient with fatal massive hemoptysis resulting from erosion of the pulmonary artery was seen 10 days after implantation [42]. Latter complications strongly suggest that Gianturco stent insertion in its present form cannot be advised in bronchostenosis following lung transplantation.

Conclusion

When facing respiratory distress from either benign or malignant causes, the indication for endoprosthesis implantation is clear because dyspnea is relieved almost instantly. However, we must choose between a temporary silicone prosthesis or a permanent, auto-expandable metallic prosthesis.

Although silicone prostheses can actually be removed, they have many disadvantages as described earlier (*eg*, more traumatic installation with general anesthesia and rigid bronchoscope; regular follow-up required to detect and possibly treat complications; and migration with secondary obstruction).

Theoretic advantages of metallic prostheses are: 1) ease of insertion under local anesthesia; 2) lower risk of obstruction when the prosthesis is covering a distal bronchus, allowing the treatment of lesions more distally located; and 3) lower complication rate, implying that less endoscopic follow-up is required.

The clinical studies demonstrate that self-expandable endoprostheses can be very attractive solutions to the treatment of stenoses and of long, noninflammatory, tracheobronchial dyskinesias; they offer a good alternative to surgical correction of extrinsic compressions in inoperable patients.

Again, given its very large diameter, the Gianturco stent seems well suited for the management of tracheomalacia lesions. However, migration and fractures have been observed in early clinical trials.

The Wallstent allows for very accurate placement and conforms extremely well to the bronchial anatomy, making it very suitable for this indication as well. Wallstent insertion appears to be a safe procedure and is a good alternative to silicone-stent insertion for the treatment of malacic or purely fibrous stenosis.

The major disadvantage of expanding metal stents is that they cannot be removed endoscopically. No major problems have appeared thus far with the use of the Wallstent, based on a mean follow-up of 10 months. Although the possibility of this stent eroding into the mediastinum is unclear at this time, it is hoped that this kind of stent can be left in place for years without major complications.

It was recently proposed that until a longer follow-up has been studied, the use of these stents should be limited to patients with recurrent bronchial stenosis

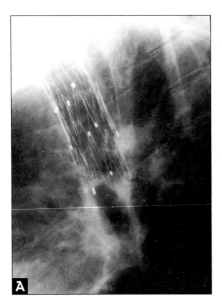
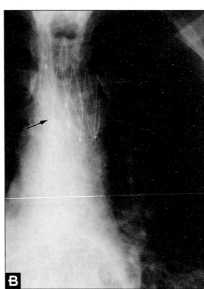

FIGURE 13-10.

A, The Gianturco stent seems well suited to tracheomalacias. **B,** In this case, breaks in the filament branches with migration (potentially leading to obstruction or wall perforation) were observed 3 months later (*arrow*). This patient had to undergo endoscopic extraction of the prosthesis.

resistant to treatment by other techniques, such as simple dilatations, laser therapy, or silicone stents. This issue specifically regards the Gianturco stents [46].

However, in other recent reports, the Wallstent was successfully used as a first-line treatment in miscellaneous causes of malignant or benign tracheobronchial strictures, including those following lung transplantation [27••, 34•,44••]. Although silicone stents remain valuable for the treatment of inflammatory bronchial stenosis, early clinical results from different studies indicate that the combination of balloon dilatation and Wallstent prosthesis insertion may be considered in selected patients as a first-line treatment for inflammatory granulomatous lesions.

In malignant stenoses to date, indications are restricted to extrinsic compression waiting for results on the effectiveness of silicone- or dacron-covered, auto-expandable metallic endoprostheses with wall invasion [48].

The ultimate role of these stents in tracheobronchial pathology will be better defined with time. However, we speculate that in the future the use of selected self-expanding metal stents will be extended to various conditions including benign stenosis and diskinesia of the tracheobronchial tree in emphysematous processes. Such prospects are currently under investigation at our institution.

References and Recommended Reading

Recently published papers of particular interest have been highlighted as:
• Of interest
•• Of outstanding interest

1. Grillo HC, Mathisen DJ: Surgical Management of Tracheal Strictures. *Surg Clin North Am* 1988, 68:511–524.

2. Landa L: The Tracheal T-tube in Tracheal Surgery. In *International Trends in General Thoracic Surgery*, vol 2. Edited by Grillo HC, Eschapasse H. Philadelphia: WB Saunders; 1987:124–213.

3. Cohen MD, Weber TR, Rao CC: Balloon Dilatation of Tracheal and Bronchial Stenosis. *AJR* 1984, 142:477–478.

4. Carlin BW, Harrell JH, Moser KM: The Treatment of Endobronchial Stenosis Using Balloon Catheter Dilatation. *Chest* 1988, 93:1148–1151.

5. Fowler CL, Aaland MO, Harris FL: Dilatation of Bronchial Stenosis with a Gruentzig Balloon. *J Thorac Cardiovasc Surg* 1987, 93:308–315.

6. Homasson JP, Renault P, Angebault M, *et al.*: Bronchoscopic Cryotherapy for Airway Strictures Caused by Tumors. *Chest* 1986, 90:159–164.

7. Schafers HJ, Haydock DA, Cooper JD: The Prevalence and Management of Bronchial Anastomotic Complications in Lung Transplantation. *J Thorac Cardiovasc Surg* 1991, 101:1044–1052.

8. Toohill RJ: Autogenous Graft Reconstruction of the Larynx and Upper Trachea. *Otolaryngol Clin North Am* 1979, 12:909–917.

9. Neel B: GoreTex Implants. *Arch Otolaryngol* 1983, 109:427–433.

10. Greve H: Substitution of the Wall of the Trachea by Absorbable Synthetic Material. *Thorac Cardiovasc Surg* 1988, 36:20–26.

11.• Dumon JF: A Dedicated Tracheobronchial Stent. *Chest* 1990, 97:328–332.
Although the use of silicone stents in bronchial obstructive lesions is safe, these prostheses are found to be poorly tolerated in the long term and may cause complications.

12.• Gaer JA, Tsang V, Khagiani A, *et al.*: Use of Endotracheal Silicone Stents for Relief of Tracheobronchial Obstruction. *Ann Thorac Surg* 1992, 54:512–516.
This study is comparable to the information presented in Dumon [11•].

13. Cooper JD, Pearson FG, Patterson GA, *et al.*: Use of Silicone Stents in the Management of Airway Problems. *Ann Thorac Surg* 1989, 47:371–378.

14.• Oturanlar D, Klepetko W, Grimm M, *et al.*: Management of Severe Bronchial Ischemia After Bilateral Sequential Lung Transplantation. *Ann Thorac Surg* 1992, 54:1221–1222.
Another study reviewing the efficacy of silicone stents in bronchial lesions.

15. Belsey R: Resection and Reconstruction of the Intrathoracic Trachea. *Br J Surg* 1951, 38:200.

16. Bucher RM, Busnett WE, Rosemond GP: Experimental Reconstruction of Tracheal and Bronchial Defects with Stainless Steel Wire Mesh. *J Thorac Surg* 1951, 21:572.

17. Pagliero KM, Shepherd MP: Use of Stainless Steel Wire Coil in Treatment of Anastomotic Dehiscence After Cervical Tracheal Resection. *J Thorac Cardiovasc Surg* 1974, 67:932–935.

18. Wallace MJ, Charnsangavej C, Ogawa K, *et al.*: Tracheobronchial Tree: Expandable Metallic Stents Used in Experimental and Clinical Applications. *Radiology* 1986, 158:309–312.

19. Rauber K, Franke C, Rau WS: Self-expanding Stainless Steel Endotracheal Stents: An Animal Study. *Cardiovasc Intervent Radiol* 1989, 12:274–276.

20. Rousseau H, Dahan M, Bilbao I, *et al.*: Use of Self-expandable Prostheses in the Tracheobronchial Tree (abstract). *Cardiovascular and Interventional Radiological Society of Europe*, Oslo, Norway, 1991.

21. Rousseau H, Joffre F, Puel J, *et al.*: A New Type of Self-expanding Endovascular Stent Prosthesis: Experimental Study. *Radiology* 1987, 164:709–714.

22. Milroy EJG, Shappler CR, El-Din A, Wallsten H: A New Stent for the Treatment of Urethral Strictures. Preliminary Report. *Br J Urol* 1989, 63:392–396.

23. Salomonowitz EK, Antonnucci F, Heer M, *et al.*: Biliary Obstruction: Treatment with Self-expanding Metal Prostheses. *JVIR* 1992, 3:365–370.

24. Uchida BT, Putnam JS, Rosch J: Modifications of Gianturco Expandable Wire Stents. *AJR* 1988, 150:1185–1187.

25. Petri F, Ewert R, Romberg B, *et al.*: Intermediate Tracheobronchial Stenting (Strecker Device) by Fibrebronchoscopy in Combination with Irradiation in Patients Suffering From Severe Tumorous Obstruction of Central Airways (abstract). *Eur Res J* Firenze, Italy, 1993.

26. Varela A, Maynar M, Irving D, *et al.*: Use of Gianturco Self-expandable Stents in the Tracheobronchial Tree. *Ann Thor Surg* 1990, 49:806–809.

27.•• Rousseau H, Dahan M, Lauque D, *et al.*: Self-expandable Prostheses in the Tracheobronchial Tree. *Radiology* 1993, 188:199–203.
The authors prefer the use of these prostheses to the use of silicone stents in the treatment of tracheomalacia. In this study, 49 of 55 patients showed improvement in respiratory status and a good tolerance of the device.

28.•• Sawada S, Tanigawa N, Kobayashi M, *et al.*: Malignant Tracheobronchial Obstructive Lesions: Treatment with Gianturco Expandable Metallic Stents. *Radiology* 1993, 188:205–208.
An increase in tracheal and bronchial diameter was observed in this study of 14 patients treated with the Gianturco stent. Clinical improvement was noted in 12 of these patients.

29. Hind CRK, Donnelly RJ: Expandable Metal Stents for Tracheal Obstruction: Permanent or Temporary? A Cautionary Tale. *Thorax* 1992, 47:757–758.

30.•• George PJ, Irving JD, Manell BS, *et al.*: Covered Expandable Metal Stents for Recurrent Tracheal Obstruction. *Lancet* 1990, 335:581–582.
The authors report their experience with silicone-covered metallic stents in preventing endotracheal tumor proliferation or (when the stent is placed in the esophagus) treating esophageal fistulas caused by tracheal tumor invasion.

31.•• Colt HG, Meric B, Dumon JF: Double Stents for Carcinoma of the Esophagus Invading the Tracheo-bronchial Tree. *Gastrointest Endosc* 1992, 38:485–489.
These authors report similar results as in George *et al.* [30••] in their study of esophageal fistulas and tracheobronchial tumors.

32. Song HY, Lee BH, Kim KH, *et al.*: Esophagorespiratory Fistula Associated with Esophageal Cancer Treatment with a Gianturco Stent Tube. *Radiology* 1993, 187:673–677.

33. Dumon JF, Reboud E, Garbe L, *et al.*: Treatment of Tracheobronchial Lesions by Laser Photoresection. *Chest* 1982, 81:278–284.

34.• Tsang V, Goldstraw P: Self-expanding Metal Stents for Tracheobronchial Strictures. *Eur J Cardiothorac Surg* 1992, 6:555–560.
The authors report their experience with Wallstents for the treatment of 12 tracheobronchial strictures due to either benign or malignant processes.

35. Simons AK, Irving JD, Clarke SW, Dick R: Use of Expandable Metal Stents in the Treatment of Bronchial Obstruction. *Thorax* 1989, 44:680–681.

36. Couraud L, Nashef SAM, Nicolini PH, Jougon J: Classification of Airway Anastomotic Healing. *Eur J Cardiothorac Surg* 1992, 6:496–497.

37. Bonnette P, Bisson A, Ben El Kadi N, *et al.*: Bilateral Single Lung Transplantation. Complications and Results in 14 Patients. *Eur J Cardiothorac Surg* 1992, 6:550–554.

38. De Hoyo AL, Patterson GA, Maurer JR, *et al.*: Pulmonary Transplantation. Early and Late Results. *J Thorac Cardiovasc Surg* 1992, 103:295–306.

39. Patterson GA, Todd TR, Cooper JD, *et al.*: Airway Complications After Double Lung Transplantation. *J Thorac Cardiovasc Surg* 1990, 99:14–21.

40. Shennib H, Noirclerc M, Ernst P, *et al.*: Double-lung Transplantation for Cystic Fibrosis. *Ann Thorac Surg* 1992, 54:27–32.

41.• Keller C, Frost A: Fiberoptic Bronchoplasty: Description of a Simple Adjunct Technique for the Management of Bronchial Stenosis Following Lung Transplantation. *Chest* 1992, 102:995–998.
The authors report their experience with balloon dilatation for the treatment of benign bronchial stenoses.

42. Nashef SAM, Dromer C, Velly JF, *et al.*: Expanding Wire Stents in Benign Tracheobronchial Disease: Indications and Complications. *Ann Thorac Surg* 1992, 54:937–940.

43. Brichon PY, Blanc-Jouvan F, Rousseau H, *et al.*: Endovascular Stents for Bronchial Stenosis After Lung Transplantation. *Transplant Proc* 1992, 24:2656–2659.

44.•• Carré P, Rousseau H, Didier A, *et al.*: Balloon Dilatation and Self-expanding Metallic Wallstent Insertion for Bronchostenosis Following Lung Transplantation. *Chest* 1994, 105:343–348.
These authors report their strategy for preparing patients with inflammatory stenoses for subsequent stenting using the Wallstent and balloon dilatation or silastic and metallic stents.

45.•• Tsang V, Williams A, Goldstraw P: Sequential Silastic and Expandable Metal Stenting for Tracheobronchial Strictures. *Ann Thorac Surg* 1992, 53:856–860.
A review of silastic and metallic Wallstents and balloon dilatation for patients with tracheobronchial strictures.

46. Spatenka J, Khaghani A, Irving D, *et al.*: Gianturco Self-expanding Metallic Stents in Treatment of Tracheobronchial Stenosis After Single Lung and Heart and Lung Transplantation. *Eur J Cardiothorac Surg* 1991, 5:648–652.

47. Audry G, Balquet P, Vazquez MP, *et al.*: Expandable Prosthesis in Right Post Pneumonectomy Syndrome in Childhood and Adolescence. *Ann Thorac Surg* 1993, 56:323–327.

48. Kishi K, Kobayashi H, Suruda T, *et al.*: Treatment of Malignant Tracheobronchial Stenosis by Dacron Mesh-covered Z Stents. *Cardiovasc Intervent Radiol* 1994, 17:33–35.

Select Bibliography

Fraser RG, Pare JAP, Genereaux GP: Diseases of the Airways. In *Diagnosis of Diseases of the Chest*, vol 3, edn 3. Philadelphia: WB Saunders; 1990:1969–2005.

Irving JD, Goldstraw P.: Tracheobronchial Stents. *Semin Intervent Radiol* 1991, 8:295–304.

Mathisen DJ: Surgical Management of Tracheobronchial Diseases. In *Clinics in Chest Medicine*. Edited by Buchalter SE, McElvein RB. Philadelphia: WB Saunders; 1992:151–171.

Percutaneous Fluoroscopic Gastrostomy and Gastrojejunostomy: Current Status of the Technique

Stuart D. Bell
Eugene Y. Yeung
Chia-Sing Ho

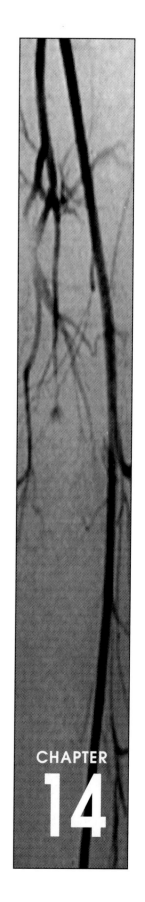

Percutaneous gastrostomy and gastrojejunostomy have become standard interventional radiologic techniques over the past 10 years, largely replacing the previously used surgical methods of gastrostomy. The fluoroscopically guided percutaneous technique was first described in 1983 and is now performed routinely in many radiology departments [1,2]. It is a safe, effective, and inexpensive procedure often performed within 15 to 20 minutes.

Clinical Indications and Contraindications

CLINICAL INDICATIONS

The majority of patients are referred for gastrostomy and gastrojejunostomy as a route for enteral feeding. Although short-term enteral feeding may be given via fine-bore nasojejunal tubes, there is a high incidence of complications related to gastroesophageal reflux with their long-term use [3]. Whenever possible, the enteral route of feeding is favored over the parenteral route because of more efficient assimilation of nutrients, lower complication rates, and lower costs. Enteral feeding is most commonly indicated in patients with cerebrovascular accident, head and neck carcinoma, or esophageal carcinoma. Another group of patients commonly referred for percutaneous gastrostomy are those requiring gastric decompression because of gastroparesis, paralytic ileus, or mechanical small-bowel obstruction related to advanced abdominal malignancy [4,5].

Newer indications include patients with neurologic damage following head injury and patients with short-gut syndrome [6,7]. The latter group has been previously managed with total parenteral nutrition, but more recent reports suggest that in some patients adequate absorption may be achieved with an elemental diet given via a jejunally placed feeding catheter. The current indications for percutaneous gastrostomy are listed in Table 14-1.

CONTRAINDICATIONS

If the air-filled distended stomach does not extend below the costal margin or if that part of the stomach that does is covered by the transverse colon or left lobe of the liver, it is sometimes not possible to safely perform a percutaneous gastrostomy. This most commonly arises in patients postpartial gastrectomy when the stomach remnant may be high under the left costal margin.

Massive ascites, including those in patients receiving continuous ambulatory peritoneal dialysis, are also a contraindication and although lesser degrees of peritoneal fluid are not an absolute contraindication, some method of percutaneous gastropexy is required to keep the anterior wall of the stomach adjacent to the abdominal wall [5].

The procedure should not be undertaken in patients with an increased risk of hemorrhage. This includes patients with an uncorrected bleeding diathesis, most commonly caused by anticoagulant therapy, as well as patients with local causes such as severe gastritis or gastric varices.

INTERNATIONAL VARIATIONS IN PRACTICE

There is considerable variation between North American and European practice regarding the accepted indications for feeding gastrostomy insertion. In the United Kingdom, it is not normal practice to insert gastrostomies in patients following stroke, but this is likely the single most common indication in North America. This is resulting from a difference in approach to the management of these patients—in particular, a different appreciation of a reasonable

Table 14-1. Indications for Gastrostomy

Enteral nutritional therapy
  Dysphagia
    Cerebrovascular accidents
    Other neuromuscular causes of swallowing problems
    Head and neck and esophageal carcinoma
    Dementia
    Trauma victims
    Comatose patients
  Small-bowel disease
    Crohn's disease
    Short-gut syndrome
  Anorexia group
    Anorexia nervosa
    Severe depression
    Advanced malignancy
Upper gastrointestinal decompression
  Gastroparesis
  Paralytic ileus
  Mechanical obstruction in advanced malignancy

quality of life. Recently, reports of the use of percutaneous gastrostomy are appearing in literature from European centers [8,9]. This may indicate a change in practice that will lead to a more uniform global use of the procedure.

Technique

SUMMARY OF EQUIPMENT
Puncture Needles

We prefer an 18-gauge, 15-cm, two-part trocar needle (Cook, Bloomington, IN) for the initial puncture (Fig. 14-1). The blunt outer cannula of this needle is useful to direct the guidewire and to aid in pyloric canal canalization. Some groups prefer to use a smaller-caliber needle for the initial puncture, such as a 22-gauge Chiba needle (Cook, Bloomington, IN), and then to dilate the initial tract with a coaxial system allowing the passage of a straight-tipped, 1-mm guidewire. Several such systems are available, including the Mitty-Pollack needle (Cook, Bloomington, IN), which consists of a 14-cm, 18-gauge cutting needle mounted over a 22-cm, 22-gauge needle. The extra precaution in making the initial puncture with a small-caliber needle is not considered necessary when performing percutaneous gastrostomy because of the large target size of the distended stomach. Its use may be reserved for the less-experienced operator.

Wires, Catheters, and Dilators

A 1-mm, (0.038 inch) straight-tipped, 145-cm guidewire is almost invariably all that is required for the procedure. Occasionally, a stiffer wire such as an Amplatz extra stiff (Cook, Bloomington, IN) may be required. This is particularly true if a less-rigid catheter, such as a multipurpose catheter (Cook, Bloomington, IN), is used for manipulation through the pylorus. The use of a straight-tipped wire is preferred as it advances more easily through the pylorus. A standard 9-French tapered dilator (Cook, Bloomington, IN) is used to both dilate the tract and, if necessary, to use as a guiding catheter simply by bending the distal 2 to 3 cm to an angle of approximately 60 ° (Fig. 14-1).

Feeding Catheters

Our preferred catheter for initial insertion is the 60-cm long Cope loop gastrojejunostomy catheter (Cook, Bloomington, IN) (Fig. 14-2). It has a locking pigtail at the distal end of the catheter and is available in sizes from 10.2- to 14-French. Many other variations of catheter design are available including the Gray-St. Louis gastrojejunostomy catheter (Cook, Bloomington, IN) with the retaining loop positioned centrally along the catheter length, forming within the proximal duodenum or stomach [10]. The disadvantage we have

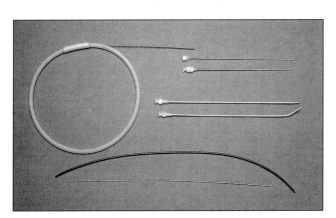

FIGURE 14-1.

Equipment used for gastrojejunostomy catheter insertion. A two-part, 15-cm, 18-gauge puncture needle and straight and curved-tipped, 9-French dilators are shown. The guidewire is a straight-tipped, 1-mm wire and below is a 9-French Kifa catheter and metal stiffener.

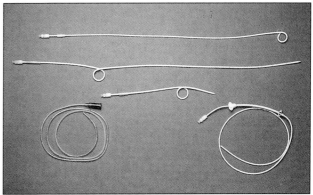

FIGURE 14-2.

Some of the various types of gastrojejunostomy and gastrostomy catheters are shown. At the top is the Ho gastrojejunostomy catheter with a retaining Cope loop at the catheter tip. Below this is a Gray-St. Louis catheter with a centrally placed Cope loop. Below this is the shorter Wills-Oglesby gastrostomy catheter. At the bottom left is an Argyle nasogastric catheter that can be used as a replacement gastrojejunostomy feeding catheter. On the bottom right is a Carey-Alzate-Coons gastrojejunostomy catheter that has a Malecot-type expansion to be positioned in the stomach.

found with this design is that the straight, rather soft catheter tip has a tendency to curl back on itself, pointing proximally within the duodenum. This catheter also has multiple sideholes positioned along its distal 17 cm, and unless the infusion rate of feeds is fast, there is a tendency for all of the feed to leave from the first sidehole and the distal segment of the catheter to become blocked [11]. The ideal design is to have one large endhole, and if sideholes are present, they should be clustered nearer to the catheter tip.

Standard Kits

We do not favor the use of standard kits for interventional radiologic procedures, as each case may have different requirements. Kits are thus either incomplete or wasteful. They also inhibit the constant testing of new ideas and new equipment needed to optimize and develop new techniques.

PATIENT PREPARATION

Informed Consent

Fully-informed written consent should be obtained from all patients. When a patient is unable to comprehend the procedure, consent should be obtained from the next of kin.

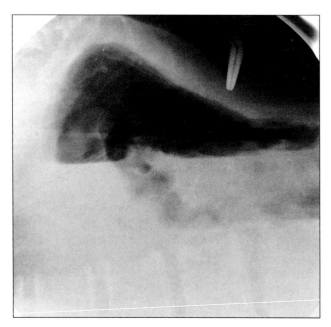

FIGURE 14-3.

A supine lateral radiograph of the epigastrium showing an air-filled distended stomach and its relation to the proposed cutaneous puncture site.

Preprocedural Requirements

Whenever possible, patients should arrive in the department having had a nasogastric tube passed. If attempts to pass a nasogastric tube have failed, it is nearly always possible to pass a Bilbao-Dotter small-bowel enema tube (Cook, Bloomington, IN) with an accompanying large-caliber guidewire through the narrowest of esophageal strictures under direct fluoroscopic guidance. As an alternative, a 7-French multipurpose angiographic catheter (Cook, Bloomington, IN) and straight-tipped guidewire may also be useful in crossing tight esophageal strictures.

Debate remains as to whether patients who do not receive anticoagulants and have no clinical evidence of a bleeding disorder require preprocedural blood work such as prothrombin and partial thromboplastin times and platelet count [12]. The expense of routine blood tests has been recently estimated, and despite the high cost and low positivity rate, they are still often performed [13]. Unfortunately, they are often used as a substitute for adequate patient clinical history.

Fasting for 6 to 8 hours prior to the procedure is recommended for all patients.

Liver Edge and Transverse Colon Localization

Ultrasound of the upper abdomen is initially performed to localize the inferior border of the left lobe of the liver. When the liver is enlarged, it is normal for the stomach to be displaced inferiorly, but on occasion the body of the stomach may come to lie deep to the left lobe. If the stomach cannot be distended below the inferior margin of the liver, this precludes a percutaneous approach.

Fluoroscopy of the abdomen is used to localize the gas-filled transverse colon that is typically seen inferior to the antrum of the stomach. Air is introduced via the nasogastric tube to fully distend the stomach, which then usually displaces the transverse colon inferiorly, bringing the body of the stomach below the costal margin and left lobe of the liver. If the colon is not visible, it may be helpful to fluoroscope the patient laterally depressing the anterior abdominal wall at the proposed entry point to the stomach (Fig. 14-3). The air-filled stomach is easily identified and there should be no intervening loops of bowel between the skin and the anterior wall of the stomach. If doubt remains, air or dilute contrast may be introduced rectally [14]. This is of particular importance in infants and young children where the gas pattern of the colon and small bowel are difficult to distinguish [15].

Patient Sedation and Monitoring

It is not routinely necessary to sedate adult patients as long as adequate local anesthesia is used. The occasional anxious patient may require some parenteral sedation with a short-acting benzodiazepine such as midazolam (Versed; Hoffmann-La Roche, Nutley, NJ). It is more common following stroke that patients are restless, poorly orientated, and do not understand the importance of the procedure. These patients are best managed by appropriate physical restraint bands rather than pharmacologic sedation, which is not without risk. Any patient who receives parenteral sedation should be monitored with a pulse oximeter and be observed by a nurse or physician dedicated to that duty [16]. Older patients or those with respiratory disease receiving sedation should also routinely receive oxygen by nasal prongs or mask.

STANDARD TECHNIQUE

Fluoroscopically Guided Percutaneous Gastrostomy

The patient is positioned supine on the fluoroscopy table and the upper abdomen prepared and draped in a sterile fashion. The stomach is inflated with air via the nasogastric tube. The surface marking of the puncture point over the midgastric body, avoiding the vascular greater curve, is then marked on the skin using fluoroscopy (Fig. 14-4). The skin and subcutaneous tissues are infiltrated with local anaesthetic. When infiltrating the deeper subcutaneous tissues with a 22-gauge needle, it is normal to be able to enter the gastric lumen and aspirate air; this confirms a good location for gastric puncture. An appropriately sized skin incision is then made. The chosen puncture needle, typically an 18-gauge, 15-cm, two-part trocar needle (Cook, Bloomington, IN), is then advanced vertically into the stomach under direct fluoroscopic visualization. To avoid irradiating the operator's hands, the radiographic tube can be obliqued from the vertical. As the needle is advanced, the stomach wall is initially indented and pushed away. The needle is then advanced with a sharp vertical motion and is seen to enter the gastric lumen (Fig. 14-5A). The tip of the needle will now move freely within the distended stomach. Any resistance suggests that both walls of the stomach have been punctured. The needle can then be

easily withdrawn into the gastric lumen. If doubt remains as to the location of the needle tip, a small volume of water-soluble contrast medium may be injected after removal of the central trocar. If posterior to the stomach, the contrast will pool at the needle tip; if within the gastric lumen, the contrast will flow away from the needle and outline gastric rugae. A straight-tipped, 1-mm guidewire is then advanced through the outer cannula of the needle into the stomach lumen (Fig. 14-5B). The needle can then be angled toward the antrum or fundus and the guidewire advanced into a secure position within the stomach.

Pyloric Canal Cannulation

Following a successful percutaneous gastrostomy, the needle is angled toward the gastric antrum to direct the guidewire to the pylorus. It may also be advantageous to advance the rigid-blunt outer cannula of the needle over the guidewire further into the stomach to aid manipulation of the wire through the pylorus. It is normal with appropriate manipulation of the wire and needle cannula to be able to advance the wire through the pylorus. It is often most effective to angle the cannula slightly inferiorly, allowing the guidewire to follow the greater curvature of the antrum superiorly toward the pylorus (Fig. 14-5C). If this is not successful, it may be helpful to inject a small amount of water-soluble contrast medium through the needle to

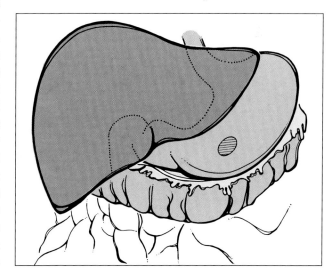

FIGURE 14-4.

The epigastrium showing the relationship of the costal margins, the liver, and the transverse colon to the proposed gastric puncture site (*hatched area*).

better outline the position of the pylorus and proximal duodenum, as this may vary between individuals. If success is still not achieved, some form of rigid angle-tipped catheter may be required to better direct the wire. We favor the use of a 9-French dilator (Cook, Bloomington, IN) with its tip bent to an angle of approximately 60° (Fig. 14-5D). The rigidity of the catheter system chosen is essential to prevent the guidewire looping within the stomach, keeping a straight line between the stomach entry point and the

pylorus. Once the floppy tip of the straight guidewire passes into the duodenum, it will often get caught in one of the circular duodenal folds and form a wide-angle J. The wire may then be advanced further in this shape; if resistance is met, the wire should be withdrawn to straighten the J loop and then readvanced. This push-pull technique (Fig. 14-5E) is repeated until the wire reaches, or preferably passes beyond, the ligament of Treitz into the proximal jejunum. This can nearly always be achieved with the needle cannula or

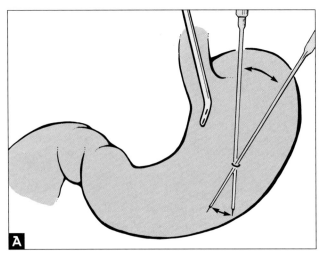

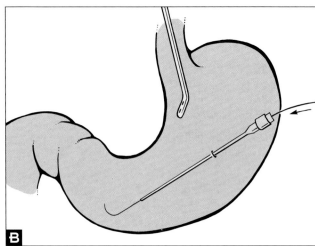

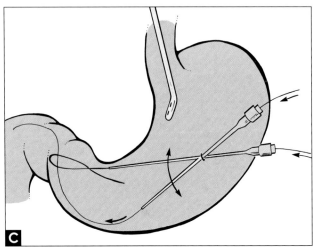

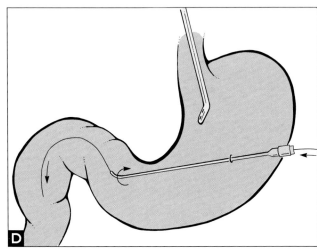

FIGURE 14-5.

The technique for percutaneous gastrojejunostomy catheter placement. **A**, Vertical needle puncture into the gastric lumen with an 18-gauge, two-part needle; after puncture, the needle tip is freely mobile in the gastric lumen. **B**, After withdrawal of the central trocar, the outer cannula of the needle has been angled toward the pylorus and then a straight-tipped, 1-mm guide-wire advanced into the gastric lumen. The needle cannula is then advanced over the wire for a more secure position. **C**, The cannula is then used to help direct the guide-wire through the pylorus. **D**, An angled dilator or catheter is used to direct the guidewire through the pylorus. (***continued***)

angled dilator positioned at the pylorus. Occasionally a longer catheter system, such as a black 9-French Kifa (Elema, Stockholm, Sweden) with a steam-curved tip and central metal stiffener or a 7-French multipurpose catheter (Cook, Bloomington, IN) may be required.

Catheter Insertion

Once the guidewire has been advanced into the stomach for gastrostomy and to the proximal jejunum for transgastric jejunostomy, the needle cannula is removed over the wire and the tract into the stomach serially dilated to a size appropriate for the final catheter to be placed. Entry of each dilator into the

stomach should be confirmed fluoroscopically following the initial tenting of the anterior gastric wall. Apposition of the stomach to the anterior abdominal wall by further air insufflation, and advancing each dilator with a rotatory motion ease the process of tract dilatation.

For initial gastrojejunostomy catheter placement, we use a 10.2-French Cope loop catheter (Cook, Bloomington, IN) (Fig. 14-2). It is usually only necessary to pass a single 9-French dilator into the stomach prior to catheter placement. The Cope catheter is mounted on a metal stiffener that is advanced with the catheter preloaded over the guidewire to the level of the pylorus. The line between the gastric puncture point and the pylorus should again be kept straight; this may require withdrawal of some of the guidewire to remove any loop within the stomach. The catheter is then detached from the stiffener and advanced over the guidewire, holding the stiffener and wire steady (Fig. 14-5F). Fluoroscopy should be centered on the pylorus as the catheter will naturally follow the guidewire as long as the stiffener remains in position at the pylorus. Final catheter position in the proximal jejunum is confirmed by injection of a water-soluble contrast media (Fig. 14-6).

If only gastrostomy placement is required, a shorter 25-cm nephrostomy Cope loop catheter (Cook, Bloomington, IN) is used. Again, the stiffener and

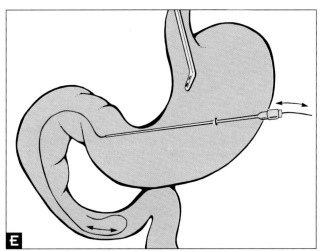

FIGURE 14-5. (CONTINUED)

E, The guidewire is advanced through the duodenum using a push-pull technique. **F**, A Cope loop catheter and stiffener have been advanced over the wire to the pylorus and the catheter is then further advanced to the doudenal-jejunal flexure.

catheter are advanced into the stomach before the catheter is advanced off of the stiffener, over the guidewire, and into the gastric lumen. Problems may be encountered inserting the final catheter despite adequate tract dilatation. In this situation, the use of a peel-away sheath (Cook, Bloomington, IN) will allow easier catheter placement. Except for the initial insertion of catheters above 18-French in size, it is uncommon to require the use of a peel-away sheath.

Skin Fixation and Dressings

The principle requirements of skin fixation for a gastrostomy tube are similar to those for any other percutaneously placed tube such as a nephrostomy, a biliary drain, or an abscess-drainage catheter. The method we use has been described previously but will be outlined here [17]. A rectangular piece of Elastoplast (Smith & Nephew, Hull, United Kingdom) with an attached silk suture is stuck to a similar-sized piece of Stomadhesive (Convatec, Princeton, NJ) that is then applied to the patient's skin. The suture is tied securely to the catheter. The Elastoplast is then covered with a waterproof, clear Opsite (Smith & Nephew, Hull, United Kingdom) dressing. A further sandwich of Opsite (20 × 14 cm) is used to secure the catheter to the skin (Fig. 14-7). The catheter entry site is finally covered by a small gauze dressing. This system allows

easy inspection of the wound and has proven both secure and relatively resistant to problems associated with leakage around the catheter.

AFTERCARE

Vital signs should be monitored regularly for the first 6 hours with particular attention to the development of any clinical signs of peritonism. If the patient is well, the nasogastric tube can be removed after 24 hours and feeding may be permitted 4 hours following a gastrojejunostomy and 24 hours following a gastrostomy. If abdominal pain and peritonism develop at any stage, feeding should be stopped immediately and the nasogastric tube left to free drainage and broad-spectrum parenteral antibiotics administered.

Complications

The results from the four largest published series have been collated and are presented in Table 14-2 [18–21]. The 30-day mortality rate of the technique is variable and relates to the population of patients on whom the procedure was undertaken, ranging from 11% to 26% [18]. Major and minor complications have been previously defined by Shellito and Malt [22]. Major complications include peritonitis requiring laparotomy, gastrointestinal hemorrhage requiring transfusion,

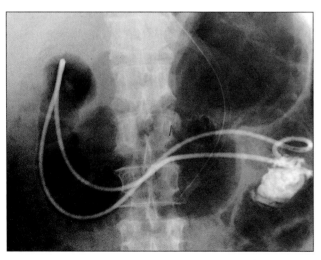

FIGURE 14-6.

A radiograph showing the final position of a gastrojejunostomy feeding catheter, with contrast injection through the catheter into the proximal jejunum.

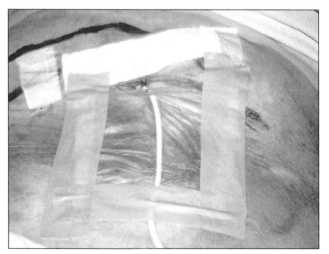

FIGURE 14-7.

Method of securing the catheter without suturing to the skin. The catheter has been tied with a silk suture previously sewn to a piece of Elastoplast that is stuck to a similar-sized piece of Stomadhesive applied to the skin. Opsite dressings then cover both the Elastoplast and the catheter.

deep stomal infection, external stomal leakage, and tracheal aspiration. The overall incidence of major complications ranges from 0% to 6%. The minor complications include peritonism, superficial stomal infection, and pneumoperitoneum. The frequency of these complications ranges from 4.4% to 15%.

TECHNICAL PROBLEMS AND PITFALLS

Gastric Wall and Abdominal Wall Apposition

This is the most common cause of difficulty encountered during the procedure. The body of the stomach is freely mobile within the peritoneal cavity. The upper gastrointestinal tract is fixed at the esophageal hiatus in the diaphragm and at the retroperitoneal portion of the duodenum. Thus, there is a tendency for the stomach to be pushed away from the anterior abdominal wall during attempts to advance a catheter or dilator. If attempts to advance a relatively nontapered feeding catheter over a wire are made prior to adequate tract dilatation into the stomach, the catheter will displace and invaginate the stomach but not enter the gastric lumen (Fig. 14-8). Viewing this in the anteroposterior plane fluoroscopically may lead to the mistaken impression that the catheter has entered the gastric lumen. Further catheter advancement will lead to recoil of the wire and loss of access to the stomach, with the catheter being left within the peritoneal cavity.

Table 14-2. Mortality and Morbidity Related to Percutaneous Fluoroscopic Gastrostomy*	
	Occurrence, %
Procedure-related mortality	0.8
30-day mortality	14.2
Major complications	5.2
Peritonitis requiring laparotomy	0.8
Gastrointestinal hemorrhage requiring transfusion	0.9
Deep stomal infection	0.5
External stomal leakage	1.4
Aspiration	1.6
Minor complications	5.0
Peritonism	2.8
Superficial stomal infection	1.6
Pneumoperitoneum	0.3
Erosion of catheter through viscus	0.3

*Data from Hicks et al. (18), Saini et al. (19), Halkier et al. (20), and O'Keefe et al. (21).

Despite adequate tract dilatation with tapered dilators, the mobile stomach may still be pushed away from the anterior abdominal wall during attempts at catheter advancement. In this situation, apposition of the anterior wall of the stomach and the anterior abdominal wall is facilitated by keeping the stomach well distended with air and by intermittently placing traction on the catheter before further advancement. In some patients it may be helpful to paralyze the stomach with glucagon to allow adequate distention with air. Occasionally, it may also be necessary to perform more gradual stepwise

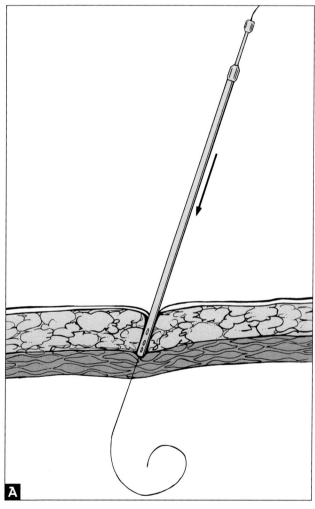

FIGURE 14-8.

Demonstration of invagination of the stomach wall leading to peritoneal placement of the final catheter. **A,** Catheter and stiffener reach but never enter the gastric lumen because of inadequate dilatation of the stomach wall. Note the wire safely coiled in the gastric lumen and good initial apposition of stomach and abdominal walls. (***continued***)

dilatation of the tract into the stomach. This problem may be compounded in patients with ascites in whom the stomach is separated from the anterior abdominal wall by fluid. In this situation, gastropexy with suture anchors may be required.

Intragastric Wire and Catheter Loops

If a wire or catheter is advanced forcefully against a resistance within the duodenum, there is a tendency for the wire to back up in the stomach or peritoneum and form a loop (Fig. 14-9A). If this is not corrected, continued advancement will cause the catheter and wire to recoil back into the gastric lumen. If the loop forms in the peritoneum, access to the stomach may be lost. It is thus important to make sure the line of the

wire and catheter is kept straight within the stomach during advancement of the wire through the duodenum. This is aided by the use of either the outer metal cannula of the puncture needle (Fig. 14-9B) or a rigid catheter.

Variations in Technique

PHARMACOLOGIC GASTROPARESIS

The use of gastric paralysis is not routinely recommended. On occasion, the stomach may not adequately distend with air, because of rapid loss into the upper small bowel. However, this is uncommon unless related to previous pyloroplasty. A single dose of 0.5 mg intravenous glucagon is adequate to paralyze the

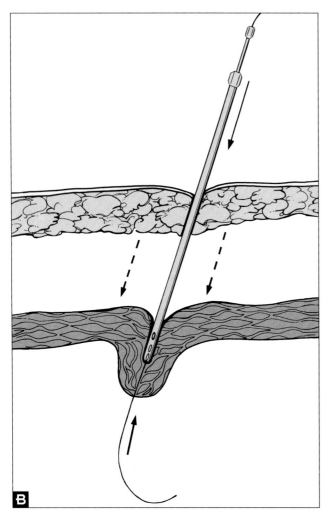

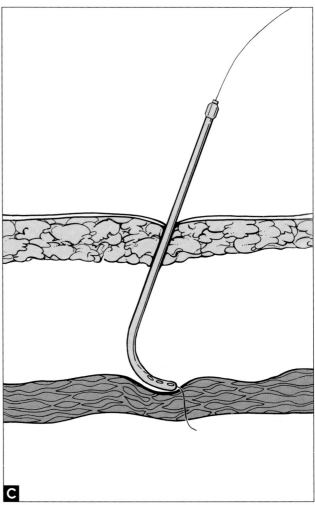

FIGURE 14-8. (CONTINUED)

B, Advancement of the catheter off of the stiffener leads to displacement of the stomach away from the anterior abdominal wall and to invagination of the wall of the

stomach. C, The catheter is deployed within the peritoneal cavity and the wire recoils out of the gastric lumen.

stomach for 15 to 20 minutes. Unfortunately, this has the disadvantage of making it slightly more difficult to cannulate the pylorus, because of the absence of peristalsis that normally assists the passage of the guidewire. Pharmacologic paralysis is also recommended when the stomach is unusually mobile and when a direct percutaneous jejunostomy is being performed.

Draining Gastrostomy

Effective decompression of the upper gastrointestinal tract via a percutaneous gastrostomy requires the placement of a large-caliber catheter. Some authors suggest above 24-French in size [21]. Such large-caliber drainage catheters require placement via a peel-away sheath. As it may not be necessary in all cases to have such a large-sized catheter and the theoretic risks of peritoneal leakage are greater, initial insertion of an 18-French catheter is suggested. If necessary, this can be exchanged for a larger catheter at a second procedure.

DIRECT PERCUTANEOUS JEJUNOSTOMY

This is a more difficult technique that is only occasionally performed [23]. Enteral feeding may be required in patients who have previously had total or partial gastrectomy, or when the stomach is inaccessible, resting high under the costal margin, behind the colon, or behind the left lobe of the liver [24•]. Accurate localization of the transverse colon is essential. A nasojejunal

tube is passed just beyond the ligament of Treitz and a combination of water-soluble contrast and air are infused to opacify the proximal jejunal loops. Peristalsis is then paralyzed with glucagon. Using a C-arm, a proximal and anteriorly placed jejunal loop is identified fluoroscopically. Two suture anchors are then used to fix the chosen loop to the anterior abdominal wall prior to catheter placement distally in the lumen of the jejunum. Some groups advocate the use of a balloon catheter passed transorally into the proximal jejunum. The balloon can then be inflated with contrast and located fluoroscopically for direct puncture.

USE OF ULTRASOUND AND COMPUTED TOMOGRAPHY FOR GUIDANCE OF PERCUTANEOUS GASTROSTOMY

If a nasogastric tube cannot be passed into the stomach because of complete pharyngeal or esophageal obstruction, direct percutaneous puncture of the collapsed stomach with a 22-gauge needle is used to inflate the stomach prior to definitive gastrostomy. When there is complete esophageal obstruction, it is common for there to be no gastric air shadow. In this situation, either ultrasound or computed tomography (CT) may be used to direct a needle into the stomach [25]. A 22-gauge Chiba needle is preferred and it is normal to perform a double-wall puncture of the collapsed stomach. Under direct fluoroscopic vision, the needle is then withdrawn slowly when injecting small

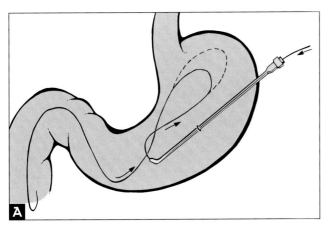

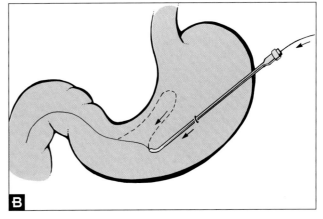

FIGURE 14-9.

Demonstration of intragastric loop formation and method of loop removal. **A**, Advancement of a guidewire against resistance within the duodenum will lead to the formation of a loop within the stomach and eventually to recoil of the guidewire back into the stomach. **B**, The guidewire is withdrawn through the guiding catheter or needle cannula until the loop is removed. The catheter can then be advanced over the wire, keeping a straight line between the gastric puncture point and the pylorus. The wire can then be further advanced into the duodenum by the push-pull technique.

amounts of water-soluble contrast medium. When the needle enters the gastric lumen, the contrast flows away from the needle tip outlining gastric rugae. Air is then injected through the needle until the stomach is adequately distended. Ultrasound is preferred over CT because the collapsed stomach is often above the left costal margin, requiring a cephalad angulation of the Chiba needle. Ultrasound also has the advantage of being portable and more easily available in the same room as fluoroscopy.

Computed tomography has also been used to guide direct puncture of the retroperitoneal portion of the duodenum via a right-lumbar approach for insertion of a feeding catheter in a patient on continuous ambulatory peritoneal dialysis and with a diabetic gastroparesis [26].

SUTURE ANCHORS

Although some authors use suture anchors routinely, we feel that their use is only indicated in specific situations and that routine gastrostomy and gastrojejunostomy can nearly always be performed without the need for gastropexy [27•]. There are several anchoring device designs currently available for performing gastropexy prior to percutaneous gastrostomy. We favor the Cope gastrointestinal suture anchor (Cook,

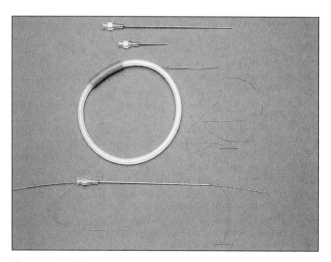

FIGURE 14-10.

The Cope gastrointestinal suture anchor. The kit contains a puncture needle preloaded with a suture, a second suture, a loading guide for reloading the second suture, and a straight-tipped guidewire for displacing the T-suture from the needle into the gastric lumen. The needle is shown with the guidewire displacing a suture anchor from the needle.

Bloomington, IN) (Fig. 14-10) [28]. The stomach puncture site is selected with fluoroscopy and the skin around a slightly wider area infiltrated with local anesthetic. The preloaded, single-piece needle is advanced vertically into the gastric lumen with a sharp stabbing motion (Fig. 14-11A). A straight guidewire is passed through the central lumen of the needle and pushes the preloaded T-suture into the stomach (Fig. 14-11B). The puncture needle is withdrawn over the thread and suturing needle. The thread is then pulled tight, causing the T-piece to pull the stomach up against the anterior abdominal wall (Fig. 14-11C). The suture needle is used to stitch the thread to the skin. It is normal to place between two and four suture anchors approximately 2 to 3 cm apart and perform the gastrostomy puncture centrally between them. When the tract has matured sufficiently and the stomach is fixed to the anterior abdominal wall, the sutures may be cut allowing the T-pieces to fall into the gastric lumen.

CONVERSION OF GASTROSTOMY TO GASTROJEJUNOSTOMY

Conversion of gastrostomy to gastrojejunostomy may be indicated if the patient is unable to tolerate feeds because of gastric outlet obstruction or reflux with the associated risks of aspiration. The procedure is usually easily performed, although may be more difficult if the original gastrostomy was placed endoscopically or surgically and the tract angled cephalad toward the fundus [29•]. The stomach is initially inflated with air via the indwelling catheter and the gastrostomy catheter is exchanged over a wire for a rigid steerable catheter. We prefer to use a 9-French Kifa catheter (Elema, Stockholm, Sweden) with a central metal stiffener, although others advocate the use of a sheath and dilator, a malleable steel cannula, or even a pediatric endotracheal tube [29•,30–32]. The steam-curved tip of the Kifa catheter can be used to direct the guidewire toward the pylorus and if necessary, the whole axis of the stomach may be rotated with the stiffener. Once the pylorus is cannulated, the procedure is the same as inserting a new percutaneous gastrojejunostomy feeding tube. On the rare occasion that the tract cannot be redirected toward the pylorus, a new puncture may be performed. This may also be indicated if there is early proximal migration of the catheter back into the fundus of the stomach, despite successful repositioning of the feeding catheter in the jejunum [29•].

Infracolonic Approach

When the transverse colon covers the inflated stomach, it usually precludes the percutaneous approach for gastrostomy. On occasion, it may be possible to inflate the stomach allowing the antrum and lower gastric body to hang below the inferior border of the transverse colon. It is then possible to perform an infracolonic puncture of the stomach [33].

Further Management

It is the responsibility of the physician inserting a tube or catheter to be familiar with and to provide a service for the further management of the tube and any associated complications.

Frequency and Indications

Routine prophylactic exchange of long-term gastrostomy catheters should be performed every 6 months to prevent catheter stiffening or disintegration. Indications for earlier catheter exchanges are catheter blockage, displacement, leakage, and damage. If a catheter blocks, it should be exchanged for a new catheter two French sizes larger. Catheter blockage is often related to the administration of crushed tablets through the tube. Particular care must be taken to adequately crush and preferably dissolve any medication prior to administration. Catheter blockage is much less common for catheters 14-French or larger.

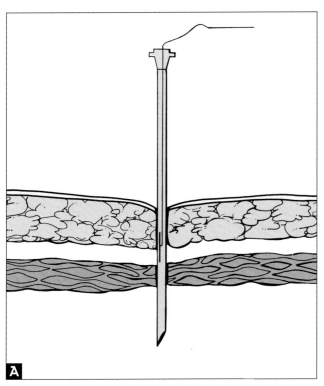

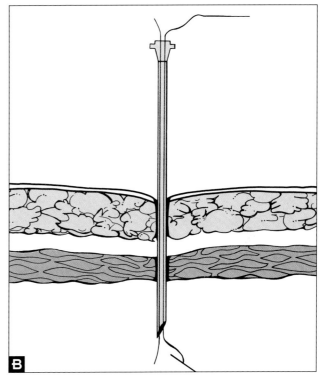

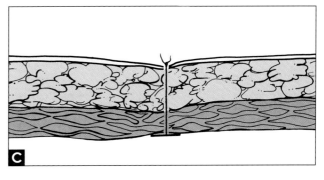

FIGURE 14-11.

Diagrams outlining the method of insertion of the Cope suture anchor. **A,** The preloaded suture anchor and needle are advanced vertically into the distended gastric lumen. **B,** The guidewire is then advanced through the needle and displaces the T-piece into the gastric lumen. Following removal of the wire, the needle is removed over the suture leaving the T-piece free within the gastric lumen. **C,** The suture thread is pulled tight, causing the stomach to be closely apposed to the anterior abdominal wall. The suture needle is then used to secure the thread to the skin.

Technique

A water-soluble contrast medium is initially injected to confirm correct catheter location prior to exchange over a 145-cm, straight-tipped, 1-mm guidewire. If it is not possible to pass a standard guidewire through a blocked catheter, it is worth trying an Amplatz extra-stiff wire. The alternative is to pass a peel-away sheath over the outside of the blocked catheter as far as the gastric antrum and then withdraw the feeding catheter back through the sheath, automatically undoing the retaining Cope loop. Access to the stomach is maintained by the sheath, the pylorus renegotiated, and a new catheter inserted. Exchange of percutaneous gastrojejunostomy feeding catheters requires fluoroscopy; other groups suggest that gastrostomy catheters may be exchanged at the bedside, although correct positioning of the new tube should be checked radiographically before recommencement of feeding.

For catheters that have fallen out completely, it is usually possible to renegotiate the tract into the stomach with a straight-tipped, 1-mm guidewire as long as the catheter has been in position for at least 1 week and the patient is referred within 48 hours of catheter displacement. With very mature tracts, renegotiation may be achieved even when the catheter has been dislodged for a week or more.

Catheter Type and Use of Argyle Catheters

We have found that standard nasogastric-type Argyle catheters (Sherwood Medical, St. Louis, MO) make excellent and inexpensive replacement catheters. They are designed with an endhole and a few large sideholes near to the tip, making catheter blockage a less-common problem than with standard Cope loop-type feeding catheters. For patients with mature tracts, the Argyle catheter can be easily advanced over a straight-tipped, 1-mm guidewire into the proximal jejunum. If any difficulty is encountered, a metal stiffener can be positioned within the Argyle catheter to the level of the pylorus prior to advancing the catheter to the proximal jejunum over the guidewire.

SKIN CARE

Problems with skin irritation and infection are far less common with percutaneously placed tubes compared with surgically placed tubes, because of the substantial reduction in peristomal leakage of gastric contents onto the skin. If leakage does occur, exchange of the catheter for a larger size may be helpful to tamponade the leak. The dry gauze dressing covering the catheter entry site should ordinarily be changed weekly, but if there is leakage around the entry site the dressing must be changed more frequently to keep the skin dry. Skin may also be protected from local irritation by gastric contents with the use of a barrier cream.

Frank skin sepsis is best treated by a course of oral antibiotics in combination with a topical antibacterial preparation such as a polymyxin-B antibacterial ointment (Polytopic; Technilab, Montreal, Quebec, Canada). The development of granulation tissue around the skin entry site of the catheter may cause significant discomfort and bleeding and is easily treated by cauterization with topical silver nitrate.

CATHETER REMOVAL

Any tube with a self-retaining mechanism, such as a Cope loop, is best removed under direct fluoroscopic vision with a guidewire to straighten the loop and avoid disrupting the tract. As long as a good tract is present, there is no risk of peritonitis. If a gastrostomy catheter falls out or requires removal within a week of insertion, a nasogastric tube should be inserted to provide gastric drainage for 24 hours.

Current Controversies

GASTROSTOMY OR GASTROJEJUNOSTOMY

Placement of a percutaneous gastrojejunostomy catheter beyond the ligament of Treitz has the advantage of almost eliminating the risk of gastroesophageal reflux compared with direct intragastric feeding, which is associated with a high incidence of esophageal reflux [34, 35••]. Many of the patients receiving enteral nutrition are unable to protect their airways and are at constant risk of aspiration if they develop reflux.

In selected patients, it may be more convenient to feed directly into the stomach. This allows for bolus feeds where a large volume is instilled over a short period of time, allowing the patient to be freely mobile between feeds with a capped-off tube. In the majority of patients undergoing enteral feeding, particularly those with stroke, this is not of practical importance. However, in patients who are otherwise mobile, being attached to a continuous-drip feed for several hours at a time may significantly reduce their quality of life. In these patients it may be preferable to perform a gastrostomy only. If the patient develops problems with reflux, the catheter can be easily advanced to the proximal jejunum. Shorter gastrostomy catheters also have a theoretically lower rate of blockage compared with a longer gastrojejunostomy catheter of the same internal diameter [35••].

It has been recently reported that percutaneously placed gastrostomy tubes in adults do not cause reflux [34]. Despite this, the population of patients referred for gastrostomy has an incidence of reflux of up to 46% [35••]. We feel that in the vast majority of patients it is worth the extra few minutes required to insert a gastrojejunostomy feeding catheter because of the lower incidence of the potentially serious complications related to aspiration. The alternative approach of initially assessing patients for the presence of reflux with a radionuclide study has been suggested [35••]. No test for reflux can be 100% sensitive because it is typically an intermittent problem, and we believe that this approach is still likely to leave a number of patients at risk for aspiration.

FLUOROSCOPIC, ENDOSCOPIC, OR SURGICAL PLACEMENT

The results of surgical and fluoroscopic and of surgical and endoscopic gastrostomy placement have been previously compared [36,37]. There has been no direct comparison of endoscopic and fluoroscopic techniques. It is well established that the nonsurgical techniques have lower mortality and morbidity rates when compared with the original surgical method (Table 14-3). Surgical gastrostomy is now rarely performed as an isolated procedure. Complications of the surgical procedure relate to the need for a general anesthetic because aspiration is caused by gastric placement of the tube, general anesthesia, and a high incidence of pericatheter leakage and associated skin infection [22,38].

The endoscopic technique has a lower mortality rate and a reduced complication rate compared with the surgical procedure, but can still result in a higher skin infection rate than the percutaneous fluoroscopic method, because of the transoral route of catheter placement (Table 14-3) [37–42]. The incidence of aspiration is also higher in the endoscopic technique because of the intravenous sedation used during the procedure and the usual intragastric position of the final tube. Initial attempts at inserting jejunal feeding catheters via an endoscopically placed percutaneous gastrostomy proved both ineffective and time consuming [43]. More recently, the technique of percutaneous endoscopic jejunostomy has met with some technical success, although its effectiveness at reducing the incidence of aspiration is still unclear [44–48]. The endoscopic method has the advantage of being able to be performed at the bedside in the intensive care unit, but cannot be performed in patients with esophageal obstruction [6]. In some centers (including three in Canada) where both endoscopic and fluoroscopic techniques are available, the referring physicians have

Table 14-3. Comparative Mortality and Morbidity of Surgical, Endoscopic, and Fluoroscopic Gastrostomy

Study	Patients, n	30-day mortality, %	Procedure-related mortality, %	Morbidity, %		
				Total	Major	Minor
Surgical						
Shellito and Malt (22)	424	–	0.5	13.2	6.6	6.6
Ruge and Vasquez (38)	163	10.4	1.8	13.5	–	–
Endoscopic						
Larson *et al.* (39)	314	16.0	1.0	16.0	3.0	13.0
Foutch *et al.* (40)	120	4.1	0.8	16.8	4.4	12.4
Miller *et al.* (41)	316	17.0	0.6	5.7	2.1	3.6
Fluoroscopic						
Halkier *et al.* (20)	252	14.2	0.8	6.0	1.6	4.4
O'Keefe *et al.* (21)	100	15.0	0.0	15.0	0.0	15.0
Saini *et al.* (19)	125	11.0	0.0	11.1	1.6	9.5
Hicks *et al.* (18)	158	26.0	1.9	18.0	6.0	12.0

opted for the fluoroscopic technique and endoscopic gastrostomy is rarely performed [49] (Chait, personal communication; Simons, personal communication).

Initial reports of laparoscopic techniques for the placement of both gastrostomy and jejunostomy feeding catheters are encouraging [50,51]. However, these are new techniques and no comparative study has been performed to assess where their specific clinical uses may lie.

THE POSSIBILITY OF GASTROPEXY

Both the surgical and endoscopic methods of gastrostomy are dependent on performing gastropexy. Although up until a mature tract has formed there is a theoretic risk of peritoneal leakage around a percutaneously placed catheter, this does not appear to be of practical concern. There is no increased incidence of peritonitis following percutaneously placed gastrostomies compared with surgically or endoscopically placed tubes. It has been shown in an experimental animal model that significant leakage of gastric contents does not occur through holes up to 18-French size in the stomach wall [52]. Further experimental evidence using endoscopically placed gastrostomies and fluoroscopically placed gastrostomies suggests that tract formation occurs as early as 1 week after catheter placement [9,53]. In addition, there are some apparent disadvantages of performing gastropexy. It has been shown that patients with gastropexy performed at the same time as percutaneous endoscopic gastrostomy have a higher incidence of leakage around the catheter both onto the skin and into the peritoneal cavity [54]. It is hypothesized that this relates to gastric-wall ischemia resulting from traction on the stomach. Therefore, gastropexy is not routinely recommended when performing gastrostomy or gastrojejunostomy [27•].

However, there are specific situations when gastropexy is indicated prior to percutaneous gastrostomy. Patients with a moderate amount of ascites, patients with a partial gastrectomy, those undergoing direct percutaneous jejunostomy, and pediatric patients all may require gastropexy [5,15,23,24•].

Conclusion

Fluoroscopically guided gastrostomy and gastrojejunostomy are simple, safe, and effective procedures for the provision of enteral feeding or upper gastrointestinal decompression. The radiologic techniques are of comparable simplicity and efficacy when compared with endoscopically guided gastrostomy and jejunostomy. In addition, they have the advantage of lower stomal infection rates and successful placement in patients with esophageal obstruction.

The already varied indications for enteral nutrition continue to expand, providing an increasing referral source of patients. However, without good comparative data between the endoscopic, radiologic, and laparoscopic methods, the selection of the best technique will continue to be influenced by subjective bias including self-referral. This places an extra burden on the radiologist to familiarize the referring clinicians with the advantages of the fluoroscopic technique.

References and Recommended Reading

Recently published papers of particular interest have been highlighted as:
• Of interest
•• Of outstanding interest

1. Ho C-S: Percutaneous Gastrostomy for Jejunal Feeding. *Radiology* 1983, 149:595–596.

2. Wills JS, Oglesby JT: Percutaneous Gastrostomy. *Radiology* 1983, 149:449–453.

3. Miller KS, Tomlinson JR, Sahn SA: Pleuropulmonary Complications of Enteral Tube Feedings, Two Case Reports: Review of the Literature and Recommendations. *Chest* 1985, 88:230–233.

4. Yeung EY, MacPhadyen N, Ho C-S: Intractable Gastroparesis: Treatment with Percutaneous Fluoroscopically Guided Gastrostomies. *Am J Gastroenterol* 1992, 87:651–654.

5. Lee MJ, Saini S, Brink JA, *et al.*: Malignant Small Bowel Obstruction and Ascites: Not a Contraindication to Percutaneous Gastrostomy. *Clin Radiol* 1991, 44:332–334.

6. Kirby DF, Clifton GL, Turner H, *et al.*: Early Enteral Nutrition After Brain Injury by Percutaneous Endoscopic Gastrojejunostomy. *J Parenter Enteral Nutr* 1991, 15:298–302.

7. Nightingale JM, Lennard-Jones JE: The Short Bowel Syndrome: What's New and Old? *Dig Dis* 1993, 11:12–31.

8. Lycke KG, Bernland P, Henriksson O, *et al.*: Percutaneous Non-endoscopic Placement of 24-French Gastric Feeding Tubes. *Eur Con Radiol* 1993, 244.

9. Lindberg CG, Ivancev K, Kan Z, *et al.*: Percutaneous Gastrostomy. A Clinical and Experimental Study. *Acta Radiol* 1991, 32:302–304.

10. Gray RR, St Louis EL, Grosman H: Modified Catheter for Percutaneous Gastrojejunostomy. *Radiology* 1989, 173:276–278.

11. Gehman KE, Elliott JA, Inculet RI: Percutaneous Gastrojejunostomy with a Modifed Cope Loop Catheter. *AJR* 1990, 155:79–80.

12. Silverman SG, Mueller PR, Pfister RC: Hemostatic Evaluation Before Abdominal Interventions: An Overview and Proposal. *AJR* 1990, 154:233–238.

13. Murphy TP, Dorfman GS, Becker J: Use of Preprocedural Tests by Interventional Radiologists. *Radiology* 1993, 186:213–220.

14. Ignotus P, Gray RR, Pugash R: Infracolonic Percutaneous Gastrojejunostomy [Letter]. *Radiology* 1992, 183:583.

15. King SJ, Chait PG, Daneman A, *et al.*: Retrograde Percutaneous Gastrostomy: A Prospective Study in 57 Children. *Pediatr Radiol* 1993, 23:23–25.

16. McDermott VGM, Chapman ME, Gillespie I: Sedation and Patient Monitoring in Vascular and Interventional Radiology. *Br J Radiol* 1993, 66:667–671.

17. Sheridan J, Yeung E, Ho C-S, *et al.*: Skin Fixation of Percutaneous Drainage Catheters. *J Intervent Radiol* 1993, 8:57–59.

18. Hicks ME, Surratt RS, Picus D, *et al.*: Fluoroscopically Guided Percutaneous Gastrostomy and Gastrojejunostomy: Analysis of 158 Consecutive Cases. *AJR* 1990, 154:725–728.

19. Saini S, Mueller PR, Gaa J, *et al.*: Percutaneous Gastrostomy with Gastropexy: Experience in 125 Patients. *AJR* 1990, 154:1003–1006.

20. Halkier BK, Ho C-S, Yee ACN: Percutaneous Feeding Gastrostomy with the Seldinger Technique: Review of 252 Patients. *Radiology* 1989, 171:359–362.

21. O'Keefe F, Carrasco CH, Charnsangavej C, *et al.*: Percutaneous Drainage and Feeding Gastrostomies in 100 Patients. *Radiology* 1989, 172:341–343.

22. Shellito PC, Malt RA: Tube Gastrostomy: Technique and Complications. *Ann Surg* 1985, 201:180–195.

23. Gray RR, Ho C-S, Yee A, *et al.*: Direct Percutaneous Jejunostomy. *AJR* 1987, 149:931–932.

24. • Stevens SD, Picus D, Hicks ME, *et al.*: Percutaneous Gastrostomy and Gastrojejunostomy After Gastric Surgery. *JVIR* 1992, 3:679–683.

The conclusion of this study is that previous gastric surgery need not be a contraindication to percutaneous fluoroscopic gastrostomy tube placement. Thirty patients with various types of gastric surgery all successfully underwent percutaneous gastrostomy. Variations from the basic technique are described.

25. Sanchez RB, van Sonnenberg E, D'Agostino HB, *et al.*: CT Guidance for Percutaneous Gastrostomy and Gastrojejunostomy. *Radiology* 1992, 184:201–205.

26. Koolpe HA, Dorfman D, Kramer M: Translumbar Duodenostomy for Enteral Feeding. *AJR* 1989, 153:299–300.

27. • Deutsch LS, Kannegieter L, Vanson DT, *et al.*: Simplified Percutaneous Gastrostomy. *Radiology* 1992, 184:181–183.

This paper provides evidence that gastropexy is not routinely required when performing a percutaneous gastrostomy, even when inserting very large caliber catheters. The study of 68 patients only has short-term follow-up but both 30-day mortality (12%) and morbidity (12.5%) are similar to previously published series.

28. Coleman CC, Coon HG, Cope C, *et al.*: Percutaneous Enterostomy with the Cope Suture Anchor. *Radiology* 1990, 174:889–891.

29. • Lu DS, Mueller PR, Lee MJ, *et al.*: Gastrostomy Conversion to Transgastric Jejunostomy: Technical Problems, Causes of Failure, and Proposed Solutions in 63 Patients. *Radiology* 1993, 187:679–683.

This paper deals with the radiologic technique for conversion of gastrostomy to gastrojejunostomy. The results are given for 63 patients in whom there were 11 failures, nearly all due to a fundal angulation of the initial gastrostomy tract. This problem only occurred with surgically or endoscopically placed catheters. In eight of 52 successful conversions, the jejunally placed tube recoiled into the stomach. It was concluded that when an unfavorable fundal angulation of the tract is present, a fresh percutaneous gastrostomy puncture should be considered.

30. Kerns SR: Conversion of Gastrostomy Tube to Gastrojejunostomy Tube by Using a Peel-away Sheath [Letter]. *AJR* 1993, 160:206–207.

31. Cope C: Directable Cannula for Gastrojejunal Catheterization. *AJR* 1989, 152:1346.

32. Bar-Maor JA, Sweed Y, Shoshany G, *et al.*: The Uses of Endotracheal Tubes to Assist in Manipulation of Esophageal Strictures, in Elongation of the Esophagus in Esophageal Atresia, and in Gastrojejunal Feeding Tube Placement. *J Pediatr Surg* 1992, 27:652–653.

33. Mirich DR, Gray RR: Infracolonic Percutaneous Gastrojejunostomy. *Radiology* 1990, 12:340–341.

34. Gustke RF, Varma RR, Soergel KH: Gastric Reflux During Perfusion of the Proximal Small Bowel. *Gastroenterology* 1970, 59:890–895.

35. •• Olson DL, Krubsack AJ, Stewart ET: Percutaneous Enteral Alimentation: Gastrostomy Versus Gastrojejunostomy. *Radiology* 1993, 187:105–108.

The presence of reflux was evaluated by a scintigraphic technique immediately prior to and 1 week following gastrostomy insertion. The important findings of this study are that the incidence of reflux is high (46%) in the patient population referred for gastrostomy and that gastrostomy tube placement did not influence the rate of reflux. It was also observed that gastrojejunostomy tubes block more frequently than gastrostomy catheters of the same caliber (58% vs 8.3%).

36. Ho C-S, Yee ACN, McPherson R: Complications of Surgical and Percutaneous Nonendoscopic Gastrostomy: Review of 233 Patients. *Gastroenterology* 1988, 95:1206–1210.

37. Grant JP: Comparison of Percutaneous Endoscopic Gastrostomy with Stamm Gastrostomy. *Ann Surg* 1988, 207:598–603.

38. Ruge J, Vazquez RM: An Analysis of the Advantages of Stamm and Percutaneous Endoscopic Gastrostomy. *Surg Gynecol Obstet* 1986, 162:13–16.

39. Larson DE, Burton DD, Schroeder KW, *et al.*: Percutaneous Endoscopic Gastrostomy. Indications, Success, Complications and Mortality in 314 Consecutive Patients. *Gastroenterology* 1987, 93:48–52.

40. Foutch PG, Woods CS, Talbert GA, *et al.*: A Critical Analysis of the Sacks-Vine Gastrostomy Tube: A Review of 120 Consecutive Procedures. *Am J Gastroenterol* 1988, 83:812–815.

41. Miller RE, Castlemain B, Lacqua FJ, *et al.*: Percutaneous Endoscopic Gastrostomy: Results in 316 Patients and Review of the Literature. *Surg Endosc* 1989, 3:186–190.

42. Yeung EY, Ho C-S: Percutaneous Radiologically-guided Gastrostomy: An Under-utilised Technique? *J Intervent Radiol* 1991, 6:43–49.

43. DiSario JA, Foutch PG, Sanowski RA: Poor Results with Percutaneous Endoscopic Jejunostomy. *Gastrointest Endosc* 1990, 36:257–260.

44. MacFadyen BV Jr, Catalano MF, Raijman I, *et al.*: Percutaneous Endoscopic Gastrostomy with Jejunal Extension: A New Technique. *Am J Gastroenterol* 1992, 87:725–728.

45. Shike M, Wallach C, Likier H: Direct Percutaneous Endoscopic Jejunostomies. *Gastrointest Endosc* 1991, 37:62–65.

46. Adams DB: Feeding Jejunostomy with Endoscopic Guidance. *Surg Gynecol Obstet* 1991, 172:239–241.

47. Kadakia SC, Sullivan HO, Starnes E: Percutaneous Endoscopic Gastrostomy or Gastrojejunostomy and the Incidence of Aspiration in 79 Patients. *Am J Surg* 1992, 164:114–118.

48. Montecalvo MA, Steger KA, Farger HW, *et al.*: Nutritional Outcome and Pneumonia in Critical Care Patients Randomized to Gastric Versus Jejunal Tube Feedings. *Crit Care Med* 1992, 20:1377–1387.

49. Watkinson AF, Fache JS, Burhenne HJ: Percutaneous Gastrostomy: Experience in 100 Cases. *Eur Con Radiol* 1993,245.

50. Murphy C, Rosemurgy AS, Albrink MH, *et al.*: A Simple Technique for Laparoscopic Gastrostomy. *Surg Gynecol Obstet* 1992, 174:424–425.

51. Morris JB, Mullen JL, Yu JC, *et al.*: Laparoscopic Guided Jejunostomy. *Surgery* 1992, 112:96–99.

52. Moote DJ, Ho C-S, Felice V: Fluoroscopically Guided Percutaneous Gastrostomy: Is Gastric Fixation Necessary? *Can Assoc Radiol J* 1991, 42:113–118.

53. Mellinger JD, Simon IB, Schlechter B, *et al.*: Tract Formation Following Percutaneous Endoscopic Gastrostomy in an Animal Model. *Surg Endosc* 1991, 5:189–191.

54. Chung RS, Schertzer M: Pathogenesis of Complications of Percutaneous Endoscopic Gastrostomy: A Lesson in Surgical Principles. *Am Surg* 1990, 56:134–137.

Select Bibliography

Ho C-S, Yeung EY: Percutaneous Fluroscopically Guided Gastrostomy. In *Margulis and Burhenne's Alimentary Tract Radiology*, edn 5. Edited by Freeny PC, Stevenson GW. Philadelphia: Mosby; 1994:2011–2019.

Ho C-S, Yeung EY: Percutaneous Gastrostomy and Transgastric Jejunostomy. *AJR* 1992, 158:251–257.

Yeung EY, Ho C-S: Percutaneous Radiologic Gastrostomy. In *Bailliere's Clinical Gastroenterology*, vol 6, no 2. London: Bailliere Tindall; 1992:297–317.

The Use of Articulated Catheters for Biliary and Pancreatic Obstructions and Difficult T-tube Placements

Richard D. Shlansky-Goldberg

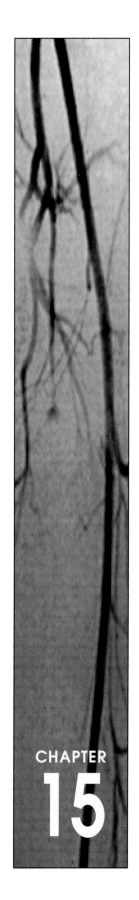

CHAPTER

15

Single conventional catheters are ideal for simple biliary drainages involving common bile duct obstructions, but may not suffice in providing adequate drainage for complex lesions. Hilar cholangiocarcinoma may require two or three catheters to adequately drain the isolated areas but these are often difficult for the patient to tolerate [1]. In addition, if multiple catheters share the same tract, bile may leak around the tubes and create problems in the long-term care of the patient. Other alternatives for drains are permanent internal metal stents that can be introduced through a single tract to stent multiple regions without the need for external tubes. Unfortunately, metal stents may not uncommonly become occluded and they often require reintervention to obtain adequate secondary patency rates [2,3,4•]. In addition, there are a group of patients who are not suitable for internal stenting because of benign disease or the possibility of transcatheter brachytherapy.

One solution for the treatment of these patients is the use of an articulated stent catheter. First described

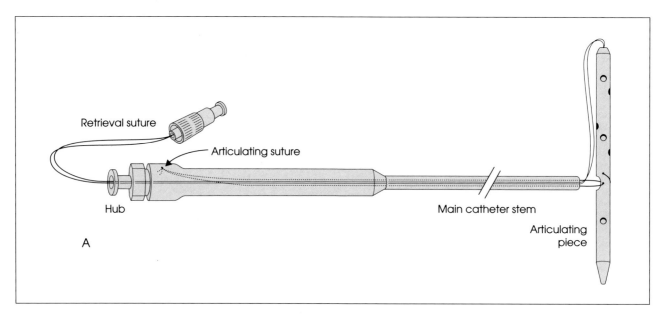

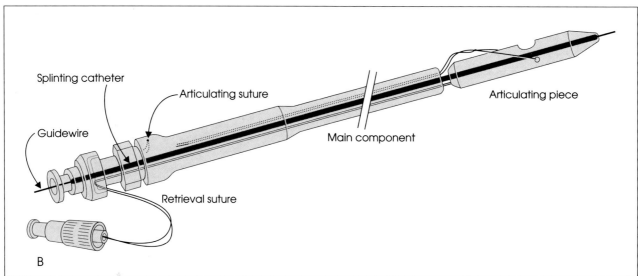

FIGURE 15-1.

Stages of catheter deployment. **A,** Fully deployed configuration of an articulated stent. **B,** Articulated stent predeployment, mounted on a wire and a splinting catheter.

by Cope and Gensburg [5••] in 1990 and Scotti [6••] in 1991, an articulated stent catheter is uniquely suited to provide drainage from more than one area.

An articulating catheter is made from different catheter components that are held together by a suture. The articulating suture usually attaches to the midportion of the shorter catheter piece and holds it to the distal end of the main catheter to form a T. An additional suture is attached to the end of the catheter crosspiece for retrieval and passes through the main catheter (Fig. 15-1A). For introduction, the main stem of the catheter and connecting piece are held in line by a splinting catheter and advanced over a guidewire past the lesion to be stented (Figs. 15-1B and 15-1C). The guidewire and the splinting catheter are removed and the articulating suture is tightened to pull the crosspiece and main catheter together (Fig. 15-1D). An alternative configuration not requiring a retrieval suture is seen in Figure 15-1E. The articulated catheter

is extremely useful because it can be easily introduced through difficult tracts and can easily stent multiple areas within the biliary system. For drainage catheter placement in complex lesions, the articulating fragment may be positioned over a different wire than the one used to place the main catheter. This is helpful in tight hilar obstructions where the catheter crosspiece must be inserted through a high-grade malignant stricture high in the left duct and may not have enough room to form the catheter in the conventional method.

Articulated catheters are also useful where proximal and distal control of a drainage site is necessary to prevent leakage, promote drainage, or maximize retention of the catheter. Examples of these clinical situations include articulated catheter use in the common bile duct after T-tube removal when an adequate tract has not formed (*eg*, in liver transplant patients or in treating external pancreatic duct fistulae that would usually require additional endoscopic therapy) [7,8•,9•].

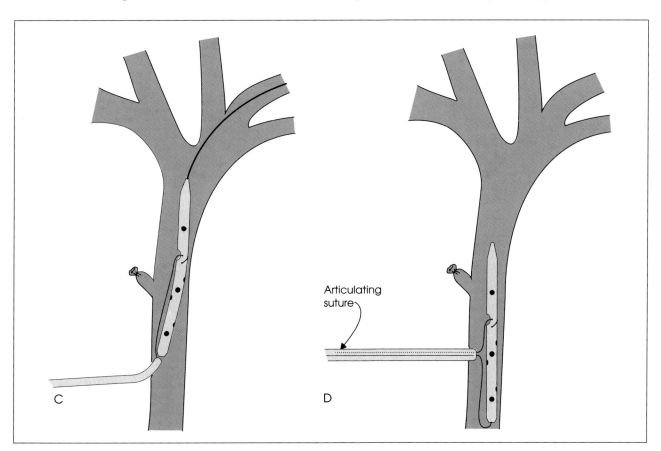

FIGURE 15-1. (CONTINUED)

C, Introduction of the articulated catheter into the biliary system over the wire and splinting catheter. D, Catheter

articulating within the biliary tree. The articulating suture is pulled tight to draw the components together.

Surgically placed T-tubes are usually replaced according to the technique described by Crummy and Turnipseed [10] that requires the folding of a T-tube limb against the drain stem. This results in tract dilation, a doubling in tract size, and potential tract disruption which may then lead to bile leakage. This is particularly a problem in liver transplant patients who have delayed healing caused by immunosuppressive drugs. In addition, latex T-tubes are generally difficult to insert or replace over a wire because of friction.

For use in conventional T-tube percutaneous replacement after common duct exploration for stones, commercially available articulated tubes (Cook, Bloomington, IN) may be used. These are available in various diameters (8- to 12-French) and crosspiece lengths (Fig. 15-2).

These premade devices are useful for temporary drainage of the common duct but may also be used for more complex intrahepatic obstructions of hilar lesions in the right and left ducts.

Articulated Catheter Design

For more complex catheter placement (*eg*, hilar lesions), the articulated components must be crafted from conventional catheters to fit the pattern of occlusive lesions found in the patient. The affected bile ducts should be measured by placing a guidewire through the catheters draining the lesion and then bending it to the precise length required to stent the region (Fig. 15-3). After measuring, radio-opaque catheter segments of similar diameter can be obtained from standard drain tubes such as 8- to 14-French polyurethane C-flex (Cook, Bloomington, IN) or Percuflex (Medi-Tech and Boston Scientific, Watertown, MA). The short articulating fragment or crosspiece should be tapered on one end to ease insertion. Depending on the length needed, the proximal few centimeters of a Cope-style biliary catheter or proximal loop catheter work well as the articulating piece (Fig. 15-3A). The distal stem of the drainage catheter can be formed from a 25- to 35-cm nephrostomy- or biliary-type catheter with the curved portion cut off. After the length of the articulating fragment is determined, the distance from the end of the main catheter to the exit site from the skin must be measured (Fig. 15-3B). Additional sideholes should be added to the component pieces as needed to adequately drain the ducts. The position of the hole in the transverse catheter piece that aligns with the end of the main catheter must also be measured (Fig. 15-3C).

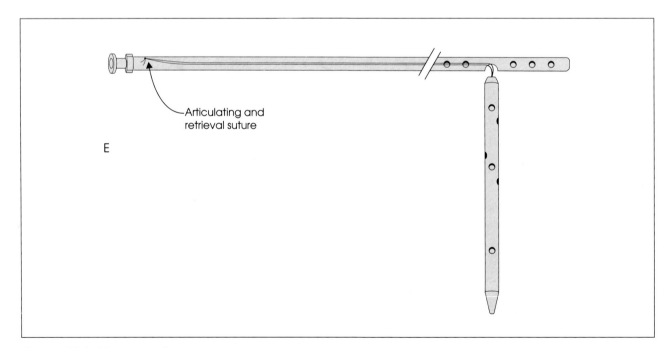

Articulating and retrieval suture

E

FIGURE 15-1. (CONTINUED)

E, An alternative configuration of the catheter with the end of the catheter piece connecting with the side of the main catheter, eliminating the need for a retrieval suture.

In conceiving the catheter design, the method of articulation placement must be determined to properly drain several ductal stenoses from one drainage site. In general, the articulated catheter can manage the problem in two configurations: the main long stem with extra sideholes can drain the right duct and extend into the duodenum, and the articulating piece can extend into the left duct. An alternate drainage pattern consists of the main component extending from the right to the left ducts and the articulating piece extending into the common bile duct. These different configurations are depicted in Figure 15-4. The three factors that influence this decision are: 1) geometry of the lesion facilitating deployment; 2) maximum drainage; and 3) catheter extraction. If it is more difficult to cross the left lesion, it may be easier to place the main catheter right to left and place the articulating fragment down into the common bile duct. This arrangement would maximize the external drainage for the right and left ducts if the articulating fragment became occluded, and would make for simpler construction and removal. For complicated deployments, the main stem and articulating piece should be introduced over separate guidewires to ease placement (Fig. 15-5).

Articulated Catheter Construction

If a premade catheter is not adequate, the catheter must be constructed. Generally, all but the simplest of catheters must be built to best fit the duct, adding the appropriate sideholes. After the catheter fragments are

cut to the appropriate size, sideholes are added on the articulated fragments as needed. A larger, approximately 3-mm hole is placed at the point of conjunction with the longer main stem component. A 20-gauge, 20-cm needle is introduced into the side of the main catheter and advanced to the open end (Fig. 15-6). Following attachment of a 3-0 Tevdek II suture (Deknatel, Floral Park, NY) to the articulating piece as seen in Figure 15-6, the two ends of the suture are introduced into the needle protruding from the end of the main stem catheter and pulled through the sidehole. An additional Tevdek suture should be tied to the end of the fragment as a retrieval suture and again brought out through the end of the main catheter. If the main catheter is a Cope-style loop biliary or nephrostomy catheter, the existing anchoring suture that exits from the portion of the catheter near the hub can be tied to this retrieval suture and pulled through or used for the articulating suture (Fig. 15-7). A retrieval suture is not needed if the end of the articu-

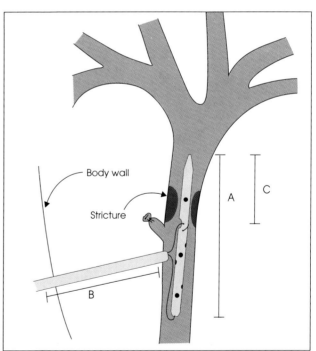

FIGURE 15-3.

The different measurements that are needed to properly tailor an articulated stent. **A,** Length of the articulating piece. **B,** Length of the catheter outside of body to locate exit of the articulating suture outside of the patient and length of the main catheter. **C,** Position of the articulating hole with the suture to allow the articulating piece to form in the proper position.

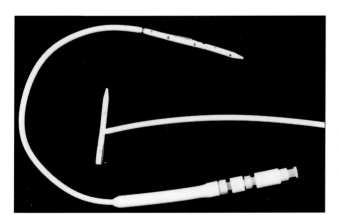

FIGURE 15-2.

A nondeployed and deployed commercially available Cope-style articulated catheter.

lating piece is to connect with the side of the main catheter. The final catheter is seen in Figure 15-8.

Articulated Catheter Placement

As previously described, the articulated catheter may be placed over a single wire. This is usually used for simple T-tube placements in the common bile duct through an existing tract. The commercially available tubes are always placed with a single-wire technique. Once in position, the articulating suture is pulled and the catheter is reformed. At times, the articulating fragment may not disengage properly and may require nudging by the main catheter tip to help it advance into the duct. The catheter may also be manipulated back and forth when retracting the

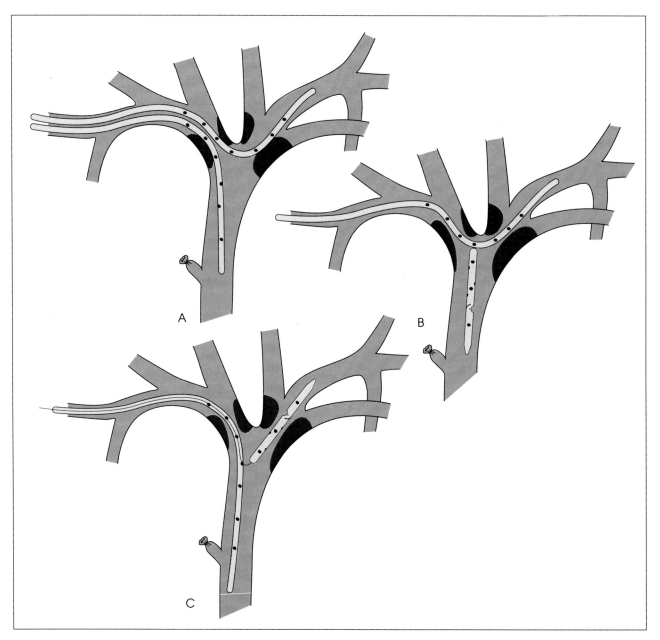

FIGURE 15-4.

Different configurations possible in a complex lesion. **A**, Two-catheter technique in a hilar lesion. **B**, An articulated catheter with the catheter piece inserted down into the common duct. **C**, The catheter piece inserted into the left duct with the main catheter set in the common bile duct.

suture to permit the two pieces to approximate each other. The articulating suture is tightly secured to the main catheter by wrapping it around the catheter body and covering it with surgical tape to prevent bile leakage. The retrieval suture is loosely wrapped at the proximal end for later use during the removal procedure.

The two-wire technique performed with a custom-made catheter, is used for complicated lesions with a custom-made catheter. The articulating fragment is first placed over one wire with a pusher catheter and then the main catheter is placed over an additional wire. If more than one area must be drained, an additional catheter piece can be added to stent any duct.

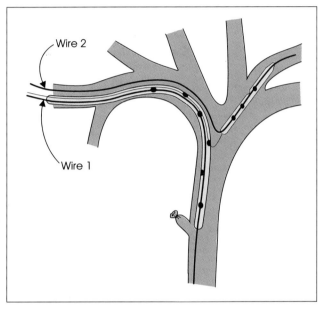

FIGURE 15-5.

The two-wire technique with the articulating piece of one wire inserted into the left duct and the main catheter on an additional wire running into the common bile duct.

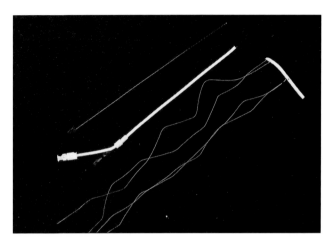

FIGURE 15-6.

A 20-gauge, 20-cm needle advanced from the proximal end of the catheter (measured from a point previously measured to be outside of the patient) to draw the sutures for the articulating piece through the main catheter. The articulating suture can be seen attached to the middle, and the retrieval suture attached to the end of the short catheter piece.

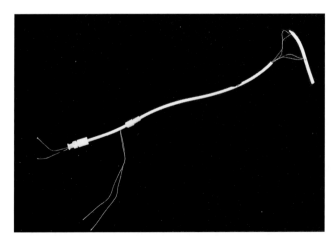

FIGURE 15-7.

The sutures pulled through the main catheter.

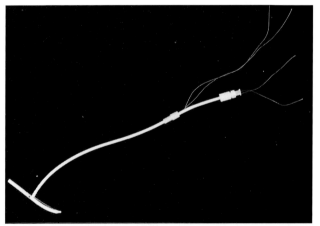

FIGURE 15-8.

The formed articulated T-tube with the retrieval suture at the proximal end and the articulating suture situated in the middle.

Articulated Catheter Removal

To remove the catheter, a guidewire is placed through the main catheter excluding the fragment. The articulating suture is then released and the retrieval suture is pulled, aligning the articulating fragment with the main

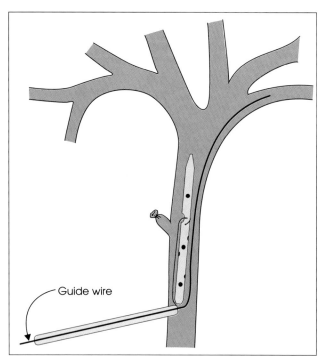

FIGURE 15-9.

The removal of the articulated catheter over a guidewire.

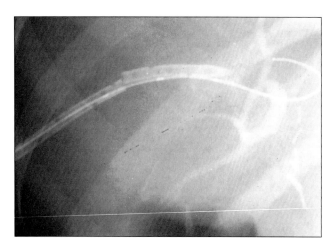

FIGURE 15-10.

The articulated catheter being removed from a patient.

catheter. The two components are removed, leaving the wire behind for additional access or tube replacement as demonstrated in Figures 15-9 and 15-10. For fragments that articulate from the side of main catheter, the articulating suture is used for removal. Occasionally, the fragment will not disengage adequately from the main catheter. In this case, the main catheter is removed and a new catheter is introduced over the suture to pull the articulated fragment out.

Clinical Experience

The articulated catheter has been very useful, particularly in treating liver transplant patients whose T-tube tracts are poorly formed as a result of chronic use of steroids. They are additionally useful in patients who have had a small T-tube placed after common duct exploration for retained stones. In these cases, premade commercial tubes work well and alleviate the usual struggle in attempting to advance a larger catheter

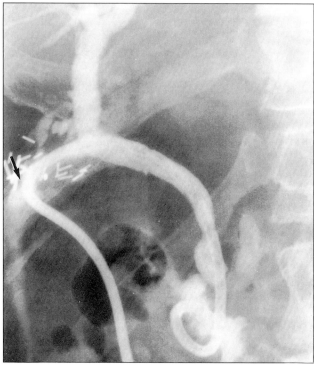

FIGURE 15-11.

A loop catheter enters the T-tube tract, advanced into the bile duct through the ampulla. The tube has pulled back, causing the sidehole to appear within the tract; contrast leaks into the patient's separate cutaneous fistula (*arrow*).

through a small tract. Patients with transperitoneal T-tubes who have retained stones and ampullary stenoses are more easily managed with an articulated T-tube. Figure 15-11 demonstrates a patient who had a retained stone in addition to a stricture of the ampulla

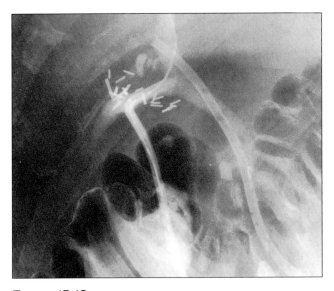

FIGURE 15-12.

An articulated catheter deployed into the common bile duct.

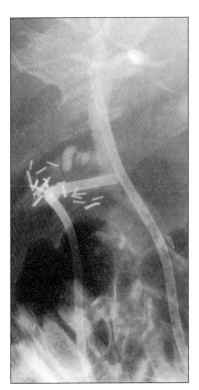

FIGURE 15-13.

The articulated catheter in place.

and a cutaneous fistula from the T-tube tract to the anterior abdominal wall. Initially, the stone was snared and the ampulla dilated. A nephrostomy loop catheter was placed through the tract with sideholes in the distal duct and with the loop through the ampulla. With time, the catheter would pull out of the tract and the sideholes would enter the tract, leaking bile into the fistula. An articulated tube was formed with a long distal limb and sideholes extending through the ampulla. The main portion of the catheter had no sideholes. The method of deployment is seen in Figure 15-12. With this construction, the ampulla was stented and the sideholes could not slip back into the tract (Figs. 15-13 and 15-14). The fistula healed after several weeks and the tube was removed.

Transhepatic articulated catheters are usually constructed the day following the initial procedure, depending on the complexity of drainage. Figures 15-15 and 15-16 demonstrate a patient with a cholechojejunostomy due to a laparoscopic cholecystectomy injury. The patient not only had an obstruction at the anastomosis, but also developed a stricture and a stone in the left duct. After initially receiving two drainage tubes, the patient was converted to an articulated tube with the main catheter placed right to left and the artic-

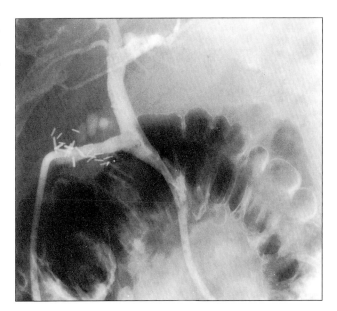

FIGURE 15-14.

The articulated catheter with the tip stenting the ampulla. Contrast injection does not leak into the patient's cutaneous fistula because there are no holes in the main catheter.

ulating piece running down through the anastomosis. This procedure was used because of the difficulty in crossing the stricture past the stones. After stone removal and several weeks of stenting, the tube was removed and the patient improved.

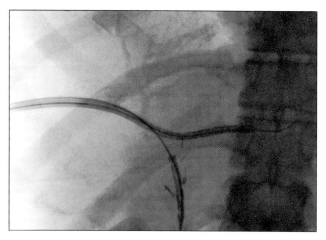

FIGURE 15-15.

The deployment of an articulated tube using the two-wire technique in a patient with a choledochojejunostomy performed after a laparoscopic cholecystectomy injury. The articulating fragment extends into the anastomosis.

Patients with cholangiocarcinoma or liver metastasis undergoing transhepatic drainage usually require both the right and left ducts to be catheterized. We have had one patient with metastatic colon carcinoma to the liver with biliary obstruction in whom we initially did not want to use metal stents. This patient had both anterior and posterior right duct strictures and a left duct stricture requiring required two articulations with two catheter pieces connected to the main stem component.

We have also used articulated catheters in a novel manner to stent two patients with pancreaticocutaneous fistulae. One of these patients, as seen in Figure 15-17, had a chronic fistula to skin with no communication with the proximal pancreatic duct. The patient was too poor a surgical risk to undergo distal pancreatectomy. After months of external drainage, a small communication developed from the distal duct to the jejunum that we dilated with a balloon catheter and then placed an articulated stent from his distal pancreatic duct to the jejunum. After several months we removed the stent and the fistula healed without recurrence or further episodes of pancreatitis.

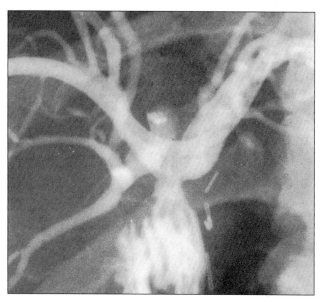

FIGURE 15-16.

Good filling of the ducts and anastomosis with both the anastomotic and left duct stricture stented by one tube.

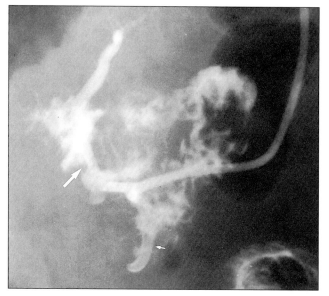

FIGURE 15-17.

The tip of the stem portion of the catheter is situated in the isolated distal pancreatic duct (*large arrow*). The articulating portion of the catheter is situated in the jejunum (*small arrow*). The articulating catheter stents the pancreatic-jejunal fistula in internal drainage.

Conclusion

The articulated catheter has many advantages over conventional T-tubes such as ease of insertion through a small tract and the ability to stent multiple regions. In complex biliary cases for which the commercially available tube is not applicable, the operator must take time to construct and custom fit his own device. In patients with hilar obstruction, we prefer to use two catheters initially if necessary and then bring the patient back to convert them to a single articulated tube. Potential problems that can occur with the articulated tubes include difficulty in removing the crosspiece or separation of the crosspiece due to breakage of the articulating suture. In both cases, the catheter segment can be easily retrieved with a snare or basket. Articulated catheters represent a novel approach in the management of difficult biliary and pancreatic drainages, especially in light of the limited patency of metal stents and the problems associated with multiple catheters.

References and Recommended Reading

Recently published papers of particular interest have been highlighted as:

• Of interest

•• Of outstanding interest

1. Ring EJ: Radiologic Approach to Malignant Biliary Obstruction: Review and Commentary. *Cardiovasc Intervent Radiol* 1990, 13:217–222.

2. Lameris JS, Stoker J, Nijs HGT, *et al.*: Malignant Biliary Obstruction: Percutaneous Use of Self-expandable Stents. *Radiology* 1991, 179:703–707.

3. Adam A, Chetty N, Roddie M, *et al.*: Self-expandable Stainless Steel Endoprotheses for Treatment of Malignant Bile Duct Obstruction. *AJR* 1991, 156:321–325.

4.• Rossi P, Bezzi M, Rossi M, *et al.*: Metallic Stents in Malignant Obstruction: Results of a Multicenter European Study of 240 Patients. *JVIR* 1994, 5:279–285.
Review of a large number of patients with different types of stents.

5.•• Cope C, Gensburg RS: Drainage of Bile Ducts with an Articulated T-tube. *JVIR* 1990, 1:113–116.
Good paper describing technical aspects of building and using an articulated T-tube for biliary lesions. Nicely describes the advantages of an articulated tube.

6.•• Scotti DM: Simplified T-tube Replacement with Two-Piece Retrievable Catheters. *JVIR* 1991, 2:393–399.
Another excellent paper describing clinical uses of articulating T-tubes in multiple clinical cases. Drawings depict different T-tube configurations that can be built.

7. Letourneau JG, Castaãneda-Zuãniga WR: The Role of Radiology in Diagnosis and Treatment of Bilary Complications After Liver Transplantation. *Cardiovasc Intervent Radiol* 1990, 13:278–282.

8.• Gomes AS: Diagnosis and Radiologic Treatment of Bilary Complications of Liver Transplantation. *Semin Intervent Radiol* 1992, 9:283.
Good review of the different types of complications associated with liver transplants.

9.• Saeed ZA, Ramirez FC, Hepps KS: Endoscopic Stent Placement for Internal and External Pancreatic Fistulas. *Gastroenterology* 1993, 105:1213–1217.
Novel endoscopic therapy for external pancreatic fistulae.

10. Crummy AB, Turnipseed WD: Percutaneous Replacement of a Biliary T-tube. *AJR* 1977, 128:869–870.

Interventional Management of Recurrent Pyogenic Cholangitis

Joon Koo Han
Jae Hyung Park
Byung Ihn Choi

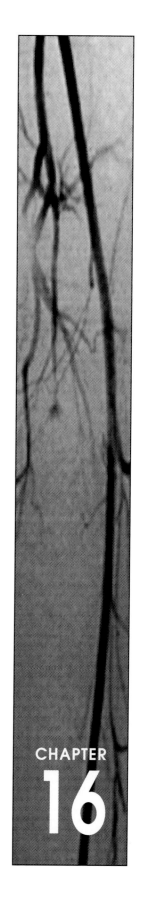

Recurrent pyogenic cholangitis (RPC) also known as oriental cholangiohepatitis, primary cholangitis, recurrent pyogenic cholangiohepatitis, and intrahepatic pigment stone disease, is a distinct clinical entity characterized by repeated attacks of bacterial infection to the biliary tree. The intra- and extrahepatic ducts may show dilatation and stricture, and they may contain calculi, debris consisting mainly of bile pigments, epithelial cells and mixed exudates, and sometimes frank pus. Intrahepatic stones are usually multiple, soft, muddy, and often tenaciously adherent to duct walls. These stones lead to progressive biliary obstruction and recurrent infection, resulting in the formation of multiple cholangitic abscess, biliary strictures, and eventually severe liver destruction, cirrhosis, and portal hypertension [1••].

As the name implies, the disease is prevalent in the Oriental populations. The incidence of RPC is reported as high as 20% in Taiwan and 15% in Korea [2,3]. Although the exact cause is not known, it is postulated that portal bacteremia, metabolic derangement caused by low socioeconomic status, poor hygiene, and dietary insufficiency result in cholangitis and stone formation. In some countries, infestation of *Clonorchis sinensis* or *Ascaris lumbricoides* may play some role [4,5]. As there has been marked improvement in the standard of living in east Asian countries, a decrease in the incidence of RPC has been reported [2,6].

Patients usually experience several attacks of fever, chills, and jaundice before seeking medical attention. Two thirds of the patients present with acute cholangitis,

and others complain of abdominal pain, pancreatitis, jaundice, or abnormal liver biochemistry. Patients with acute cholangitis are managed conservatively with intravenous broad-spectrum antibiotics. Emergency procedures, either surgical or interventional, are performed when these patients do not respond to conservative management. Patients should undergo radiologic examinations to evaluate the extent and the severity of the disease (*ie*, number and location of stones, strictures, lobar atrophy, secondary biliary cirrhosis, or associated cholangiocarcinoma). Then, surgical treatment is planned according to the extent of the disease [1••].

Cholecystectomy, choledochotomy, hepaticodochotomy and stone extraction, or biliary-drainage procedures such as choledochojejunostomy are usually performed. However, because of the multiplicity of stones and associated biliary strictures, the complete removal of intrahepatic stones is not always possible. Partial hepatectomy is the treatment of choice for those patients who have severely damaged liver segments (particularly the left lobe) with localized intrahepatic stones. The rate of residual stones after the surgery is very high, ranging from 42% to 77%, despite recent advances in surgical techniques and the increased use of the operative flexible choledochoscope [1••,3,6].

There are also several factors that preclude further surgical treatment. The morbidity and the mortality rate of a repeated surgical procedure is higher and the procedure more difficult because of dense adhesion compared with the primary procedure. In some patients, poor liver

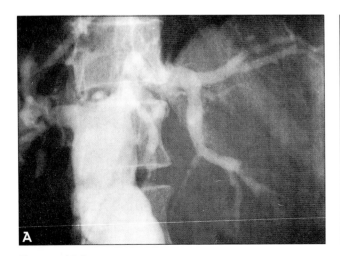

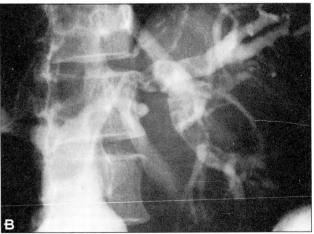

FIGURE 16-1.

Recurrence of stones after initial complete removal. **A,** Cholangiogram after the end of the first surgery and percutaneous stone removal. There is no residual stone in the left intrahepatic duct. **B,** Cholangiogram obtained 9 months later reveals multiple recurrent stones in the left intrahepatic duct.

function caused by parenchymal destruction and secondary biliary cirrhosis preclude general anesthesia and further surgical treatment. In addition, there is a repeated recurrence of intrahepatic stones after complete removal in 15% of patients (Fig. 16-1) [1••]. Appropriate management for these patients is nonsurgical removal of retained or recurrent stones and nonsurgical management of associated biliary strictures.

Removal of Retained Stones

Roentgenologic techniques of nonoperative stone extraction in the ambulatory patient represent a significant improvement in postoperative medical management. Trans-T-tube catheterization using standard vascular catheters and guidewires has been used to dislodge sediment and blood clots to re-establish drainage [7,8]. Removal of the T-tube is indicated to extract retained stones through the tract, with the tube left in place for 4 to 5 weeks after the operation to establish a fibrous tract. In 1962, Mondet [9] extracted stones through a mature T-tube tract with specially designed forceps. Margarey [10] used the Dormia ureteral basket and a small angiographic catheter. Burhenne [11] developed a special steerable catheter and reported excellent results in the treatment of retained common duct stones.

Although the use of the steerable catheter yielded excellent results in extrahepatic bile ducts, it was difficult to use in the relatively small, tortuous, and angulated intrahepatic bile ducts. Chen and colleagues [12] used a fiber optic choledochoscope and Park and colleagues [13] used individually fitted, preshaped angulated catheters to negotiate the tortuous intrahepatic ducts.

Each procedure has its own advantages and disadvantages. In general, better results have been reported with choledochoscopy. However, the use of choledochoscopy requires expensive devices, well-trained personnel, and yields a higher complication rate. The removal of the stone with the preshaped angulated catheter is relatively simple and economic. Such a catheter can better negotiate acute angles and strictures of the bile duct so that it can approach the stone in small peripheral ducts. The catheter technique has a lower success rate than choledochoscopy because it lacks the effective means of crushing large stones by intracorporeal shock wave lithotripsy [14,15••]. It is also responsible for a high radiation exposure to both

the patient and hand of the operator. In one report, the patient received about 350 mR per minute of fluoroscopy time at the entry skin on the table top and the radiologist received 1.9 to 4.1 mR per minute at the dorsum of right hand, and 0.6 to 1.2 mR per minute at the waist level outside his apron [11]. To minimize the radiation exposure, the radiologist should reduce the size of the fluoroscopic field by tight collimation. The T-tube should be inserted in such a way as to exit the right lateral abdominal wall, permitting the radiologist to work away from the radiation field.

TECHNIQUES

Fluoroscopically Guided Stone Removal

Generally, the procedure begins 4 to 6 weeks following surgery to allow the maturation of the fibrous T-tube tract. In patients who suffer from severe biliary strictures, patulent sphincter of Oddi, or in those who have undergone previous drainage procedures, a nonenhanced computed tomography (NECT) of the liver should first be obtained.

This procedure is very important because T-tube cholangiography may miss stones because of the presence of air, or the inability to fill all air ducts with contrast medium. Following sterile preparation and administration of 50 mg of pethidine intramuscularly and broad-spectrum antibiotics, the tube is extracted and replaced over a guidewire with a 30-cm long, 9-French polyethylene catheter. Several types of catheters with different angles of distal tips can be made beforehand; the most appropriate one is selected according to the anatomy and branching angle of the bile duct (Fig. 16-2).

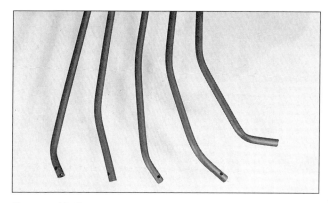

FIGURE 16-2.

Frequently used preshaped catheter. If any of these catheters did not fit the angle of the bile duct, a new catheter was made according to the anatomy of the bile duct.

Selective cholangiography of individual ducts is performed to demonstrate all strictures and impacted stones. NECT can be used as a road map in selection of individual ducts. After the thorough evaluation of the course taken by the bile ducts and location of stones, a preshaped catheter is inserted into the periphery of a stone-bearing duct. A Dormia stone basket (Medi-Tech, Watertown, MA) is inserted through the catheter beyond the stone, expanded and rotated to trap the stone that is then extracted through the tube tract (Fig. 16-3). Dormia baskets measuring 9 to 15 mm in diameter are preferred, but larger sizes up to 25 mm may be required on occasion. If the trapped stone is too large to be extracted, it can be broken up by repeatedly opening and closing the basket through the catheter. Intrahepatic stones are usually friable and easily

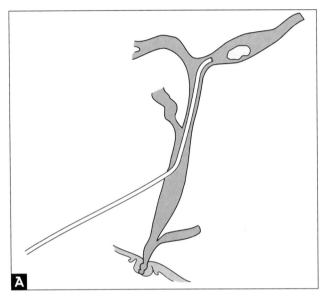

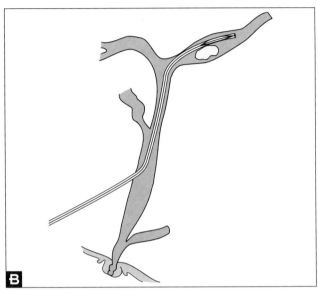

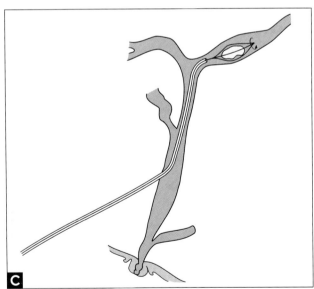

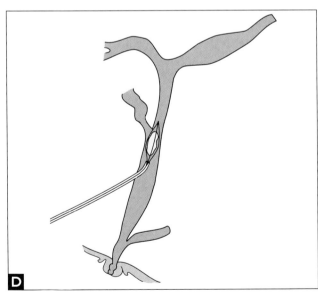

FIGURE 16-3.

The technique used during percutaneous catheter removal of intrahepatic stones. **A**, The stones are localized by cholangiography after removal of the T-tube. **B**, The preshaped catheter is advanced to the distal intrahepatic duct beyond the stone. A Dormia stone basket is inserted through the catheter beyond the stone. **C**, The basket is expanded by withdrawing the catheter, and the stone is trapped by rotation of the basket. **D**, The stone is extracted through the T-tube tract or crushed by strong pulling of the basket when the catheter is held tightly.

crushed. Fragments are extracted separately by basketing or removal by repeated irrigation and suction. A large Nelaton rubber tube (16- to 20-French outer diameter, 30-cm long) with many sideholes is then inserted into the biliary tree through the T-tube tract for repeated infusion and aspiration with saline. Small particles are either aspirated or passed into the duodenum; if larger fragments are impacted within the drainage holes of the tube, they are removed with continuous negative pressure.

Large stones that cannot be trapped with a Dormia basket can sometimes be snared and crushed with the use of specially designed mechanical lithotriptor basket (Cook, Bloomington, IN). When there are severe strictures that impede the passage of the 9-French catheter, ductoplasty can be performed by inflating a 5- to 7-French, 6- to 10-mm angioplasty balloon catheter for 1 to 3 minutes at 5 to 10 atmospheres, following instillation of 5 to 10 mL of 2% lidocaine into the bile ducts (Fig. 16-4).

Multiple small stones in nonstenotic peripheral ducts can be retrieved into the common duct with a 10-mm Fogarty (Arrow International, Reading, PA) or occlusion balloon catheter. Residual stones in the common duct will usually pass spontaneously into the bowel, or can be flushed down with saline injection (Fig. 16-5).

Percutaneous transhepatic biliary drainage (PTBD) should be performed with an 8- to 9-French catheter to remove otherwise unreachable peripheral impacted stones. The catheter is inserted into the duct that contains stones, and the stones are trapped and crushed or displaced to a more central duct where they can be easily extracted. Generally, larger stones should not be extracted intact through a small PTBD tract, because the procedure is too traumatic and may result in loss of access; instead, the stones should be crushed into smaller particles and removed with the irrigation and suction technique [13, 14,15••].

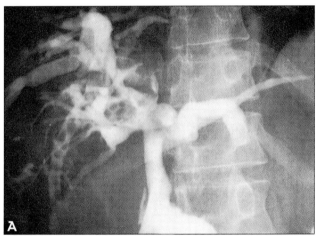

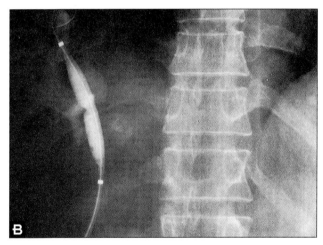

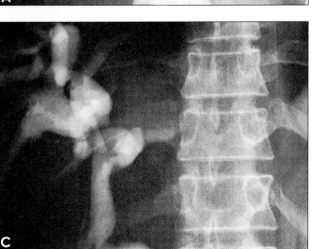

FIGURE 16-4.

Complete removal of right intrahepatic duct stones with multiple sessions of ESWL and ductoplasty to relieve the stricture of the bile duct. **A,** Selective cholangiogram reveals multiple intrahepatic stones in the right lobe of the liver. There is a tight stenosis at the orifice of the right intrahepatic duct. **B,** The stricture is dilated with a balloon angioplasty 3 mm in diameter and 4 cm in length. **C,** After six ESWL sessions and percutaneous stone removal, all stones in the right intrahepatic ducts were completely extracted. The patient was observed for 2 years, with no recurrent symptoms found.

Because the size of the stone that can be extracted depends on tract size, it is recommended that surgeons use large-bore T-tubes to facilitate postoperative percutaneous removal. The course of the tube should extend from a lateral stab wound straight across to the common ducts [11]. Recently, a transjejunal tube approach was described to remove large stones that cannot be extracted through the T-tube tract [16].

Extracorporeal Shock-Wave Lithotripsy of Retained Stones

Extracorporeal shock-wave lithotripsy (ESWL) is a new procedure that can be used for the nonsurgical treatment of retained bile-duct stones when conventional stone extraction methods are unsuccessful. Even then, failure can occur with the use of laser lithotripsy and direct electrohydraulic lithotripsy because of the inability to maneuver an endoscope close enough to the stones [17–19]. Because the piezoelectric lithotriptor has low energy per pulse, high pressure gain, and small focal volume, it causes less pain and induces minimal tissue damage. This technique may be the most appropriate form of equipment for ESWL of intrahepatic stones [20•].

Intrahepatic stones are initially localized with a real-time sonographic probe before the patient is placed on the lithotriptor. The position of the patient depends on the location of the stones and on the sonic window that will permit the safest and best visualization of the stones. Targeting of the stones is performed by means of an in-line transducer with continuous ultrasound monitoring.

With the piezoelectric lithotriptor (EDAPLT.01; EDAP, Croissy Beaubourg Marine La Val, France), the shock waves are given at a rate of 5 impulses per second at 30% to 50% power. Each session lasts 30 to 60 minutes (9,000 to 18,000 shock waves). A selective cholangiogram is obtained 1 day after ESWL. To facilitate early fragmentation and to attain better visualization and localization of the stones, normal saline can be dripped into the bile duct through the T-tube or PTBD tube during ESWL. If unsuccessful, the ESWL procedure is repeated 1 week later until successful fragmentation is achieved. Fragmentation of intrahepatic stones does not need to be as fine as does lithotripsy of gallbladder stones because large fragments that cannot pass spontaneously can be removed with a basket. Even when stones are not grossly fragmented by ESWL, they may become more fragile or displaced to a more favorable location so that they may be accessible by mechanical extraction if possible (Figs. 16-6 and 16-7).

Although the piezoelectric lithotriptor causes the least pain and tissue damage compared with the other types of lithotriptors, it does cause some parenchymal damage in the liver and gallbladder in animal experiments [21]. So far, there have been no reports of significant adverse reactions in patients as a result of piezoelectric ESWL.

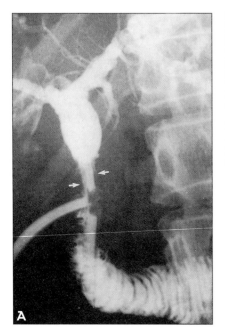 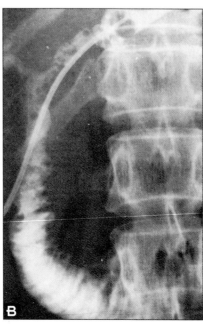

FIGURE 16-5.

Complete removal of left intrahepatic stones by sweeping with a Fogarty balloon. **A,** Cholangiogram shows multiple stones in the peripheral branch of left intrahepatic duct. Note that the T-tube is inserted from the jejunum (*arrows*) and the upper limb is placed within the common bile duct. **B,** With a Fogarty balloon of 1 cm in diameter, stones are displaced to a more central duct. As the T-tube is inserted from the jejunum, stones can be displaced into the jejunum and extraction is not necessary.

Postoperative Flexible Choledochoscopy and Intracorporeal Electrohydraulic Lithotripsy for Retained Biliary Stones

This procedure is performed 4 weeks after the surgical exploration under no sedation or mild parenteral diazepam sedation. General anesthesia is only used if complex and traumatizing maneuvers are planned. Antibiotics are given to all patients for 3 to 5 days following the procedure. The access route most commonly used is the T-tube tract, but the PTBD tract

or a Roux-en-Y hepaticojejunostomy with the blind loop attached to the anterior abdominal wall can also be used. The jejunostomy offers the advantage of a permanent percutaneous route to the biliary tract which can be utilized for choledoscopic removal of stones in patients with complex biliary problems [22•].

The choledochoscope Olympus CHF type T20, (Olympus Optical, Tokyo, Japan) has a steerable tip and channel for saline irrigation (6-mm outer diameter, 2.6-mm instrument channel) or for passage of

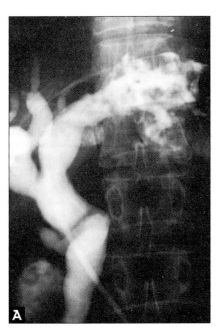
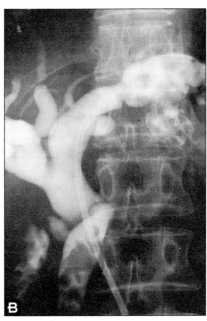

FIGURE 16-6.

Complete removal of left intrahepatic stones with multiple ESWL sessions and percutaneous extraction in 52-year-old woman. **A,** Selective cholangiogram reveals numerous impacted stones in the left intrahepatic duct. **B,** After 11 ESWL sessions, some stones were displaced to the common bile duct and the impaction in the left intrahepatic duct was relieved. All stones were removed from left intrahepatic duct after 22 sessions of percutaneous removal.

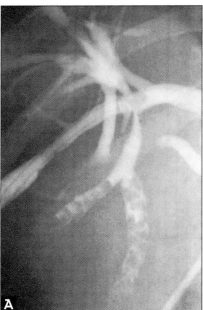
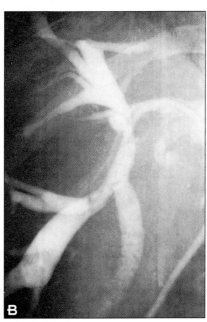

FIGURE 16-7.

Complete removal of right intrahepatic stones with one ESWL session and irrigation in a 38-year-old man. **A,** Initial selective cholangiogram of the right hepatic duct shows multiple intrahepatic stones in the posterior segment of the right hepatic lobe. **B,** After one ESWL session, stones were broken down into numerous tiny fragments that were completely removed by irrigation instead of the more traumatic basket extraction.

various instruments such as grasping forceps, stone baskets, balloon catheters, or irrigation catheters. The flexibility of the catheter permits complete visualization of extrahepatic ducts as well as the secondary or tertiary radicals of intrahepatic ducts. Mud and small grains are removed with saline irrigation. When a stone is snared, it is removed together with the endoscope. The balloon catheter is used to dislodge stones impacted in the smaller ducts. Large stones are broken up with stone-crushing baskets or biopsy forceps, and are then removed with the basket or the grasping forceps. Intracorporeal electrohydraulic lithotripsy is performed with a flexible 5-French electrode under direct visualization [17,18]. The electrode should contact the stone for best results; it should also protrude at least 2 cm beyond the tip of the choledochoscope and should not touch the bile duct wall during sparking, to prevent damage or injury. Preliminary trapping of stones is not usually necessary, as the impacted stones are stationary and not likely to be repelled by the shock wave.

When a stricture is encountered, the duct is dilated with an angioplasty balloon to permit the passage of the endoscope and remove distal retained stones. For a severe stricture that precludes the passage of the balloon or choledochoscope, PTBD is performed distal to the stricture. This allows an angled, hydrophilic, coated guidewire to be inserted and maneuvered through the stricture under fluoroscopic guidance. The guidewire can then be grasped using transendoscopic biopsy forceps, and pulled out through the T-tube tract. The stricture can now be dilated after passing an angioplasty balloon catheter antegradely over the wire. This rendezvous technique will then allow the cholangioscope to be inserted beyond the stricture [23].

Before and after each session of choledochoscopy, a cholangiogram is taken. The whole procedure is repeated for 5 to 7 days until all the stones have been cleared as demonstrated by both the cholangiogram and the choledochoscopy. When a hepaticocutaneous jejunostomy is used for choledochoscopy, the jejunostomy is closed with one seromuscular layer of interrupted suture with the patient under local anesthesia after all stones are removed [24,25].

RESULTS

The rate of successful removal of retained stones depends on several factors: 1) the number and location of residual stones; 2) the presence and degree of biliary strictures; and 3) the anatomy of the bile ducts. Excellent results are reported for the removal of extrahepatic bile duct stones (95% to 100%) [13,14,15••,24]. On the other hand, intrahepatic stones can be completely removed in only 50% of patients. A further 20% can be rendered asymptomatic following incomplete stone extraction, yielding a total success rate of approximately 70%. The average number of sessions required is 3.7 ± 2.9, ranging from 1 to 22 [15••]. In choledochoscopically guided removal, complete removal is possible in 82% to 90% of patients. The average number of sessions required here is 4, ranging from 1 to 22 [1••,24,25]. Severe angulation deformities, strictures of the bile duct that impede the passage of guidewires or devices, and impacted stones are the most frequently encountered problems (Table 16-1). With the recent additional use of extracorporeal shock-wave lithotripsy, these problems can often be solved, provided the stones can be targeted safely. In our experience at Seoul National University Hospital, percutaneous fluoroscopically guided removal of stones combined with ESWL resulted in complete removal of retained stones in 25 patients and partially successful removal in 5 of 35 patients treated in the past 2 years. The complete success rate was 71.4% and the overall success rate was 85.7%. When combined treatment was used, the number of ESWL sessions was 8.3 ± 5.7 and the number of stone-removal sessions was 5.9 ± 4.1.

Long-term follow-up results after successful stone removal are reported in small groups. Stones recurred

Table 16-1. Causes of Failure for Stone Removal in 170 Patients*

Causes	Patients, n
Angulation	14
Strictures	24
Impacted stones	16
Large stones	2
Tortuous tracts	2
Stones in short peripheral duct	1
Too many stones	1
Refusal to follow-up	5
Total†	65

*From Choi et al. (15••); with permission.
†Some patients had more than one cause of failure.

in 3% of extrahepatic stone patients and 15.8% of intrahepatic stone patients [1••,25].

COMPLICATION AND PREVENTION

Minor acute complications include right upper quadrant pain, nausea, vomiting, and limited hemobilia following balloon dilatation that subsides under observation or with analgesics. Fever and chills caused by periprocedural sepsis are controlled with oral antibiotics and subside in 2 to 3 days. In our 10-year experience with 170 patients, two patients developed abscesses of the liver and T-tube tract, respectively, and one patient experienced hemobilia, requiring transfusion after traumatic catheterization. There were no procedure-related deaths [15••].

The complication rate of choledochoscopic removal is higher than that of fluoroscopically guided catheter removal. Gandini and colleagues [25] report three deaths and 13 reports of complications in 97 patients. In this series, there were cases of pancreatitis (n=4), acute tubular necrosis caused by contrast media (n=1), subphrenic fluid collection treated by percutaneous catheter drainage (n=4), intestinal perforation (n=1), asymptomatic dissection of the main bile duct that resolved spontaneously by maintaining internal drainage for 3 days (n=2), and persistent hemobilia that required a blood transfusion (n=1).

The operator should be very gentle to avoid injury to the bile duct and tract. Catheters should always be advanced over a guidewire. Forceful injection of saline or contrast material into strictured bile ducts can result in bacteremia or liver abscess. It is recommended that a safety guidewire be used when instrumenting transhepatic or potentially immature T-tube tracts.

Interventional Procedures During Acute Cholangitis

Approximately two thirds of the patients who present with acute cholangitis respond well to conservative management. The rest require percutaneous interventional treatment, which is generally more safe than surgery (0.7% mortality rate) [26]. The mortality rate after the emergency surgical treatment is 8% compared with 1.9% after elective surgery [3]. Also, 21% of the patients require a second elective surgery after the initial emergency surgery [1••].

Recent reports reveal that the success rate of complete stone removal through a PTBD tract in RPC is as high as 78% [27]. Stones can be removed earlier through PTBD tracts because the transhepatic tracts mature approximately 2 to 3 weeks earlier than surgical T-tube tracts.

Selection of the proper duct from the percutaneous transhepatic cholangiogram is the most important factor determining the final outcome. PTBD is selectively performed with an 8.5-French tube in stone-bearing or strictured ducts. Stones are trapped and crushed with a 9-French preangulated catheter and flushed into the duodenum. In general, large stones should not be removed or pulled out through small PTBD tracts for fear of accidental loss of tract or excess bleeding (Fig. 16-8). Associated liver abscess can be treated with ultrasound-guided aspiration or catheter drainage.

Management of Biliary Strictures

Intrahepatic biliary strictures are found in approximately 90% of the patients with RPC and are a main cause for treatment failure in conventional surgery, postoperative stone removal, and stone recurrence. Clinically, biliary strictures are characterized by repeated episodes of cholangitis with sepsis or progressive fibrosing inflammation of the involved bile ducts, leading to biliary cirrhosis. To prevent the progression of inflammation and to minimize the recurrence of stones, it is mandatory to dilate the strictures and to extract the associated stones [28•].

Recent data suggest that surgical reconstruction is the initial choice for most physicians treating patients with primary postoperative benign strictures of extrahepatic bile ducts. Balloon dilatation is reserved for anastomotic strictures after biliary reconstruction for hilar strictures [29]. For multifocal intrahepatic strictures, dilatation with balloon angioplasty is the only possible option other than liver transplantation.

Balloons (6 to 10 mm in diameter) are introduced through T-tube or PTBD tracts. The balloon is inflated and maintained under pressure for approximately 1 minute. Broad-spectrum antibiotics (eg, ampicillin 500 mg orally, every 6 hours) are prescribed for 3 days afterward. Dilatation of intrahepatic biliary strictures greatly facilitates removal of retained stones proximal to the stricture. After complete removal of stones, the stricture is stented with a small diameter silastic catheter (size ranging from 8- to 12-French, depending on location of the stricture) which is left in place for 4 to 8 weeks, or longer if necessary. The most frequent complication developing from balloon dilatation is transient hemobilia [28•,29].

Although long-term follow-up results for balloon dilatation of intrahepatic strictures are not available, current data suggest that cumulative probability of stricture recurrence is 4% at 2 years, 6% at 2.5 years, and 8% at 3 years [28•]. However, the progression of the benign stricture might be slow, and partial obstructions are sometimes completely asymptomatic for long periods. Longer follow-up is required to appraise the efficacy of balloon dilatation in the treatment of biliary strictures.

Self-expandable metallic stents have been used recently to treat intractable benign strictures, with favorable initial results. However, with longer follow-up, more cases of delayed obstruction or stenosis of metallic stents are reported. Sung and colleagues [30] report 18.7% of stent obstruction in 16 patients with hepatolithiasis after a median follow-up of 18 months (with a range of 10 to 29 months). Although obstructed metallic stents can be managed with the internal deployment of other stents, the first stent may hinder further interventional procedures.

We should bear in mind that during the management of this disease, some biliary strictures may be malignant. Cholangiocarcinoma is found in 2% to 10% of patients with RPC [31••,32]. The tumor can spread intra- or periductally, appearing as a localized mass that can be easily diagnosed with ultrasound or CT. It is quite difficult to differentiate the benign stricture from infiltrating cholangiocarcinoma based on radiologic findings alone.

Exfoliative cytology or brush biopsy has a low sensitivity (approximately 40%) and high specificity. However, three consecutive negative results greatly reduce the likelihood of cholangiocarcinoma [33]. The use of biopsy forceps through an endoscope will provide better tissue samples for a histologic diagnosis.

Conclusion

Despite the need for multiple sessions to manage RPC, the outcome is unsatisfactory. With better methods for crushing stones and the combined use of all instrumental modalities, it is hoped that better results will be achieved in the future. The experimental use of expanding metallic stents to treat benign intractable strictures in this disease has not been as favorable as initially expected. For patients with recurrent cholangitis and severe parenchymal damage, liver transplantation constitutes a new treatment option.

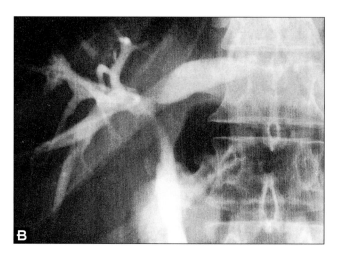

FIGURE 16-8.

Incomplete removal of multiple intrahepatic stones through the PTBD tract in a 26-year-old man who presented with symptoms of acute cholangitis. **A**, An initial tubogram after PTBD revealed multiple stones in both lobes of the liver and common duct. There were also strictures at the level of the right, left, and common hepatic duct (*arrows*). **B**, Through the PTBD tract, stones in the right posterior segment and left lobe of the liver are completely cleared. However, because of the acute angle, stones in the right anterior segment could not be removed. The PTBD was removed after balloon dilatation of the stricture and stenting for 2 months. The patient was free of complications for 15 months.

References and Recommended Reading

Recently published papers of particular interest have been highlighted as:

• Of special interest

•• Of outstanding interest

1.•• Fan ST, Choi TK, Lo CM, *et al.*: Treatment of Hepatolithiasis: Improvement of Results by a Systematic Approach. *Surgery* 1991, 109:474–480.
The authors give an extensive review of their experience in surgical and postoperative management of hepatolithiasis as well as preoperative evaluation of the patients.

2. Su CH, Lui WY, Peing FK: Relative Prevalence of Gallstone Disease in Taiwan: A Nationwide Cooperative Study. *Dig Dis Sci* 1992, 37:764–768.

3. Kim SW, Park YH, Choi JW: Clinical and Epidemiological Analysis of a 10 Year Experience with 1719 Gallstone Patients (in Korean). *Korean J Gastro* 1993, 25:159–167.

4. Ong GB: A Study of Recurrent Pyogenic Cholangitis. *Archives Surg* 1962, 84:63–89.

5. Wenn CC, Lee HC: Intrahepatic Stones: A Clinical Study. *Ann Surg* 1972, 175:166–177.

6. Chang TM, Passaro E: Intrahepatic Stones: The Taiwan Experience. *Am J Surg* 1983, 146:241–244.

7. Margulis AR, Newton TH, Najarian JS: Removal of Plugs From a T-tube by a Fluoroscopically Guided Catheter: Report of a Case. *AJR* 1965, 93:975–977.

8. Short WF, Howard JM, Diven WF: Trans T-tube Catheterization. *Arch Surg* 1971, 102:136–138.

9. Mondet A: Technica de la Extraccion Incruenta de Los Calculos la Litiasis Residual del Coledoco. *Bol Soc Cir Air* 1962, 46:278–290.

10. Margarey CJ: Non-surgical Removal of Retained Biliary Calculi. *Lancet* 1971, 1:1044–1046.

11. Burhenne HJ: Nonoperative Retained Biliary Tract Stone Extraction. *AJR* 1973, 117:388–399.

12. Chen MF, Chou FF, Wang CS, *et al.*: Postoperative Choledochofiberscopic Removal of Intrahepatic Stones. *J Formos Med Assoc* 1980, 79:700–705.

13. Park JH, Choi BI, Han MC, *et al.*: Percutaneous Removal of Residual Intrahepatic Stones. *Radiology* 1987, 163:619–623.

14. Han JK, Choi BI, Park JH, *et al.*: Percutaneous Removal of Retained Intrahepatic Stones with a Pre-shaped Angulated Catheter: Review of 96 Patients. *Br J Radiol* 1992, 65:9–13.

15.•• Choi BI, Han JK, Han MC: Percutaneous Removal of Retained Intrahepatic Stones Utilizing a Combination of Techniques with Emphasis on a Preshaped Angulated Catheter: Review of 170 Patients. *Eur J Radiol* 1992, 2:199–203.
The authors describe various techniques used in fluoroscopically guided percutaneous stone removal and the results. Also, they discuss advantages and disadvantages of fluoroscopically guided intervention compared with choledochoscopic stone removal.

16. Lee Y, Choi BY: Percutaneous Transjejunal T-Tube Approach (A New Method for Extraction of Residual Biliary Stones in Roux-en-Y Biliary Jejunal Anastomosis). *Sejong Med J* 1988, 5:237–243.

17. Picus D, Weyman PJ, Marx MV: Role of Percutaneous Intracorporeal Electrohydraulic Lithotripsy in the Treatment of Biliary Tract Calculi. *Radiology* 1989, 170:989–993.

18. Fan ST, Choi TK, Wong J: Electrohydraulic Lithotripsy for Biliary Stones. *Aust NZ J Surg* 1989, 59:217–221.

19. Dawson SL, Mueller PR, Lee MJ, *et al.*: Treatment of Bile Duct Stones by Laser Lithotripsy: Results in 12 Patients. *AJR* 1992, 158:1007–1009.

20.• Choi BI, Han JK, Park JH, *et al.*: Retained Intrahepatic Stones: Treatment with Piezoelectric Lithotripsy Combined with Stone Extraction. *Radiology* 1991, 178:105–108.
ESWL was performed in 11 patients with retained intrahepatic stones that were difficult to extract by conventional methods of fluoroscopically guided techniques. The overall success rate in this selected group was 82%. Difficulty in targeting stones and severe strictures and deformities of intrahepatic ducts were the factors responsible for failure. There were no significant complications.

21. Ell CH, Kerzel W, Heyder N, *et al.*: Tissue Reaction Under Piezoelectric Shock Wave Application for the Fragmentation of Biliary Calculi. *Gut* 1989, 30:680.

22.• Fan ST, Mak F, Zheng SS, *et al.*: Appraisal of Hepaticocutaneous Jejunostomy in the Management of Hepatolithiasis. *Am J Surg* 1993, 165:332–335.
In 41 patients who underwent this procedure for removal of intrahepatic stones, the presence of the cutaneous stoma facilitated postoperative choledochoscopy for dilatation of biliary strictures and extraction of residual stones. In addition, for patients who have recurrent symptoms, a cutaneous stoma can be reconstructed easily under local anesthesia. The overall complication rate related to the cutaneous stoma was 15%.

23. Maetani I, Hoshi H, Ohashi S, *et al.*: Cholangioscopic Extraction of Intrahepatic Stones Associated with Biliary Strictures Using the Rendezvous Technique. *Endoscopy* 1993, 25:303–306.

24. Choi TK, Lee M, Lui R, *et al.*: Postoperative Flexible Choledochoscopy for Residual Primary Intrahepatic Stones. *Ann Surg* 1986, 203:260–265.

25. Gandini G, Righi D, Regge D, *et al.*: Percutaneous Removal of Biliary Stones. *Cardiovasc Intervent Radiol* 1990, 13:245–251.

26. Günther RW, Schild H, Thelen M: Review Article: Percutaneous Transhepatic Biliary Drainage; Experience with 311 Procedures. *Cardiovasc Intervent Radiol* 1988, 17:65–71.

27. Ryeon HK, Sim JI, Park AW, *et al.*: Percutaneous Transhepatic Removal of Biliary Stones: Clinical Analysis of 16 Cases (in Korean). *J Kor Radiol Soc* 1993, 29:1234–1239.

28.• Jeng KS, Yang FS, Ohta I, *et al.*: Dilatation of Intrahepatic Biliary Strictures in Patients with Hepatolithiasis. *World J Surg* 1990, 14:587–593.
In 57 consecutive patients with biliary strictures associated with hepatolithiasis, balloon dilatation was performed to relieve the strictures. The cumulative probability of restricture was low (6% at 2.5 years). The authors also discuss the similar and different aspects of recurrent pyogenic cholangitic strictures and postoperative strictures.

29. Millis JM, Tompkins RK, Zinner MJ, *et al.*: Management of Bile Duct Strictures: An Evolving Strategy. *Arch Surg* 1992, 127:1077–1084.

30. Sung KB, Song HY, Kim MW, *et al.*: Occlusion of Metallic Stents Used for Benign Biliary Strictures. Paper Presented At the Annual Meetings of the Korean Radiology Society, October 1993.

31. •• Fan ST, Wong J: Complications of Hepatolithiasis. *J Gastroenterol Hepatol* 1992, 7:324–327.
The authors review various complications and treatments of recurrent pyogenic cholangitis.

32. Chen MF, Jan YY, Wang CS, *et al.*: Reappraisal of Cholangiocarcinoma in Patients with Hepatolithiasis. *Cancer* 1993, 71:2461–2465.

33. Rabinovitz M, Zajko A, Hassanein T, *et al.*: Diagnostic Value of Brush Cytology in the Diagnosis of Bile Duct Carcinoma: A Study in 65 Patients with Bile Duct Strictures. *Hepatology* 1990, 12:747–752.

Select Bibliography

Chan F, Man S, Leong L, *et al.*: Evaluation of Recurrent Pyogenic Cholangitis with CT: Analysis of 50 Patients. *Radiology* 1989, 170:165–169.

Coons H: Biliary Intervention—Technique and Devices: A Commentary. *Cardiovasc Intervent Radiol* 1990, 13:211–216.

Jeng K, Shih S, Chiang H, *et al.*: Secondary Biliary Cirrhosis: A Limiting Factor in the Treatment of Hepatolithiasis. *Arch Surg* 1989, 1301–1305.

Jeng K, Yang F, Chiang H, *et al.*: Bile Duct Stents in the Management of Hepatolithiasis with Long-Segment Intrahepatic Biliary Strictures. *Br J Surg* 1992, 79:663–666.

Lim JH, Ko YT, Lee DH, *et al.*: Oriental Cholangiohepatitis: Sonographic Findings in 48 Cases. *AJR* 1990, 55:511–514.

Index to Subjects

A

Abdomen
  abscesses and fluid collections in, postoperative, 112–122
  arteriovenous malformations of, 18–19
Abdominal pregnancy, embolotherapy in, 47
Abdominal wall apposition, percutaneous gastrostomy and, 163–164
Ablation of parathyroid adenomas, 60–64
Abscesses, intra-abdominal, postoperative, 112–122
Adenomas, parathyroid, 52–64
  ablation of, 60–64
  diagnosis of, 53–60
Alcohol ablation, direct, for parathyroid adenomas, 63–64
Amplatz mechanical thrombectomy device, 105–106
Anchoring devices for gastropexy, 166
Angiography
  diagnostic, in hemoptysis, 32–35
  over-the-wire, after renal angioplasty, 93–94
Angioplasty see also Percutaneous transluminal angioplasty
  dialysis access, early, 129–130
  intimal flap after, 71
  medial dissection after, 70
Angio-Seal Hemostatic Puncture Closure Device, 82–86
Aortogram
  flush, after renal angioplasty, 93–94
  pelvic, 40
    postpartum, 41
Argyle catheters, in percutaneous gastrostomy, 168
Arterial perforation and rupture, percutaneous transluminal renal angioplasty and, 97
Arteries see specific arteries
Arteriography, in parathyroid adenoma diagnosis, 58–60
Arteriovenous fistulae, pediatric, 19–21
Arteriovenous malformations, pediatric, 14–19
Articulated catheters, 174–183
  clinical experience with, 180–182
  construction of, 177–178
  design of, 176–177
  placement of, 178–179
  removal of, 180
Aspiration
  diagnostic
    of intra-abdominal fluid collections, 113
    of parathyroid lesions, 55
  percutaneous drainage and see Percutaneous drainage
Atherectomy
  intravascular ultrasound use during, 74–76
  of renal ostium, 96
Auto-expandable stents see Self-expanding stents

B

Balloon angioplasty see Angioplasty
Balloons, detachable, in arteriovenous fistula treatment, 19, 20
Benign obstruction, stenting for
  esophageal, 140
  tracheobronchial, 147–148
Biliary drainage, transhepatic, percutaneous, 189
Biliary obstruction, articulated catheters for, 174–183
Biliary tract, recurrent pyogenic cholangitis and, 186–194
Bleeding see also Hemorrhage
  pathophysiology of, in hemoptysis, 32
Bronchial artery
  anatomy of, 30–32
  embolization of, indications for, 30 see also Hemoptysis

Bronchial lesions, stent implantation in, 146–147 see also Self-expanding stents, in tracheobronchial stenosis treatment

C

Cannulation, pyloric canal, percutaneous fluoroscopic gastrostomy and, 159–161
Catheters see also specific disorders or procedures
  in arteriovenous fistula treatment, 19–21
  articulated, 174–183
  for percutaneous gastrostomy and gastrojejunostomy, 157, 168
    complications involving, 162–164
    exchanges of, 167–168
    insertion of, 161–162
    removal of, 168
Cavernous hemangiomas, 22
Cervical laceration, obstetric embolotherapy for, 44, 45
Cervicofacial arteriovenous malformations, 16–18
Children
  tracheobronchial lesions in, stenting for, 149
  vascular anomalies in, 12–26
Cholangiocarcinoma, articulated catheters in, 174–183
Cholangitis, pyogenic, recurrent, 186–194
Choledochoscopy, flexible, postoperative, 191–192
Circulation, uterine, 40–41
Clot-trapper device, transjugular, 109
Colon, transverse, percutaneous gastrostomy and gastrojejunostomy and, 158–159
Computed tomography
  nonenhanced, stone removal in recurrent pyogenic cholangitis and, 187–188
  in parathyroid adenoma diagnosis, 56–57
  in percutaneous gastrostomy guidance, 165, 166
Contrast agents, renal failure induced by, 97–98
Cystic fibrosis, hemoptysis in see Hemoptysis

D

Dialysis
  access maintenance for, 126–131
    early angioplasty in, 129–130
    graft hemodynamics and, 126–128
    screening criteria and, 126
  pressure measurements during, 126
Dilators, for percutaneous gastrostomy and gastrojejunostomy, 157
Direct alcohol ablation, for parathyroid adenomas, 63–64
Direct percutaneous jejunostomy, 165
Dormia stone basket, 188–189
Drainage, percutaneous
  of postoperative intra-abdominal abscesses, 112–122
  transhepatic biliary, 189
Draining gastrostomy, 165

E

Elastoy stent see Nitinol Strecker stent
Electrohydraulic lithotripsy, intracorporeal, of retained stones in recurrent pyogenic cholangitis, 190, 191
Embolization see also Macroembolization
  arteriovenous fistula, 21
  arteriovenous malformation, 16–18
  bronchial artery, 35–37
    indications for, 30
  microcholesterol crystal, percutaneous transluminal renal angioplasty and, 97

Embolization *see also* Macroembolization, *continued*
  obstetric, 40–49
  venous, 15
Emergency obstetric embolotherapy, 41–42
  indications for, 44
  results of, 43–47
Endoscopic gastrostomy, fluoroscopic placement versus, 169–170
Esophageal stents, 134–141
  for benign strictures, 140
  choice of, 135–136
  clinical reports of, 136–138
  expandable, 134–135
  insertion technique for, 136
  for malignant strictures, 138–140
  patient follow-up with, 136
Ethanol injection therapy *see* Sclerotherapy
Extracorporeal shock-wave lithotripsy, of retained stones in recurrent
      pyogenic cholangitis, 190, 191
Extremities, arteriovenous malformations involving, 18

F

Face and neck, arteriovenous malformations of, 16–18
Feeding catheters, for percutaneous gastrostomy and gastrojejunostomy,
      157–158
Fibrinolytic agents, percutaneous abscess drainage and, 121–122
Fistulae, arteriovenous, 19–21
Flap, intimal, postangioplasty, 71
Flexible choledochoscopy, postoperative, for retained biliary stones, 191–192
Fluid collections, intra-abdominal, postoperative, 112–122
Fluoroscopy
  in percutaneous gastrostomy and gastrojejunostomy, 156–170
  in prophylactic obstetric embolotherapy, 43
  retained stone removal guided by, in recurrent pyogenic cholangitis,
      187–190
Flush aortogram, after renal angioplasty, 93–94

G

Gastric wall apposition, percutaneous gastrostomy and, 163–164
Gastrointestinal tract, arteriovenous malformations of, 18
Gastrojejunostomy
  gastrostomy conversion to, 166–167
  gastrostomy versus, 168–169
  percutaneous gastrostomy and, fluoroscopic, 156–170
Gastroparesis, pharmacologic, 164–165
Gastropexy
  anchoring devices for, 166
  possibility of, percutaneous gastrostomy and, 170
Gastrostomy
  conversion to gastrojejunostomy, 166–167
  draining, 165
  gastrojejunostomy versus, 168–169
  percutaneous gastrojejunostomy and, fluoroscopic, 156–170
Gianturco stent *see also* Stents
  esophageal, 135, 139
  tracheobronchial, 145–146
    clinical results with, 151–152
Glucagon, gastroparesis induced by, 164–165
Grafts
  dialysis
    hemodynamics of, 126–128
    pressure monitoring and, 129–130
  infection of, percutaneous drainage in, 117–118

H

Hemangioendotheliomas, hepatic, infantile, 14
Hemangiomas
  cavernous, 22
  osseous, 22

Hemangiomas, *continued*
  pediatric, 13–14
Hemodialysis access, patency of, 126–131
Hemoptysis
  bleeding pathophysiology in, 32
  bronchial artery anatomy and, 30–32
  diagnosis of, 32–35
  embolotherapy in, 35–36
    complications of, 37
    indications for, 30
    results of, 36
Hemorrhage *see also* Bleeding
  obstetrical, embolotherapy in, 40–49
Hemostasis, puncture site, 82–86
Hepatic hemangioendotheliomas, infantile, 14
Hilar cholangiocarcinoma, articulated catheters in, 174–183
Hydrolyser catheter, 106–109
Hypogastric artery, obstetric embolotherapy and, 41–42 *see also* Obstetric
      embolotherapy

I

Infantile hepatic hemangioendotheliomas, 14
Infection
  graft, percutaneous drainage in, 117–118
  recurrent pyogenic cholangitis, 186–194
Inflammatory lesions, tracheobronchial, stenting for, 148
Informed consent, for percutaneous gastrostomy and gastro-
      jejunostomy, 158
Infracolonic approach, gastrostomy and, 167
Interstitial pregnancy, embolotherapy in, 44, 46
Interstitial sarcoidosis, hemoptysis in *see* Hemoptysis
Intimal dissections, detection of, intravascular ultrasound in, 73–74
Intimal flap, postangioplasty, 71
Intra-abdominal abscesses, postoperative fluid collections and, 112–122
  diagnostic aspiration of, 113
  drainage steps for, 114–115 *see also* Percutaneous drainage, of post-
      operative intra-abdominal abscesses
Intra-arterial stents, placement of, intravascular ultrasound use during,
      76–77
Intracorporeal electrohydraulic lithotripsy, of retained stones in recurrent
      pyogenic cholangitis, 191, 192
Intrahepatic pigment stone disease, 186–194
Intrahepatic portosystemic shunt, transjugular, anatomic studies of liver
      applied to, 2–9
Intrapartum hemorrhage, embolotherapy in, 40–49
Intraperitoneal abscesses, drainage of, 115–116
Intravascular ultrasonography, 68–78
  clinical applications of, 71–72
  future of, 77–78
  technical considerations in, 68–69
  unique information provided by, 69–71
  use during atherectomy, 74–76
  use during stent placement, 76–77
  use during transluminal angioplasty, 72–74
  vessel measurement using, 72

J,K,L

Jejunostomy *see also* Gastrojejunostomy
  percutaneous, direct, 165
Kasabach-Merritt syndrome, 13–14
Laceration, vaginal or cervical, obstetric embolotherapy for, 44, 45
Lithotripsy
  extracorporeal shock-wave, of retained stones in recurrent pyogenic
      cholangitis, 190, 191
  intracorporeal electrohydraulic, of retained stones in recurrent
      pyogenic cholangitis, 191–192
Liver
  abscesses of, drainage of, 117

Liver, *continued*
  anatomic studies of, applied to transjugular intrahepatic portosystemic
      shunt, 2–9
  infantile hemangioendotheliomas of, 14
  percutaneous gastrostomy and gastrojejunostomy and, 158
Lungs *see* Pulmonary entries
Lymphatic malformations, pediatric, 25–26

M

Macroembolization, percutaneous transluminal renal angioplasty
      and, 97
Magnetic resonance imaging, in parathyroid adenoma diagnosis,
      57, 58
Malignant obstruction, stenting for
  esophageal, 138–140
  tracheobronchial, 147
Medial dissection, postangioplasty, 70
Microcholesterol crystal embolization, percutaneous transluminal renal
      angioplasty and, 97

N

Neck, face and, arteriovenous malformations of, 16–18
Needles, for percutaneous gastrostomy and gastrojejunostomy, 157
Nitinol Strecker stent *see also* Stents
  esophageal, 135, 139–140
Nuclear medicine, in parathyroid adenoma diagnosis, 55–56

O

Obstetric embolotherapy, 40–49
  emergency, 41–42
    indications for, 44
    results of, 43–44, 45
  prophylactic, 42–43
    indications for, 46
    results of, 44, 46–47
  vascular anatomy and, 40–41
Occlusion, acute, percutaneous transluminal renal angioplasty and, 96–97
Oriental cholangiohepatitis, 186–194
Osseous hemangiomas, 22
Ostial lesions, renal artery, 88–101
Over-the-wire angiogram, after renal angioplasty, 93–94

P

Pancreatic fluid collections, percutaneous drainage of, 120
Pancreatic obstruction, articulated catheters for, 174–183
Parathyroid glands
  adenomas of, 52–64
    ablation of, 60–64
    diagnosis of, 53–60
  anatomic location of, 52
Pediatrics
  tracheobronchial lesions in, stenting for, 149
  vascular anomalies in, 12–26
Pelvis
  abscesses of, drainage of, 117
  arteriovenous malformations of, 18–19
  vascular anatomy of, obstetrical hemorrhage and, 40–41
Percutaneous drainage
  of pancreatic fluid collections, 120
  of postoperative intra-abdominal abscesses, 112–122
    complications of, 115
    failure of, 115
    fibrinolytic agents as adjunct to, 121–122
    graft infection and, 117–118
    hepatic, 117
    intraperitoneal, 115–116
    pelvic, 117

Percutaneous drainage, of postoperative intra-abdominal
      abscesses, *continued*
    retroperitoneal, 117
    steps for, 114–115
  of post-transplant fluid collections, 118–119
  of splenic abscesses, 120–121
Percutaneous gastrostomy and gastrojejunostomy
  CT-guided, 165, 166
  fluoroscopic
    aftercare for, 162
    catheter exchanges after, 167–168
    catheter removal after, 168
    clinical indications for, 156
    complications of, 162–164
    contraindications to, 156
    controversies in, 168–170
    endoscopic or surgical placement versus, 169–170
    equipment for, 157–158, 168
    gastropexy versus, 170
    international variations in practice of, 156–157
    management after, 167–168
    patient preparation for, 158–159
    skin care after, 168
    suture anchors in, 166
    technique for, 157–162, 164–168
  ultrasound-guided, 165–166
Percutaneous jejunostomy, direct, 165
Percutaneous thrombectomy, 104–110
  clinical devices for, 105–109
  experimental devices for, 104–105
  special devices for, 109–110
Percutaneous transhepatic biliary drainage, 189
Percutaneous transluminal angioplasty *see also* Angioplasty
  intravascular ultrasound use during, 72–74
  renal, 88–94
    balloon sizing in, 92–93
    care following, 98
    complications of, 96–98
    imaging after, 93–94
    mechanism of, 88
    patient selection for, 88
    results of, 98–101
    stenosis catheterization in, 88–92
Pharmacologic gastroparesis, 164–165
Placenta accreta, embolotherapy in
  emergency, 44, 45
  prophylactic, 46, 47
Placenta previa, embolotherapy in, 46–47
Ponomar transjugular clot-trapper device, 109
Portosystemic shunt, intrahepatic, transjugular, 2–9
Postoperative flexible choledochoscopy, for retained biliary stones, in
      recurrent pyogenic cholangitis, 191–192
Postoperative intra-abdominal abscesses, percutaneous drainage of,
      112–122
Postpartum hemorrhage, embolotherapy in, 40–49
Pregnancy
  abdominal, embolotherapy in, 47
  interstitial, embolotherapy in, 44, 46
Primary cholangitis, 186–194
Prophylactic obstetric embolotherapy, 42–43
  indications for, 46
  results of, 44, 46–47
Prostheses, endovascular, self-expanding *see* Self-expanding stents
Pulmonary arteriovenous malformations, 18
Pulmonary vasculature, hemoptysis and, 32
Puncture needles, for percutaneous gastrostomy and gastro-
      jejunostomy, 157
Puncture site hemostasis, 82–86
Pyloric canal cannulation, percutaneous fluoroscopic gastrostomy
      and, 159–161
Pyogenic cholangitis, recurrent, 186–194

R

Recurrent pyogenic cholangitis, 186–194
    acute, interventional procedures during, 193
    biliary stricture management in, 193–194
    removal of retained stones in, 187–193
        complications of, 193
Renal artery, ostial lesions in, 88–101
    angioplasty for, 88–94 *see also* Percutaneous transluminal
        angioplasty, renal
    atherectomy for, 96
    stenting for, 94–96
Renal failure, contrast-induced, 97–98
Retroperitoneal abscesses, drainage of, 117
Retroperitoneal arteriovenous malformations, 19
Rheolytic thrombectomy catheter, 105
Rotational atherectomy of renal ostium, 96

S

Saline-jet aspiration thrombectomy catheter, 109–110
Sarcoidosis, interstitial, hemoptysis in *see* Hemoptysis
Sclerotherapy
    arteriovenous malformation embolization and, 17
    for venous malformation, 22–25
Sedation, for percutaneous gastrostomy and gastrojejunostomy, 159
Self-expanding stents *see also* Stents; specific type
    esophageal, 135, 139–140
    in tracheobronchial stenosis treatment, 144–153
        background of, 144
        clinical results of, 149–152
        indications for, 147–149
        technical aspects of, 144–147
Shock-wave lithotripsy, extracorporeal, of retained stones in recurrent
    pyogenic cholangitis, 190, 191
Shunt, portosystemic, transjugular intrahepatic, 2–9
Skin care, after percutaneous gastrostomy, 168
Skin fixation, dressings and, percutaneous gastrostomy and, 162
Spasm, percutaneous transluminal renal angioplasty and, 96
Spleen, abscesses of, percutaneous drainage of, 120–121
Stenosis
    renal artery, ostial, 88–101
    tracheobronchial, self-expanding stents in, 144–153
Stents
    articulated catheter, 174–183
    esophageal, 134–141
    placement of, intravascular ultrasound use during, 76–77
    renal, 94–96
    in tracheobronchial stenosis treatment, 144–153
Stones, retained, removal in recurrent pyogenic cholangitis, 187–193
Strictures
    biliary, 193–194
    esophageal, 134–141
Surgery
    gastrostomy placement using, fluoroscopic placement versus, 169, 170
    intra-abdominal abscesses after, percutaneous drainage of, 112–122

Suture, articulating, 175
Suture anchors, percutaneous gastrostomy and, 166

T

Thallium-technetium subtraction, in parathyroid adenoma diagnosis,
    55–56
Thorax, arteriovenous malformations involving, 18
Thrombectomy, percutaneous, 104–110
Thrombosis, dialysis access, 129–130 *see also* Dialysis, access maintenance
    for
Thyroid, parathyroid adenoma within, 55 *see also* Parathyroid glands,
    adenomas of
Tracheobronchial stenosis, self-expanding stents in, 144–153
Transhepatic biliary drainage, percutaneous, 189
Transjugular clot-trapper device, 109
Transjugular intrahepatic portosystemic shunt, anatomic studies of liver
    applied to, 2–9
Transluminal angioplasty, percutaneous *see* Percutaneous transluminal
    angioplasty
Transplantation, intra-abdominal fluid collections after, aspiration and
    drainage of, 118–119
Transverse colon, localization of, percutaneous gastrostomy and
    gastrojejunostomy and, 158–159
Truncal arteriovenous malformations, 18–19
T-tubes
    articulated catheters versus, 174–183
    stone removal in recurrent pyogenic cholangitis and, 190

U

Ultrasonography
    intravascular, 68–78
    in parathyroid adenoma diagnosis, 54–55
    in percutaneous gastrostomy guidance, 165–166
Urokinase, intracavitary, as adjunct to percutaneous abscess drainage,
    121–122
Uterus, vascular anatomy of, 40–41

V

Vaginal laceration, obstetric embolotherapy for, 44, 45
Vascular anomalies, pediatric, 12–26
Vascular intervention, intravascular ultrasound in, 68–78
Venous embolization, 15
Venous malformations, pediatric, 22–25
Venous sampling, in parathyroid adenoma diagnosis, 58–60

W

Wallstent *see also* Stents
    esophageal, 135, 138–139
    tracheobronchial, 144–145
        clinical results with, 149–150
Wires, for percutaneous gastrostomy and gastrojejunostomy, 157
    complications involving, 164